second
edition

Beauty Therapy
The Basics
for NVQ 1 and 2

Maxine Whittaker
Debbie Forsythe–Conroy
Judith Ifould

second
edition

Beauty Therapy
The Basics
for NVQ 1 and 2

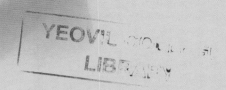

Hodder & Stoughton
A MEMBER OF THE HODDER HEADLINE GROUP

Orders: please contact Bookpoint Ltd, 130 Milton Park, Abingdon, Oxon OX14 4SB.
Telephone: (44) 01235 827720. Fax: (44) 01235 400454. Lines are open 9.00–6.00,
Monday to Saturday, with a 24-hour message answering service. You can also order
through our website www.hodderheadline.co.uk.

British Library Cataloguing in Publication Data
A catalogue record for this title is available from the British Library

ISBN 0 340 88318 9

First Edition Published 1999
This Edition Published 2004
Impression number   10   9   8   7   6   5   4   3   2   1
Year   2007   2006   2005   2004

Copyright © 2004 Maxine Whittaker, Debbie Forsythe-Conroy, Judith Ifould

Typeset by Charon Tec Pvt. Ltd, Chennai, India [www.charontec.com].
Printed in Italy for Hodder & Stoughton Educational, a division of
Hodder Headline, 338 Euston Road, London NW1 3BH

CONTENTS

In this chapter you will learn about:
- Recognising your job role
- Health and safety procedures in the salon
- The laws relating to beauty therapy practice
- Emergency procedures
- Safe working conditions
- Salon duties
- Salon hygiene procedures, including sterilisation and disinfection

In this chapter you will learn about:
- The role of a receptionist
- Interpersonal skills
- The Data Protection Act
- Reception procedures
  - dealing with clients
  - answering the telephone
  - handling enquiries
  - giving information
  - taking messages
  - making appointments
  - dealing with payments

In this chapter you will learn about:
- Marketing and promotion
- Identifying the need for additional products and services
- Ethical selling
- Legislation
- Client feedback and how to deal with it

In this chapter you will learn about:
- Working in a team
- The different roles and responsibilities of staff in the salon
- Communicating with others
- Personal development
  - job description
  - appraisal
  - setting targets
  - reviewing personal progress and development

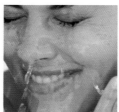
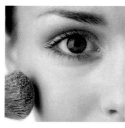
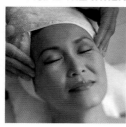
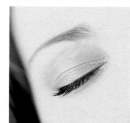

9. DEPILATORY WAXING 151

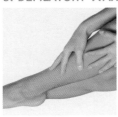

In this chapter you will learn about:
- Client consultation for safe hair removal
- Waxing products
- Preparing the work area for temporary hair removal
  - selecting products and materials for depilatory treatments
  - safety precautions
  - preparing the client for treatment
  - assessing clients and preparing a treatment plan
  - various methods of temporary hair removal
  - treatment methods for different areas of the body
  - erythema (cause and treatment)
  - aftercare advice
  - care and maintenance of equipment

10. MANICURE AND PEDICURE 169

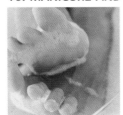

In this chapter you will learn about:
- Preparing the work area for manicure and pedicure treatment
  - tools and equipment
  - products and materials
  - hygiene procedures
  - preparation of the client
  - health and safety
  - codes of practice
- Assessing client needs by preparing a treatment plan
  - client consultation
  - types of treatments
  - contraindications
  - aftercare advice
  - client records
- Manicure and pedicure treatment methods
  - salon requirements – pricing – timing

11. NAIL EXTENSIONS AND NAIL ART 201

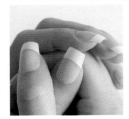

In this chapter you will learn about:
- Specialist products, chemicals, tools and equipment used in the application of nail extensions
- Health and safety
- Preparing the work area
- Assessing the needs of the client, client preferences and treatment planning
- Contraindications to the application of nail extensions
- Reasons for nail extensions
- Types of nail extensions
- Aftercare advice
- Removing artificial nails
- Contra-actions
- Nail art including preparation, techniques and design

Preface

This book has been written in line with the latest Standards for SVQ/NVQ in Beauty Therapy at Level 1 and 2 and as far as possible the language and content follow those Standards.

The book will provide the necessary essential knowledge to meet the requirements of a range of Beauty Therapy qualifications.

There are tasks within each chapter that have been designed to generate appropriate supplementary evidence for a student's portfolio as well as activities and self-assessment tests at the end of the book for students to review their own learning.

With the increasing demand for key skills to be accredited, we have written key skills tasks, which will help to identify assessment opportunities within the beauty therapy salon for key skills. The tasks should be used as examples that can be expanded upon to meet the requirements of different levels and different assessment situations as required. These can be found on page 313.

We have endeavoured to put together a book that will support students and trainees as well as tutors and trainers in their learning and teaching. We hope that *Beauty Therapy – The Basics for NVQ 1 and 2* will provide an invaluable source of practical and theoretical information to support learning, whether in the salon, college or training school.

Acknowledgements

I would like to thank my colleagues from Lincoln College for the years of work we undertook together as a team to develop NVQs in Beauty Therapy.

Their dedication to the NVQ philosophy in providing access to beauty therapy education and training for a much wider range of individuals and their hard work in adapting learning and assessment materials to meet the needs of their students and competence based assessment has inspired me to write this book.

I would like to thank Matthew Smith and Virginia Tonkin from Hodder & Stoughton for all their help and their meticulous attention to detail in making this a great 2nd edition.

Once again my thanks must go to my husband Roger who encouraged me to write the 2nd edition, for his continuing patience and tolerance as the work for this book seemed to take even longer than before!

Finally I would like to dedicate my contribution to this book to Joanie.

Maxine Whittaker

I would like to thank my colleagues at Bradford and Ilkley Community College for their inspiration, dedication and enthusiasm for Beauty Therapy. Another huge thank you for the support of my husband Chris and son Alex, my inspiration and motivation.

Debbie Forsythe-Conroy

The publishers wish to thank the following for allowing use of copyright material.

Figure 1.1 with permission from Philip Harvey/CORBIS.

Figures 2.1, 2.2, 3.1, 5.1, 9.1, 10.1, 12.1 and 13.1 with permission © Getty Images.

Figure 4.1 with permission © Jose Luis Pelaez, Inc./CORBIS

Figures 6.1 and 8.1 with permission © Thomas Schweizer/CORBIS

Figure 6.11 with permission © Photomorgana/CORBIS

Figure 7.1 with permission © Jerry Tobias/CORBIS

Figures 11.1 with permission © Ashley Karl-Alamy

Figure 12.2 with permission © Studex UK Ltd, Cambridgeshire

Figures 13.2 and 13.5 © BDI Images

Figures 13.3 and 13.4 courtesy of Saniflo & Kinedo/BDI Images Ltd

Figure 14.0 with permission © Larry Williams/CORBIS

Figures 14.29, 14.31, 14.32, 14.33 and 14.34 with permission © Wellcome

Figure 14.30 with permission © Mediscan

Figures 2.5, 5.4, 6.9, 8.4, 9.2, 10.2, 10.11, 10.13, 12.3, 12.5, 12.6 and 12.7 taken by Gary Roberts with permission from Jackie Cox, Head of the School of Hairdressing and Beauty Therapy at Basingstoke College of Technology.

Introduction

Beauty therapy is a fast-growing industry with employment opportunities in beauty therapy salons, health spas, cosmetic houses, cruise ships and working abroad. Training to a high standard is essential to enable you to access these opportunities anywhere in the United Kingdom or overseas.

National Vocational Qualifications (NVQs) are designed to assess a student's ability to do a particular job according to standards set by employers in that industry. In other words, when you have successfully completed an NVQ and apply for a job the employer will immediately know what you are capable of doing. There are other qualifications in beauty therapy besides the NVQ that are recognised by the beauty therapy industry. The information contained in this book will meet the needs of all students of beauty therapy regardless of which qualification they are working towards.

NVQs are based on assessment of **practical skills, knowledge** and **understanding** at levels 1, 2, 3 or 4. Broadly speaking, level 1 is an introduction to beauty therapy – you might be an assistant helping therapists in a salon. Level 2 includes using various practical skills to treat clients in the salon. Level 3 involves more complex treatments as well as supervising staff. Level 4 is management training for the qualified and experienced therapist.

The qualification is made up of **Units**, which describe a particular treatment or job within the salon. Each unit is made up of several **Elements** containing **Performance Criteria (PCs)**, range statements and underpinning knowledge. The awarding body will provide you with an assessment logbook that contains all the detail you require to cover the National Standards.

Before assessment can take place you must be familiar with the requirements of each unit and undertake practical and theoretical instruction either in the workplace or at a recognised training centre such as a college of further education. Your teacher will provide learning opportunities through demonstrations followed by practice on clients in the salon, as well as theory lessons to provide you with the necessary underpinning knowledge.

Assessment for an NVQ is based on you, the candidate, being able to demonstrate that you can do the job. Your skills are measured against the National Standards by a qualified assessor who is trained to make judgements about your ability.

The assessor will usually be your teacher, who will make sure that you are able to carry out treatments safely and competently before assessing you. Your assessor will advise you on assessment opportunities: observation of practical work, oral questioning, written tests, case studies and assignments. You will also compile a **portfolio**. The assessor will discuss the assessment criteria with you before an assessment takes place and agree how the assessment will be carried out. This will usually involve your assessor watching you work. This is called assessment by **observation**. The assessor will need to be sure that you understand what you are doing and why. This will involve asking you questions. This is called **oral questioning**. As most of your work involves a client this will usually be done after your client has left, unless the assessor wishes to confirm something with you during the treatment.

Portfolio evidence requires you to collect materials to confirm your skills and demonstrate your understanding. This type of evidence can be divided into **performance evidence** and **knowledge evidence**. Performance evidence includes items such as client record cards, photographs, case studies, witness testimonies, which help to confirm that you can carry out a task. Knowledge evidence will be such things as written tests and assignments, which show that you have gained knowledge of a subject.

These items are usually collected together in a portfolio (a file or folder) to form part of the assessment for each unit. You are required to provide a guide for your assessor so that the information contained in your portfolio is organised. This is called **referencing**.

Verification is a process to ensure that assessment is fair. It involves someone who is trained to observe assessments taking place and who looks at assignments and written tests. The **internal verifier** will check that the assessment processes are fair and valid and sign off your assessment logbook, before claiming certification from the awarding body. The training centre will retain your portfolio and assessment logbook for the **external verifier** who does a further check on behalf of the awarding body.

This book has been written to help you with all aspects of NVQ **levels 1 and 2 Beauty Therapy** and the range of qualifications at that level.

The book covers:

- knowledge requirements
- activities, some of which can be used to generate evidence for your portfolio
- self-assessment tasks to test knowledge and understanding (at the back of the book)
- key skills tasks, which will help to provide evidence for assessment (on page 313).

Information specific to NVQ level 1 is signposted throughout the book. However all the chapters in the book are equally relevant to beauty therapy practice.

Anatomy and physiology for all aspects of facial, nail treatments and waxing can be found in chapter 14.

Chapter 1

HEALTH AND SAFETY

LEVELS
1+2

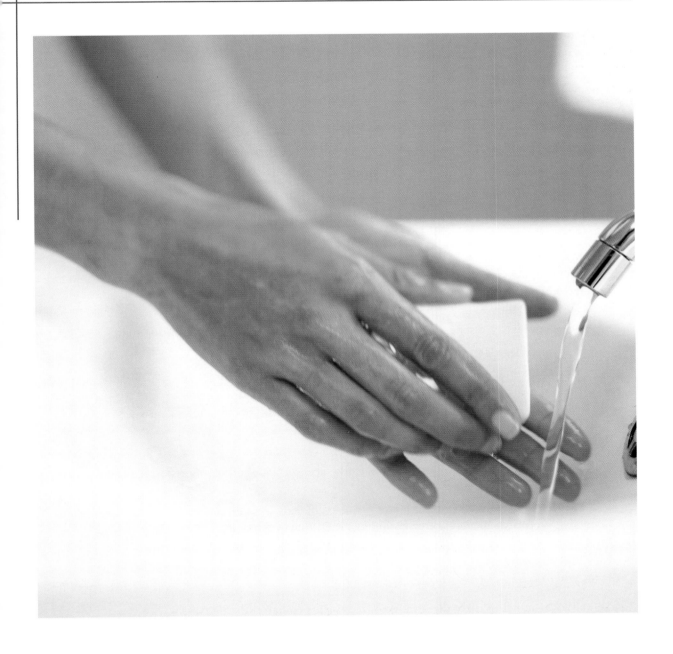

- Recognising your job role
- Health and safety procedures in the salon
- The laws relating to beauty therapy practice
- Emergency procedures
- Safe working conditions
- Salon duties
- Salon hygiene procedures, including sterilisation and disinfection

Introduction

The workplace can hold many dangers and it is everyone's responsibility to ensure that the salon is a safe and hygienic environment. The beauty therapist has additional responsibilities when working with clients. There is a **legal requirement** to ensure that the general public are not at risk when visiting the salon and receiving treatment.

Work role

The employer and/or manager

It is the responsibility of the employer to safeguard the health, safety and welfare of all in the workplace by ensuring equipment is maintained, strict hygiene procedures are followed and that there are safe working practices identified in policies and procedures.

The manager is ultimately responsible for enforcing safe working practices by ensuring that:

- health and safety legislation is in place (see page 4)
- risk assessment is in place and any hazards are kept to the absolute minimum
- all staff are trained and competent in the treatments they carry out on clients
- training for new products and treatments is available along with manufacturer's instructions.

The work role of a supervisor

A supervisor has responsibility for others in the workplace, e.g. monitoring and reporting on aspects of health and safety practice, accidents.

The supervisor may be required to train junior members of staff in salon procedures to maintain health and safety, e.g. sterilising methods, preparation of the treatment room, etc.

The supervisor may from time to time take on the responsibilities of the manager in their absence.

The work role of the therapist

The therapist is required to carry out a range of treatments competently and safely:

- take responsibility for care, maintenance and safe storage of equipment and products
- work hygienically and safely by following salon practice on preparing for treatments and clearing away after clients
- report any hazards to the designated health and safety representative (usually the owner or manager)

- ensure the treatments they carry out on their clients meet health and safety requirements, i.e. contraindications are checked before the start of the treatment
- ensure personal presentation and conduct meets salon policy.

The work role of the assistant beauty therapist

The assistant beauty therapist has responsibilities within the workplace to:

- ensure that they are aware of health and safety procedures
- carry out tasks under instruction from the therapist, supervisor or owner/manager
- be aware of the limits of their own job role and work within those limits through supervision by a senior member of salon staff
- prepare for treatments and help to maintain salon hygiene
- assist with treatments under the supervision of senior staff
- ensure personal presentation and conduct meet salon policy.

The golden rule of health and safety

It is the responsibility of all employees to work and behave in a safe manner with due consideration for everyone, i.e. fellow workers, clients and visitors to the salon.

Health and safety practice is based on assessing the risks and hazards in the salon.

The employer must make sure that they check the possible hazards and decide what the risks are to their staff and clients.

- A **hazard** is something that could possibly cause an accident and harm someone.
- A **risk** is the likelihood of the hazard harming someone.

It is important to understand the terms hazard and risk and be able to identify hazards and work towards reducing the risk to health and safety in the workplace. This is called **risk assessment**.

Possible hazards in the salon include:

- faulty electrical equipment
- trailing electrical cables
- spillages on the floor
- overheating depilatory wax
- toxic or flammable products
- poor lighting
- poor fitting carpet or flooring.

Everyone has a responsibility to work safely and not do anything that could create a health and safety risk.

Never ignore any risk but try to put things right or report it immediately to a senior member of staff if it is beyond your capabilities.

Always ask if you do not know how to do something that may put you at risk, particularly when dealing with electrical equipment, heated substances such as wax and products whose ingredients and effects you do not understand.

Always read manufacturers' instructions.

Do not attempt to do treatments that you are not fully trained to do.

Always follow strict hygiene procedures.

The law relating to beauty therapy practice
Health and Safety at Work Act 1974

This is the main Act of Parliament governing the duties and responsibilities of employers and employees while at work. The Health and Safety at Work Act (HASAW) is an 'enabling' Act that covers a whole range of legislation relating to health and safety.

The duties of the employer

The employer must:

- manage and promote safe working practices in the workplace
- provide a healthy environment through clean, tidy, well-lit and ventilated work areas
- ensure employees are adequately qualified, and provide training as necessary.

If there are more than five employees a written **Health and Safety Policy** is required.

The duties of the employee

The employee must:

- follow salon rules and regulations
- cooperate with the employer in all matters of health and safety
- follow safe working practices and attend training as required.

All individuals have responsibility for health and safety while at work.

The findings of the **Health and Safety Executive** and the demands of **European legislation** have led to a number of new laws. These are discussed in the following pages.

The Electricity at Work Regulations 1992

The beauty therapist uses a range of electrical equipment, which must be tested by a qualified electrician at least once a year. A sticker will usually be placed on each item giving the date it was tested. If not, a record of equipment inspection and servicing must be made available on request.

When using any electrical equipment you should make the following checks:

- Equipment should not be used near basins or where liquids are likely to be spilt on the appliance.
- Cables, flexes, connections, sockets and plugs must be intact, with no exposed wiring.
- The appliance should be on a level and stable trolley.
- The appliance must be switched off and disconnected from the mains when not in use.
- Cables and flexes must not be allowed to trail across the floor as they could cause someone to trip.

Remember not to touch sockets, connections, plugs or wires with damp or wet hands. If you come across faulty or damaged electrical equipment take it out of use immediately by placing a clearly written 'out of order' sign on it. Report the fault to the manager.

- Electrical equipment should be stored carefully by winding flexes and cables smoothly round the appliance.
- At the end of the working day someone must be responsible for checking that all appliances are switched off and disconnected.

Wiring a plug

It is important that all relevant staff make visual safety checks and understand the wiring of a plug.

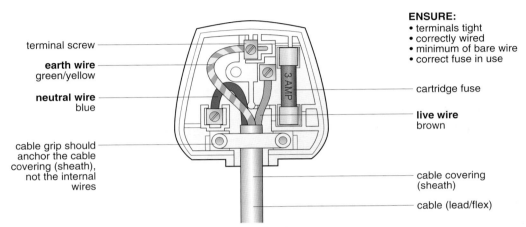

terminal screw

earth wire
green/yellow

neutral wire
blue

cable grip should
anchor the cable
covering (sheath),
not the internal
wires

ENSURE:
- terminals tight
- correctly wired
- minimum of bare wire
- correct fuse in use

cartridge fuse

live wire
brown

cable covering
(sheath)

cable (lead/flex)

3 AMP

Figure 1.1 *All salon staff should understand the wiring of a plug*

The Personal Protective Equipment at Work Regulations (PPE) 1992

The regulations state that employers must provide suitable and sufficient protective clothing and materials.

- Salon dress, aprons and disposable/latex gloves, etc., should be adequate to protect therapists.
- Protective clothing and materials should be available to protect the client.

The salon will have a uniform for all its staff, usually a white overall or jacket with trousers. The salon uniform should project a smart, clean image as well as being a means of protecting the therapist from chemicals that may be absorbed into the skin. The overall may also protect from possible cross infection. The overall should be changed daily and should only be worn in the salon, to avoid picking up odours or grime from outdoors.

It is essential that clean towels and linen are available to each client. Disposable paper such as couch role and tissues need to be readily available.

It may be in line with individual salon practice to wear latex gloves for waxing treatment.

Workplace (Health, Safety and Welfare) Regulations 1992

These regulations deal with the working environment, heating, lighting, ventilation, cleanliness and restroom facilities and the maintenance of a safe and healthy working environment.

Control of Substances Hazardous to Health Regulations 1988 (COSHH)

The employer is required to regulate employees' exposure to substances that may cause ill health or injury. The potential risks to all those working in the salon are assessed. This process is called **risk assessment** and is normally carried out by the salon manager.

Risk assessment

Risk assessment involves making a list of all the substances used in the salon or sold to clients that may be hazardous to health, because they may:

- cause irritation
- burn the skin
- give off fumes
- cause allergic reactions.

Instructions for handling and disposal of these substances are then made available to all staff, with training if required. Manufacturers will normally supply information relating to their products. See Table 1.1 for major chemical hazards.

Hazard warning symbols

These symbols appear on packaging and notices around the workplace (see Figure 1.3).

The Manual Handling Operations Regulations 1992

These regulations require everyone in the workplace to minimise risks from lifting and handling large or heavy objects. The beauty therapist must take particular care when moving equipment or boxes containing stock in the salon (see Figure 1.2).

Equipment should be fixed on a suitable trolley and free-standing equipment should be on castors for ease of movement around the salon. Trolleys must be checked regularly to ensure that they are stable and that the castors run freely. However, equipment should not be moved unnecessarily, in particular equipment containing hot liquids such as wax.

Manual tasks risk factors

Poor posture when lifting heavy items can cause injury.

Working postures for the beauty therapist can cause aches and pains and in the long term cause serious injury.

Examples of posture problems associated with treating clients

- Back bent or twisted, shoulders raised in an unnatural position when applying massage.
- Repeated movements or awkward posture over a long period of time when leg waxing.
- Back bent when doing manicure/nail art.
- Poor standing posture when applying make-up.

Awkward posture requires greater muscular effort and leads to fatigue, particularly when the position is held for a long time.

	Specification	Health hazard	Use/handling	Storage	Disposal	Caution/action
Aerosols	Hairsprays Nail dry sprays Surface cleaners	Flammable	Do not smoke. Keep away from eyes. Use in well-ventilated areas.	Cool dry place. Avoid sunlight. Avoid excessive temperatures.	Do not pierce or burn container (explosive).	In case of fire, evacuate areas known to contain aerosols.
Caustic	Cuticle remover	Substances that can burn the skin	Keep away from eyes. Do not use on sensitive skin.	Cool dry place.	Wear gloves. Mop up spills with damp cloth (rinse well).	Eye/skin contact – use eye bath or wash area with plenty of water. Ingestion – drink plenty of water.
Flammable	Acetone Astringent Eau de cologne Equipment cleaner Flowers of sulphur Nail polish remover Nail polish thinners Rose water Solvents Surgical spirit Witch hazel	Flammable vapours	Do not smoke. Label clearly. Good ventilation.	Distinguish inflammables from flammables. Store in cool place. Keep sealed. (Look at labels.)	Seek advice from EHO if disposing of large quantities.	Wash skin or eyes immediately. Remove to fresh air if inhaled.
Sensitising	Acrylic nail powder Chemical peels Equipment cleaner Gluteraldehyde solution Lash tint Nail glue Nail off remover Nail primer Resin gel	May cause allergic reaction	Wear gloves.	Cool dry place.	Use normal disposal methods or contact EHO for large amounts.	Eye/skin contact – wash immediately. Inhalation – move to fresh air. Ingestion – seek medical advice.

Table 1.1 *Major chemical hazards*

(Continued)

Health and safety

	Specification	Health hazard	Use/handling	Storage	Disposal	Caution/action
Skin bleach	All bleach products Hydrogen peroxide	May cause skin irritation	Wear gloves. Avoid inhalation.	Cool dry place.	Do not incinerate. Dilute to mop up spillage. Wash powders down drains.	Eye/skin contact – wash immediately. Inhalation – remove to fresh air, then seek medical advice.
Fine powders	Acrylic nail powder Bleaches Bronzing powder Calamine powder Face powder Flowers of sulphur Fuller's earth Kaolin Magnesium carbonate	Inhalation can cause irritation	Avoid inhalation.	Cool dry place. Closed container.	Treat as domestic waste (flowers of sulphur is a fire hazard).	Eye/skin contact – rinse immediately with water, do not inhale.

EHO – Environmental Health Officer

Table 1.1 *Major chemical hazards*

(Continued)

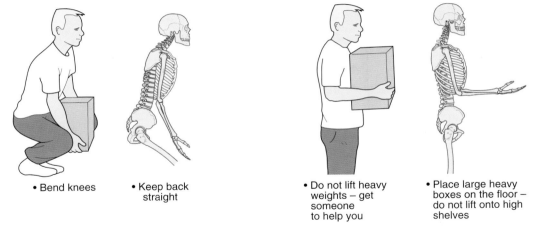

• Bend knees
• Keep back straight

• Do not lift heavy weights – get someone to help you
• Place large heavy boxes on the floor – do not lift onto high shelves

Figure 1.2 *Learn how to lift correctly, so you do not strain your back*

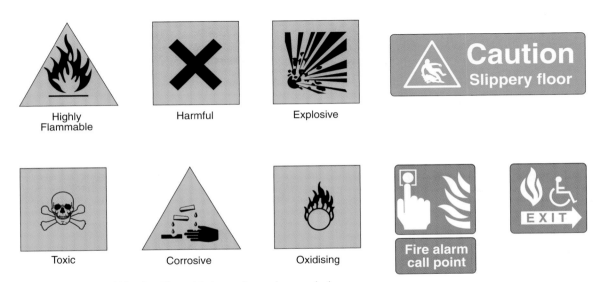

Highly Flammable

Harmful

Explosive

Caution **Slippery floor**

Toxic

Corrosive

Oxidising

Fire alarm call point

EXIT

Figure 1.3 *You should be familiar with hazard warning symbols*

The Fire Precautions Act 1971

This is concerned with fire prevention and adequate means of escape in the event of a fire. The employer must apply for a **fire certificate** if the business employs 20 or more staff and follow strict regulations on fire prevention.

Fire precautions are essential in all business premises and involve ensuring that:

▪ fire escapes are kept free of obstruction, are clearly signposted and doors can be opened easily
▪ all employees are made aware of evacuation procedures for the salon and that there is regular fire drill practice
▪ fire-fighting equipment suitable for all types of fire is easily reached and kept in good working order
▪ all staff are familiar with the salon's emergency procedures, use of fire-fighting equipment and location of the assembly point
▪ smoke alarms are fitted
▪ fire doors are fitted to help control the spread of fire.

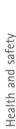

Health and safety

Fire extinguishers

Different fire extinguishers are made to deal with different types of fire. From 1997 all fire extinguishers in the UK must be coloured red except for a small band or patch of colour using the standard colour code.

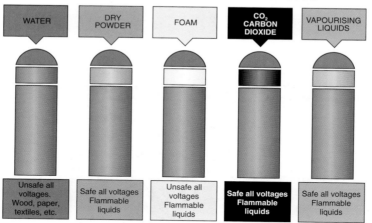

KNOW YOUR FIRE EXTINGUISHER COLOUR CODE

WATER	DRY POWDER	FOAM	CO₂ CARBON DIOXIDE	VAPOURISING LIQUIDS
Unsafe all voltages. Wood, paper, textiles, etc.	Safe all voltages Flammable liquids	Unsafe all voltages Flammable liquids	Safe all voltages Flammable liquids	Safe all voltages Flammable liquids

Figure 1.4 *Each type of fire should be dealt with using a different fire extinguisher*

Fire blanket

This is a fire-resistant material used for smothering a fire, e.g. burning wax or oil, or for wrapping around a person if their clothes are on fire.

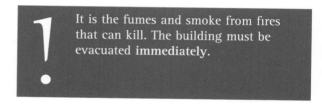

It is the fumes and smoke from fires that can kill. The building must be evacuated **immediately**.

The Local Government (Miscellaneous Provisions) Act 1982 (Local Authority Licensing)

The beauty therapist carries out some treatments such as ear-piercing, micro-pigmentation, waxing, eyebrow shaping and electrical epilation, which require particular attention to hygiene. This is due to the increased risk of cross infection from blood or body fluids coming into contact with the therapist, equipment or other clients.

Guidelines are available from the **local authority** and under the local by-laws inspection of the premises to check hygiene procedures will be necessary. When the Environmental Health Officer (EHO) is satisfied that the premises are of the required standard, the business will become registered and receive a certificate. An officer will pay particular attention to:

- cleaning and sterilising of implements
- safe working practices with materials such as disposable needles
- salon cleaning to a high standard
- therapists' personal hygiene and working practices.

Licensing by the local authority covers a range of activities including ear-piercing, electrical epilation, hairdressing/barbering and other professions such as acupuncture and tattooing.

Local authorities are not expected to assess the treatment techniques used by the therapist, however they have to ensure adequate levels of training and competence exist.

Age restrictions can be enforced under the by-laws. It is recommended that clients under 16 have a parent or guardian present and that a consent form is signed prior to treatment. A declaration and proof of age can also be insisted on under the by-law. This is a further indication of the importance of thorough and careful consultation, with fully completed records.

ACTIVITY

Working in a small group, using the Internet find your local authority local by-laws relating to the beauty therapy salon. You may find that different local authorities have different information and slightly different regulations. This is because by-laws are based on local needs and the interpretation of government guidelines may vary to meet these needs.

The Reporting of Injuries, Diseases and Dangerous Occurrences Regulations 1985 (RIDDOR)

These regulations ensure that any incident occurring in the workplace and leading to an injury or a condition resulting from a work activity is recorded in an **accident book**.

Inspection and registration

All businesses must comply with the law on health and safety. To ensure that this happens the **Environmental Health Department** of the local authority will appoint an Environmental Health Officer (EHO) to visit and inspect the premises.

This inspector has the authority to demand that any hazards identified during the inspection are dealt with by the employer within a given period of time. This is called an **improvement notice**. Should the employer not comply with the notice by removing the danger within a given period of time, closure of the business can result, with the local authority issuing a **prohibition notice**.

Insurance

Whilst every effort must be made to prevent injury and disease it may be that unforeseen circumstances will lead to accidents in the workplace. It is essential therefore that employers are covered by **insurance**.

The Employers Liability (Compulsory Insurance) Act 1969

The law requires the employer to provide insurance cover against claims for injury or illness as a result of negligence by the employer or their employees. The **certificate of insurance** must be displayed in the workplace.

Public liability insurance

The employer is not required by law to take out insurance to cover claims from the public, but is well advised to do so. It is becoming increasingly common for clients to sue businesses for damage to personal property or injury resulting from treatment in the salon.

Professional indemnity insurance

Professional indemnity insurance is part of the service offered by becoming a member of a professional organisation. Your annual subscription entitles you to liability cover against claims by clients for personal injury. Some treatments carry more risk than others, e.g. electro-epilation and ear-piercing. It is advisable to have appropriate professional indemnity insurance.

What health and safety hazards and risks are there in the salon?

The beauty therapy salon carries risks relating to the use of chemicals and electrical equipment as well as those of falling, fire, infection, scalds, burns and cuts.

ACTIVITY

Look around the salon you are working in and make a list of the hazards that could put you or your clients at risk of injury. (A list of likely hazards appears on page 3 – cross-check with our list.)

Follow emergency procedures

All staff must be prepared for emergency situations that may occur in the salon. Each person must take responsibility for the correct procedure to be carried out promptly and without panic. This can be achieved only by ensuring that everyone understands their role in an emergency and is trained to carry it out effectively. Individual members of staff should be identified as key people to handle an emergency: trained first aider, health and safety manager.

Staff training in health and safety is the responsibility of the salon owner or manager and should include:

- induction of new staff
- safe systems of work
- fire prevention
- risks and hazards found in the salon
- fire evacuation procedures
- emergency procedure in the event of an accident
- first aid.

Fire
The risk of fire in the salon

The amount of **electrical equipment** used in the salon increases the risk of electrical fire. Overloading electrical circuits or not following electrical safety procedures (e.g. ignoring worn cables) are the most common causes of electrical fires. Switching off all equipment at the mains immediately after use will help to prevent this type of fire.

Chemicals that are flammable such as nail polish remover and surgical spirit are a fire hazard and must be handled and stored in accordance with COSHH regulations (see page 6).

Depilitory wax and paraffin wax, if overheated, will give off fumes and may ignite. Thermostatically controlled heaters must be used and maintained regularly. Never leave heated wax unattended and do not carry heated wax from cubicle to cubicle.

Fires may be started by carelessness and poor working practices (i.e. drying towels over electrical or gas heaters, leaving unused appliances switched on, discarding cigarettes). A **no smoking policy** should be in force in the salon to reduce the risk of fire.

Fire prevention

- The salon should be fitted with smoke alarms.
- Fire-fighting equipment must be available and located in an easily accessible area.
- Staff should know how to use the fire-fighting equipment and be able to identify the correct type of extinguisher to use on a particular fire.
- Safe working practices must be followed at all times.
- A no smoking policy should be in force.

Emergency evacuation procedure

1. Each business premises should have an evacuation procedure that takes account of the emergency exit routes and fire escapes from the building.
2. Make sure you know where fire-fighting equipment is kept and how to use it.
3. You must take responsibility for your clients, who may be receiving treatment in different parts of the salon. Direct them to the nearest safe exit.
4. Switch off electrical equipment close by you at the mains.
5. Ensure that everyone has left the premises and is congregated well away from the building.
6. If the fire is small and can be safely tackled with a fire extinguisher this can be carried out. However, you should not take any risks and the premises must be vacated quickly, closing as many doors as possible.
7. At the earliest possible time, the emergency services should be contacted by dialling 999 (see below). Give the exact address and details of the emergency.
8. Not all emergencies are caused by fires. Bomb scares are becoming more common with the need to evacuate a premises as quickly as possible, to get well away from the building and to follow police instructions.
9. Toxic fumes or gas leaks may also require clients and employees to be evacuated from the building.
10. The salon should have regular emergency evacuation practice to familiarise staff with the procedure.

ACTIVITY

Check the emergency procedure for your salon and identify your role in an emergency.

Accidents

Emergency procedures in the event of an accident

Calling the emergency services

1. Dial 999 (check whether your phone line requires an additional number – usually 9 – to get an outside line).
2. Speak clearly, stating what the emergency is and where you are.

3. Listen carefully to any instructions you are given.

4. Return to a safe place or to the client.

Accidents in the workplace are often the result of unsafe working conditions or poor working practices. Staff may carry out treatments incorrectly or take unnecessary risks through lack of knowledge or training.

Any accident that occurs in the salon must be recorded in an **accident book**. If the accident is serious or if there are incidents of disease in the salon, **a report form** must be completed and sent to the Local Licensing Authority (see information on RIDDOR, page 11). These forms are more detailed than an accident book but fortunately are rarely required. The senior member of staff or the health and safety representative for the salon must be kept informed and take responsibility for the correct procedures being carried out.

The accident book

Keeping a record of all accidents, no matter how small, is essential. The entry in the accident book should be completed as soon as possible by a member of staff who saw the accident and can give an accurate account of what happened.

Details noted in the accident book should include:

- date
- time of the accident
- place where the accident occurred
- personal details of those involved – names, whether staff or client, contact details
- a brief description of what happened and the resulting injury
- what first aid was given
- whether the emergency services were called or the person(s) taken to hospital. If so, it is likely that the accident would be regarded as serious and an incident report form would also be required.

INCIDENT REPORT FORM		
DATE	TIME	PLACE INCIDENT OCCURRED
NAME OF INJURED PERSON	ADDRESS	TEL. NO.
DESCRIPTION OF INCIDENT:		
DETAILS OF ANY INJURY AND FIRST AID GIVEN:		
SIGNATURE OF INJURED PERSON	SIGNATURE OF PERSON ATTENDING INCIDENT	

Figure 1.5 *An incident report form*

First aid

Someone in the salon should be trained in first aid. Your local St John Ambulance (St Andrews Ambulance in Scotland) or Red Cross will be able to give you details of courses.

The first aid box

The trained first aider will have responsibility for ensuring that the first aid box is adequately stocked. The first aid box should contain:

- assorted plasters, individually wrapped
- triangular bandages
- sterile eye pads
- different sizes of sterile dressings
- safety pins
- disposable plastic or rubber gloves
- eye bath.

> **!** Painkillers should not be issued by a first aider and therefore should not be part of the first aid kit. Only a medical practitioner should issue painkillers. Antiseptics should not be part of the first aid kit because, if they have been used previously and the top not secured, they may contain germs.

First aid for minor accidents

It may be necessary for you to deal with minor accidents before calling upon the trained first aider.

- **Dizziness:** sit the person down near an open window for fresh air. Loosen clothing around the neck. Placing the head between the knees will help to bring blood to the head but care must be taken with elderly people.
- **Fainting:** as above, but if possible lie the person down with their legs raised.
- **Minor cuts:** apply pressure with clean cotton wool. Follow procedure for handling contaminated materials on page 21.
- **Epilepsy:** a person suffering from an epileptic fit may injure themselves by falling or hitting furniture during an attack. Do not try to restrain them but ensure that their airways are clear and furniture and equipment is moved away. When the attack is over, cover the person with a blanket and allow them to rest.
- **Minor burns:** hold the area under cold running water until the pain is gone.
- **Nose bleed:** bend the head slightly forward and squeeze the bridge of the nose until bleeding has stopped.
- **Electric shock:** do not touch the person but disconnect the appliance at the mains immediately. Lie the person down and check their breathing.
- **Cosmetics in the eyes:** apply cotton wool soaked in water. Allow the person to wipe their eyes. It may be necessary to use warm water in an eye bath to flush out the eyes.

Safe working conditions
Heating and ventilation

The minimum temperature in the workplace, should be 16°C (60°F). However, the temperature in the salon should be around 20–23°C (68–75°F) as clients will be removing clothing. It is essential that the client is warm to encourage relaxation. An exercise room would need to be maintained at a lower temperature, around 17°C (63°F).

Thermostatically controlled heating will ensure that the salon remains at a constant temperature. Make sure that you know how to control the heating.

Adequate ventilation is equally important. Air conditioning is the most efficient method of ensuring clean air. Extractor fans and open windows will help remove strong smells from cosmetic preparations, fumes from chemicals and stale air, which is caused by a build-up of carbon dioxide and pungent smells.

Exercise rooms and wet areas must have very efficient air circulation and good extraction systems: air conditioning is ideal. Headaches, dizziness, nausea, fainting and fatigue can be the result of poor ventilation.

Lighting

All areas of the salon should be well lit, particularly stairways and fire escapes. Treatment areas where cosmetics are used should have natural daylight to ensure that make-up colours are not distorted. Matching make-up with skin tones or the client's clothing is an important aspect of applying cosmetics. 'Daylight' lamps can substitute for poor natural light where necessary.

Lights should be checked regularly, replacing flickering fluorescent tubes or changing the angle of lights that cause unnecessary glare.

Dimmer switches in treatment rooms will enable the therapist to regulate the amount of light according to the treatment being carried out, e.g. during facial massage lights should be dimmed.

Washing and toilet facilities

The law makes it very clear that an adequate supply of clean hot and cold water should be available in the workplace, with separate washing facilities away from areas where food may be prepared or consumed.

The number of toilets is governed by the number of employees. A toilet must be available for clients. It is essential that toilets are spotlessly clean and checked regularly to ensure that there is a good supply of toilet tissue, disposable hand towels and soap and the waste bin is emptied regularly.

Salon cleaning

It is very important for the salon image, and to prevent the spread of infection, that the premises are kept very clean. Floors and windows should be cleaned once a week. This may be done by a cleaner employed out of business hours. Other daily cleaning jobs must form part of the salon routine, with all staff taking responsibility for completing jobs. This is usually done on a rota basis.

The Local Government (Miscellaneous Provisions) Act provides the local authority with powers to inspect the premises for hygiene and cleaning practices, in particular disposal of waste, cleanliness of floors, work surfaces and sterilising procedures.

ACTIVITY

It is essential that hygiene and safety tasks are carried out daily. Using the information contained in this chapter devise a salon rota to ensure that all daily tasks are completed.

Use your rota to allocate tasks to the staff (students) in the salon and check at the end of the day that the jobs have been completed to your satisfaction.

You will need to discuss the rota with the manager and the staff. Outline how the jobs should be carried out and how you intend to check at the end of the day.

Remember to give feedback on how well the duties have been carried out.

Portfolio evidence

The rota is valuable evidence for your portfolio. Remember to get your teacher or assessor to date and sign the rota, to observe you allocating jobs and monitoring that they have been carried out.

Salon duties
General cleaning

Floors may be cleaned out of business hours, however it is important that any spillages are wiped up immediately. Wet floors should have a clear sign to stop people walking over them until the surface is dry and safe to walk on. Carpets should be vacuumed as required and any worn or frayed areas secured to avoid tripping.

Laundry

There must be sufficient clean towels, sheets and headbands to supply the salon. Laundry needs to be sorted and put into machines for washing regularly throughout the day. Washed towels need to be dried, folded neatly and stacked on shelves for easy access by the therapists. There should be sufficient washing powder and fabric softener available at all times. In order for the laundry to run efficiently, the machines must be in full working order.

The salon may choose to send towels out to a commercial laundry. This will require counting soiled towels to go out and clean towels when they return. Paperwork will need to be kept up to date to check the accuracy of invoices before payment.

Waste disposal

Each work area must have a small waste bin with a lid and a foot pedal to avoid using hands to open. Used cotton wool and tissues must be placed in the bin, not left lying on the trolley, couch or floor. This bin should be emptied after each client into a large receptacle for disposal at the end of every day.

Specialist or contaminated waste such as disposable epilation probes are placed in a special yellow plastic container called a **sharps box**. This container must be handled with care and removed for incineration at appropriate intervals. Contaminated waste, i.e. with blood or serum on it, should be placed in a bin liner tied securely for incineration.

Broken glass must be disposed of carefully by wrapping in newspaper before placing in the bin.

Basins and wet areas

Blocked basins must be dealt with immediately to avoid unpleasant smells. The S-bend under the basin has a screw cap that can be opened to remove blockages. Basins and shower cubicles must be wiped down after use with disinfectant. A ceramic cleaning fluid should be used at the end of the day to remove oil and lime scale. These can accumulate, leaving unsightly stains that can harbour germs. Disinfectant should be poured down the drains at the end of every day. Saunas and steam baths require regular, thorough cleaning using disinfectant. The warmth and moisture provide the perfect breeding ground for germs.

Trolleys and work surfaces

Surfaces that are dusty and have creams, oils or wax spilt on them look unsightly, unprofessional and will harbour infection. Spillages must be wiped up immediately and all work surfaces kept clean throughout the day.

Detergent will remove oils and creams. Products like depilatory wax should be left to cool, before being picked off the surface. Wipe over with surgical spirit.

Hand mirrors are often neglected and left smeared with fingerprints. There is nothing worse than handing a dirty mirror to the client.

Equipment

Electrical equipment must be wiped over before and after use with a damp cloth to remove dust and any products that may have accumulated during treatment.

At the end of the day a final check must be made to ensure that all electrical appliances and salon equipment is switched off and disconnected.

 Remember to note any electrical faults, switch off the machine, place a clear 'out of order' sign on the machine and report the defect to the salon manager immediately.

Client refreshment facilities

Clients are often offered drinks or snacks in the salon. Hygiene procedures must be very strict when preparing food and drinks. If hot and cold drinks are supplied to the clients, they must be prepared in an area that is suitable, away from treatments and chemicals. The client should consume refreshments in a suitable room or rest area away from the treatment rooms. Disposable containers must be used if there are not adequate facilities for preparing drinks and washing up.

Sterilisation and disinfection

Everyone must be aware of the importance of carrying out strict hygiene procedures to protect themselves, other therapists and clients from infection. Guidelines laid down by the Local Government (Miscellaneous Provisions) Act (see page 10) and Beauty Therapy Codes of Practice outline hygiene procedures that are particularly important when the treatment involves skin piercing (see page 228).

The therapist must be able to recognise skin disease and disorders associated with the area of the body being treated (see chapter 14) and carry out the meticulous hygiene procedures that are outlined in this chapter.

Infection

Infection is caused by micro-organisms that invade the body and cause inflammation. These include:

- bacteria
- viruses
- fungi.

Bacteria

Bacteria that can cause disease are known as **pathogenic**; those that do not cause disease are known as **non-pathogenic**. They are categorised by their shape. Bacterial infection can usually be treated with antibiotics. Signs of bacterial infection are redness, swelling, pain and pus.

Cocci (singular = coccus)

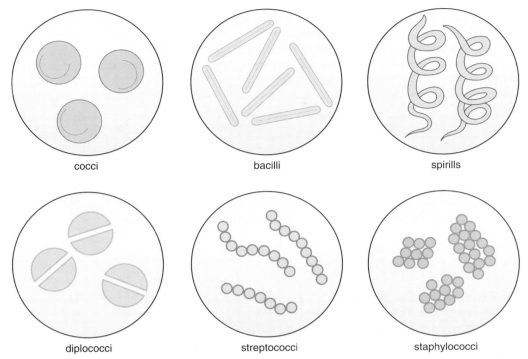

| | | |
| cocci | bacilli | spirills |

| | | |
| diplococci | streptococci | staphylococci |

Figure 1.6 *These types of bacteria can cause infection*

Fungi

Fungi that live on decaying or dead matter are known as **saprophytic**. Those that live on living matter are known as **parasitic**. Both types cause disease within the human body. For example, tinea capitis or ringworm of the scalp, athlete's foot or ringworm of the feet, and onychomycosis or ringworm of the nail.

Viruses

Viruses are smaller than bacteria and infections caused by them are more difficult to control as they are unaffected by antibiotics. Viral diseases are divided into two main groups:

Highly infectious diseases

These are transmitted by direct contact through droplets of moisture or mucus from the nose or mouth. Measles and the common cold are passed on in this way.

Infectious diseases

Here the transmission is not obvious, but can be by direct or indirect contact. Viral infections of the skin fall into this group, such as warts or herpes simplex (cold sores).

There are two serious viral diseases that a beauty therapist should be aware of. They are **Acquired Immune Deficiency Syndrome (AIDS)** and **hepatitis B**.

AIDS

The virus known as the human immunodeficiency virus (**HIV**) affects the body's natural defence or immune system, leaving it susceptible to attack from other diseases, some of which can be fatal. The virus is transmitted within body fluids, such as blood. An HIV-positive person can remain without any symptoms of AIDS for several years. In fact, in the early stages of infection the virus can be present but remain undetected when tested. It is imperative that strict hygiene precautions are followed during all beauty therapy treatments but especially when performing treatments that may involve contact with body fluids. Waxing and eyebrow tweezing, for example, can draw blood. As yet, there is no cure for HIV infection and AIDS.

Hepatitis B

This is a viral disease of the liver, which is also transmitted within body fluids. The virus is more infectious than HIV. This is because the virus is more resistant and is able to live outside the body for a considerable time. The disease is very debilitating and can be fatal. The same strict hygiene precautions should be taken with the hepatitis B virus as with HIV, to avoid cross infection.

Infestations

This is a term used to describe the transmission of diseases caused by small parasites. The most common infestation is by **head lice**. These infect the scalp and are common in small children. The condition is spread directly by contact or by the communal use of brushes or towels.

Another condition that the therapist may come across is **scabies**, where very small mites burrow through and along the epidermis to lay their eggs. The condition can appear red with the presence of swelling and fine lines indicating where the mites have burrowed.

Cross infection

Micro-organisms that cause disease are usually spread by coming into direct contact with the source. Sources include contaminated blood, body fluids, pus, sores or infected skin cells. Unclean tools, shared towels, dirty work surfaces and unwashed hands can be a source of infection in the salon.

Good hygiene procedures and the use of disposable materials will ensure that risk to yourself and others can be minimised. Cuts on your hands must always be covered by a waterproof dressing to avoid infection entering the broken skin.

Methods of sterilisation and disinfection

The terms **sterilisation** and **disinfection** are sometimes confused.

- Sterilisation destroys all micro-organisms using chemicals or high temperature.
- Disinfection inhibits the growth of disease-causing micro-organisms (except spores) using chemical agents.
- Antiseptic is a dilute disinfectant for use on the skin, which will slow the growth of bacteria.

Sterilisation methods are very harsh, using high temperature, such as boiling, or strong chemicals. Sterilisation, therefore, is not suitable for many materials. The skin cannot be sterilised without using special chemicals that would not be suitable for use in the salon. Unless items that have been sterilised are vacuum packed, they can easily be contaminated by organisms that are carried in the air.

The therapist will generally use disinfectants or antiseptics that will inhibit the growth of bacteria.

Sterilisation methods:

- The **autoclave** uses high-pressure steaming at a minimum temperature of 126°C. Autoclaves for salon use are small compact units that provide sterilisation for small metal implements. They are safe and easy to use providing the manufacturer's instructions are followed closely.

- The **bead steriliser** uses dry heat at a temperature of 200–300°C. These have limited use in the salon due to the small area available at the correct temperature for sterilisation. Because of the risk of burns when the implements are removed, they need to be used with care.

- **Ultraviolet light steriliser** uses ultraviolet rays from a quartz mercury vapour lamp. This method is very limited because of the need to turn the implements over to expose each surface to the rays. The cabinets do, however, provide a germ-free environment to store previously sterilised implements.

- **Gamma radiation** is used for epilation needles at the point of manufacture. It is used under controlled conditions when large-scale sterilisation is required.

- **Chemical agents** are available which, when diluted, can be used as sterilising fluids or disinfectants, depending on the dilution. There are implications for health and safety in the salon due to the very toxic nature of the chemicals. A COSHH risk assessment would be required to ensure that special safety precautions are followed when preparing sterilising fluid for the salon. Chemicals used are:
  - quaternary ammonium compound (QUATS)
  - gluteraldehyde
  - alcohol or surgical spirit.

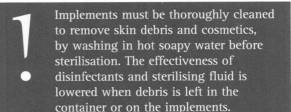

Implements must be thoroughly cleaned to remove skin debris and cosmetics, by washing in hot soapy water before sterilisation. The effectiveness of disinfectants and sterilising fluid is lowered when debris is left in the container or on the implements.

Precautions to prevent the spread of infection

1. Cover any cuts or broken skin on the hands with a waterproof dressing.
2. Wear rubber gloves when carrying out any treatment where blood may be drawn to the surface of the skin.

Bleeding may occur during treatments where the skin is pierced or a needle is inserted into the hair follicle, e.g. ear-piercing, electro-epilation.

The therapist may also cause blood spots from the hair follicle during eyebrow shaping or depilatory waxing, particularly if very coarse hair is being removed, such as with underarm or bikini-line waxing. The coarse hairs grow from follicles that are deep within the dermis and surrounded by blood capillaries (see page 288). It is these capillaries that rupture as the hair is plucked from the follicle.

Dealing with blood spots requires very strict hygiene procedures to ensure that the therapist does not come into contact with the blood, to reduce the risk of infecting the client and to ensure that contaminated materials are disposed of correctly.

Procedure for dealing with blood spots or accidental cuts during treatment

1. Soak cotton wool in antiseptic or surgical spirit and apply pressure.
2. Place contaminated cotton wool in a covered waste bin inside a securely tied bin liner.
3. Wash your hands.

The therapist may choose to take added precautions against infection by the hepatitis B virus. It is possible to be vaccinated against this disease by a doctor.

Try to extend the following list of hazards in the salon by adding your own examples.

- Slipping on wet floors or oil spilt on the floor
- Tripping over trailing wires or loose carpet
- Burns from hot wax
- Scalds from hot water or steam
- Allergic reaction to chemicals
- Electric shock from exposed wiring or poorly maintained equipment
- Cross infection from poor hygiene procedures or treating clients when infection is present
- Drowsiness and fainting due to poor ventilation or fumes from toxic chemicals (e.g. nail extension products)
- Fire from incorrect storage of flammable products or overloading of electrical circuits
- Back strain from poor posture

Hygiene checklist
Before the start of a treatment

1. Wipe the trolley with disinfectant and cover with disposable paper.
2. All tools that have been previously washed and sterilised must be placed on a clean tissue or in disinfectant on the trolley. Sponges can be placed in disinfectant such as Milton.
3. Prepare the couch with clean laundry and disposable bed paper.
4. Check your appearance and wash hands thoroughly.
5. Carry out a close inspection of the client's skin in the area to be treated to check for contraindications.

During treatment

1. Preparations are dispensed using a clean spatula onto the back of the hand or from the spatula. This is known as a **cut-out technique**. (Fingers must not be dipped into products.)
2. All waste products must be placed immediately into a closed bin, preferably using a foot pedal to open it.
3. Apply all cosmetics with disposable applicators where possible.
4. If implements fall on the floor, wipe them over with disinfectant.
5. If you need to leave the client to do another job such as answer the phone, wash your hands before returning to the client.

On completion of the treatment

1. Wash all implements in hot soapy water to remove products and skin debris.
2. Wipe over the trolley with disinfectant and prepare for the next client.
3. Wipe cosmetic jars and bottles and store in a closed cabinet.
4. Wash sponges and brushes in hot soapy water and rinse in an antiseptic solution.
5. Dispose of all waste materials from the treatment area in a lined covered bin.
6. Place soiled laundry in a basket for laundering.
7. Wash hands.

Chapter 2

SALON RECEPTION DUTIES

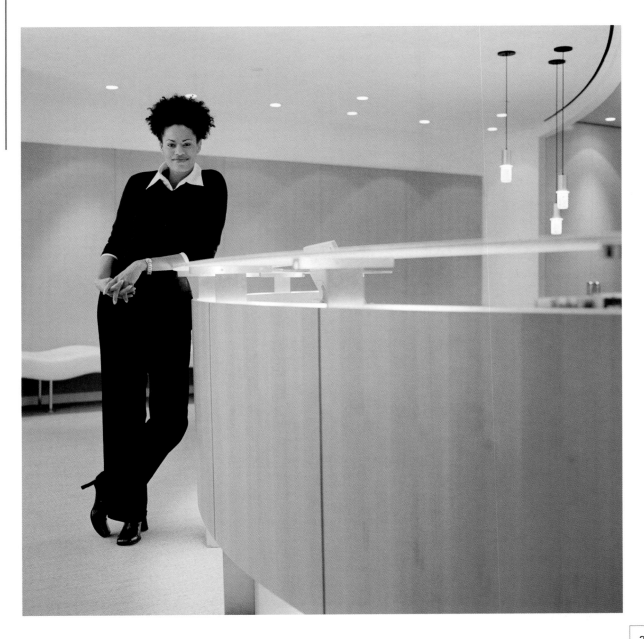

- The role of a receptionist
- Interpersonal skills
- The Data Protection Act
- Reception procedures
  - dealing with clients
  - answering the telephone
  - handling enquiries
  - giving information
  - taking messages
  - making appointments
  - dealing with payments

Introduction

Welcoming and receiving clients and visitors to the salon is an important part of the salon service. The client's **first impression** of the salon is given by the receptionist, whether on the telephone or in person.

All visitors and people making enquiries are potential clients. Therefore they must be treated in a **polite** and **helpful** manner.

The receptionist
The role of the receptionist

Clients attending a beauty therapy salon like to feel relaxed and to enjoy quality time in a pleasant environment. The receptionist can start the process the moment the client enters the salon by using their **interpersonal skills.**

- Make eye contact with the client.
- Smile and have a friendly manner.
- Be calm and gently spoken.
- Give the client individual attention and show respect.
- Show genuine interest in the client.
- Be sensitive to the needs of clients and therapists.
- Take care not to do or say anything that could offend, particularly if it involves race, gender or religion.
- Ensure client confidentiality at all times.

Everyone working in a busy salon will have to carry out reception duties from time to time. So it is important that all staff are aware of the procedures for dealing with clients and the manner in which they should be treated.

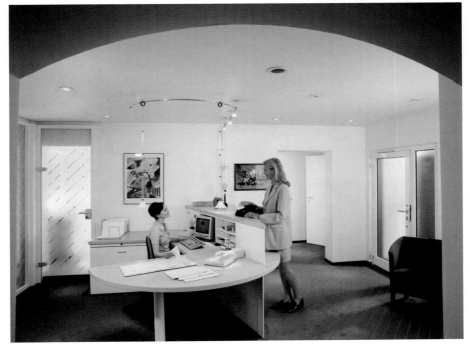

Figure 2.1 *The reception area gives the client their first impression of the salon*

The reception area

This is the first part of the salon that the client comes into contact with. It must give a good impression by providing an area that reflects the high standards of hygiene and cleanliness, personal attention, comfort and relaxation that are associated with a beauty therapy salon.

The reception area must be kept clean and tidy by ensuring that:

- carpets are vacuumed regularly
- retail displays are dusted and neatly arranged to attract the client's attention
- there is a good supply of information leaflets
- used coffee cups, etc., are removed
- flowers or plants are fresh and cared for
- magazines are kept up to date and stacked tidily.

Caring for the client
Welcome the client

The receptionist must make the client feel welcome by speaking to them as soon as they enter the salon, then helping them with their coat and offering them a seat. Magazines should be available with an offer of coffee or other beverages. A drinks machine can be a very useful asset in a reception area, allowing clients to help themselves. This can save both the receptionist and the therapist time. Information on treatments should be readily available for the client to browse through.

Dealing with delays

Should there be any delay the client must be informed as soon as possible and given an estimate of how long the delay will be.

If there is any change to the appointment, the client should be politely informed and offered alternatives.

Client records

Client records need to be available for the therapists. They should be updated by the therapist and filed after use.

Many large organisations use computer software to coordinate client appointments, client records and stock records. The receptionist in this case will be responsible for entering accurate data into the computer for each client, including:

a) client appointments
b) client's record card, including up-to-date personal data, accurate information regarding contraindications and medical history, and treatments carried out
c) products used or purchased, providing the salon manager with information for stock control.

Saying goodbye to the client

When the client is ready to leave, the receptionist must ensure that she has been offered another appointment and deal with any retail requirements. The client should be helped with their coat and thanked as they leave the salon.

Client care and communication is covered in chapter 5.

Handling enquiries and giving information

Good **communication skills** are an essential part of the beauty therapist's job and the role of the receptionist.

Communication skills are used to give and receive information. They include:

- speaking clearly
- listening
- reading and writing
- use of body language
- personal presentation.

A potential client will usually require details of treatments and products available in the salon. The receptionist should be able to explain the benefits of a treatment, how long it will take and the cost. Treatment price lists or product leaflets can be offered to the client.

Information should be as accurate and as helpful as possible. It should be offered in a caring and discreet manner. If you do not know the answer to a question, ask another member of staff. Remember that some questions from a client enquiring about treatment may be of a sensitive nature and must therefore be handled carefully and referred to the most appropriate member of staff.

Confidentiality
The Data Protection Act

The purpose of the Act is to protect people from having information about themselves freely available to others. The 1989 Act extends the 1984 Act to bring legislation in line with Europe.

The major changes that concern client records are:

- The new Act now includes manual filing of personal information.
- Only relevant personal data should be collected. This could bring into question the huge amount of information contained in some client record cards.

- Any personal information about the client must only be recorded and retained on seeking explicit permission from the client.
- The client has a right to access any information held in client record cards.
- Releasing any personal details to third parties without specific consent is not permitted.

Any organisation that keeps information on record about people (staff or clients) must:

- register with the Data Protection Registrar
- ensure that all information is accurate and up to date
- provide access to the person's own record if requested
- keep records in a safe, secure place.

ACTIVITY

Look at the client record system in your salon and evaluate whether it meets the requirements of the Data Protection Act.

Use the headings below as possible areas for discussion:

- Is there a code of practice for dealing with personal information?
- Where are records stored?
- Who has access to them?
- Do the clients sign to show they give permission for their personal details to be kept?
- Are the clients aware of their rights under the Act?

Any information given by the client, perhaps for the record card or to do with the type of treatment they request, must be treated as confidential. It should not be discussed, other than in a professional capacity, with other members of staff. Some treatments such as epilation (permanent hair removal) require detailed information on the client's health and medication. This information must be treated with sensitivity. Some clients requiring treatment for permanent hair removal may not wish other clients, who may be acquaintances, to know about it.

Some clients, wishing to be friendly, may involve you in gossip. Try to change the subject by choosing a more general topic. Never answer questions about other clients and always respond by saying that you do not have the information or that it would be inappropriate to answer the question. The best way to avoid difficult or unprofessional conversation is to remain businesslike and deal only with the reception duties.

> ! Being friendly does not require you to be familiar. Do not discuss your own personal details with the client.

Types of confidential information

- client record cards
  - name, address, telephone number
  - medical information
  - treatment information

- client's financial transactions
  - how much they spend
  - how payment is made
- information relating to the business
  - salon financial matters
  - treatment routines
  - product formulations
- staff records.

Such information must be available only to the business and its therapists. It should be kept in a locked filing cabinet or on a secure computer.

Answering the telephone

It is important to answer the telephone promptly on the second or third ring. The salon will usually have a standard response when answering the telephone. The name of the salon, your name and an offer of help should be included. You should answer with a friendly, clear and enthusiastic manner. A dull voice will give an impression of boredom and disinterest. Do not use slang and sloppy speech.

Listen carefully to what the client has to say and respond in a positive way either by making an appointment, answering a question, taking a message or offering to call back if necessary. Repeat back to the caller the main points of the conversation, such as their full name or initials (remember there are lots of Smiths), telephone number and the details of the appointment you have made for them. Always do something positive rather than say no or that you don't know. Use the client's name as you speak to them. Not only is this polite, but it will help you to remember their name in the future. Always end by thanking the client for calling.

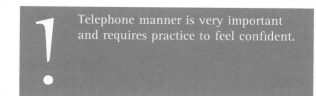
Telephone manner is very important and requires practice to feel confident.

Answering machines

An answering machine is useful for the therapist who works alone and is unable to answer the telephone during treatments. It also allows clients to contact the salon out of hours to request appointments, make enquiries or cancel appointments. All messages should be dealt with promptly and those requiring a return call must be dealt with immediately.

Electronic mail (e-mail)

E-mail has become the most widely used and efficient means of transferring information. Most large salons have a computer and when attached to the phone line with the appropriate software it is a means of storing and transferring information. E-mail allows instant responses, providing all parties are linked to the Internet.

Facsimile (FAX)

This is a very useful and quick means of transferring black-and-white documents such as invoices. The document is transmitted via the telephone line from one fax machine to another.

Taking messages

It may not be possible for a client to speak to a particular member of staff, whether on the telephone or face-to-face. A receptionist must be able to take accurate information from the client and judge the urgency of the call. A message that is clearly an emergency must be dealt with immediately. All messages must be acted upon as soon as possible. Some messages may be confidential and will therefore require direct contact with the individual therapist concerned.

A system should be in place so that no message is overlooked. You might consider using a noticeboard in the staff room or behind the reception for messages, to be displayed so that they can be seen clearly. Message pads of bright-coloured paper can be placed on the reception desk. Carbonised paper is useful as it ensures that there are two or more copies as a record of all messages received in the salon.

Dealing with problems and the dissatisfied client

The receptionist has to handle a range of problems that can affect the smooth running of the salon. Examples may include:

- a client who is late for their appointment
- a client who demands treatment that is not booked and therefore no time has been allowed
- a client who is dissatisfied with their treatment
- a therapist who is delayed taking their clients for treatment.

Each of these situations needs to be handled sensitively. Listen to the client carefully, without making judgements or excuses. In the case of a client who is late or where a treatment has been incorrectly booked, it will be necessary to speak to the therapist concerned to see if they have time to fit the client in to their appointments schedule. Do not attempt to make decisions without consulting the therapist.

If a client has a complaint about a treatment, discuss the problem with the therapist concerned or a senior member of staff straight away. Reassure the client that the matter will be dealt with. Do not try to make amends yourself by offering free treatment, for example. This would be beyond the limits of your authority. The manager will follow the salon policy on complaints and decide what action should be taken.

Your job is to keep the client calm, ensuring that they are dealt with promptly. The complaint should be logged by recording the date, time, name of client, details of the problem, how it was handled and by whom.

Providing help and support

It is sometimes necessary to provide support for the therapists when they are very busy and falling behind with their appointments. You may be required to:

- liaise with the therapist and client, keeping them both informed of any delay
- tidy or prepare work areas
- provide coffee and magazines for the client.

Booking appointments

Perhaps the most complex and important job for the receptionist is booking appointments. Mistakes can cause frustration and delay to both therapists and clients and may lead to loss of takings. There is nothing more annoying for a client than to find that the appointment they booked has not been written down or that the information on their appointment card is incorrect. Equally, the therapist will not be pleased at the disruption this may cause to other clients during the day.

Each salon will have its own system of booking appointments, but often a special printed book or loose-leaf sheets in a file are used. The appointment book is an important business record, which must be retained for auditing purposes.

The receptionist must:

- ensure that there is a good supply of pencils, pens, appointment cards, an eraser, ruler and message pads
- prepare appointment pages for several weeks in advance
- be aware of therapists' times in the salon, taking account of part-time staff, holidays and so on
- book all appointments in pencil so that they can be adjusted easily and neatly
- understand abbreviations and the timing of different treatments
- have a salon price list available
- be aware of individual clients and their special requirements
- know how to book courses of treatments and schedule follow-up appointments
- work closely with the therapists, seeking their advice on how appointments and clients should be scheduled. Remember they will know the individual needs of their clients and how long they require to carry out treatments.

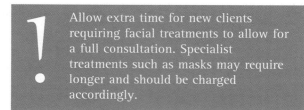

Allow extra time for new clients requiring facial treatments to allow for a full consultation. Specialist treatments such as masks may require longer and should be charged accordingly.

Use pencil to write appointments so that they can easily be changed if necessary.

Abbreviation	Meaning
DNA	did not attend
C	cancellation
✓	client arrived

Treatment	Abbreviation	Approximate Timing
Half-leg wax using warm wax	1/2/Leg cool	30 mins
Underarm wax using hot wax	U/arm hot	15 mins
Manicure with paraffin wax treatment	Man/paraffin wax	45 mins
Cleanse with evening make-up	Cleanse/eve m/up	1 hour
Eyelashes and brow tint	Lash/brow	30 mins
Full body massage	B/mass	1 hour
Eyebrow shape	E/B	15 mins
Manicure	Man	45 mins
Full leg wax, bikini, under arm	Full leg/bikini/U/arm	75 mins
Facial (deep cleanse and make-up)	Facial/m/up	45 mins
Ear-piercing	E/pierce	15 mins
Pedicure	Ped	45 mins

Abbreviations and timings used in booking appointments

AU NATURAL BEAUTY CLINIC

Date:	24 August	THURSDAY	LATE NIGHT
Time	HELEN	SUE	SOPHIE
9.00	LATE NIGHT	Nan Clancy ✔	Mrs Zaleski ✔
9.15	7.00 p.m.	man/ped	B/mass 322432
9.30			
9.45			
10.00	Mrs Hutton ✔		Sue Rossington ✔
10.15	Facial		Facial 535700
10.30		Mrs Allport ✔	e.b.
10.45		Facial	lash tint
11.00	Joan Smith ✔ 398366		
11.15	Pedicure		
11.30		Jenny Cheshire ✔	Pam ✔ 793666
11.45	Sarah O'Brien ✔	man	ear piercing
12.00	Cleanse m/up	Helen Rycroft ✔	lunch
12.15	e.b. 893883	Facial/m/up	
12.30			
12.45	Miss Briton ✔		
1.00	½ leg 614723		Tiffany **C**
1.15	LUNCH	LUNCH	lash/brow e.b.
1.30			Charlotte ✔
1.45		Mrs Marsland ✔	B/o Mass
2.00		Sauna Jan Moss ✔ e.b.	
2.15	Pam Thorpe	Full, B. Mas.	
2.30	Facial ✔		Harriet C. **DNA** 379212
2.45			3 Nails replaced
3.00			Beathem ✔
3.15	Pickford 637639		½ leg
3.30	man ✔	Mrs Albaya de Gago	Edern ✔
3.45	Beckey	Nails (full set)	man
4.00	Ear-piercing	✔	Jo Kirk ✔
4.15	✔		Ped
4.30	Janet Carter		½ leg
4.45	Facial ✔		
5.00		Sarah lash tint	
5.15		DNA	
5.30	Full leg/bikini		
5.45	Lip wax		
6.00			
6.15			
6.30			

Figure 2.2 *You must make neat entries into the appointments book*

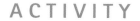

ACTIVITY

Look around your reception area and make a list of:

The things that attract clients to the
salon and make them want to return

Any improvements that could be made

ACTIVITY

Use the log below to record the range of clients and activities. This will provide evidence for your portfolio.

LOG OF VISITORS TO RECEPTION

Dates on reception

		With appointments – name	Without appointments – name	Requiring salon services	Having business with the salon
New clients and visitors	1				
	2				
	3				
	4				
	5				
	6				
	7				
Existing clients and visitors	1				
	2				
	3				
	4				
	5				
	6				
	7				
	8				

Assessor/Supervisor Signature . . . .   Student Signature . . . .

Student's log of activities while carrying out reception duties

Portfolio evidence

The telephone reception log may go towards assessment evidence for your portfolio.

Name of person requesting price lists	Name of person requiring information regarding services and products	Name of client booking a treatment	Communication with individuals on the premises
Complaints regarding services and products	Business calls from suppliers of goods and services	Person seeking employment, course details	Internal calls

Please note down the date and the person's name

Assessor/Supervisor Signature . . . .   Student Signature . . . .

Calculating and taking payments

The duties carried out by the receptionist will ultimately affect the whole business. The care required when recording information, whether it is client details on a record card, treatment information in the appointment book or accuracy in handling money, is crucial to the business. The reception desk must be fully equipped to ensure time is not wasted searching for a pen for a client to write a cheque, for example.

The salon should have a policy and procedures for dealing with customers at the payment point. Advice on dealing with different payment methods is given on page 35.

Stationery

A good supply of stationery is essential, including ballpoint pens, pencils, spare till rolls, notepads, date stamp and salon name stamp.

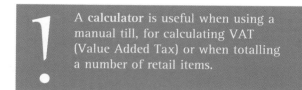

A **calculator** is useful when using a manual till, for calculating VAT (Value Added Tax) or when totalling a number of retail items.

Cash float

A cash float in the till is necessary to ensure that there is sufficient change when dealing with cash transactions. The receptionist must make sure that there is change available throughout the day. This means thinking ahead and changing notes as necessary. Change may be kept in the business safe or arrangements may have to be made for change with a bank. It can be very annoying for the client to be kept waiting while the receptionist hunts for the correct change.

The cash float may also be used as **petty cash**. Petty cash is used for small incidental items such as fresh milk, postage stamps or cleaning materials. It is essential that receipts for petty cash purchases are retained for the salon accounts.

Credit card equipment

Credit card equipment is required if a salon chooses to accept credit cards. For a small salon that only deals in small transactions, it may not be worth the fee that the credit card company requires. If the business is authorised to accept credit cards, vouchers and a transaction printer will be necessary. (See also Computerised tills below.)

The till
Computerised tills

Computerised systems that incorporate records of stock levels and clients, for example, may be used in large salons. The computer is usually attached to an automatic till that records the transaction, stores the money and produces the client receipt. Some salons may also have a facility on the till to take debit and credit payment cards.

Electric tills

An automatic electric till is used by most salons. This records the transaction on a till roll as well as producing a receipt for the client. Cashing up is automatic on the press of a key and subtotals can be made at any point in the day by pressing specific keys.

Manual tills

A manual till, which is a lockable drawer, may be all that is required in a small salon. Any transactions must be recorded by hand. It is more likely that errors will occur with this system and there is more opportunity for pilfering.

Because of the different types of tills, payment methods and salon policy, you will need to be trained in all aspects of payment procedures for your salon.

Payment

The receptionist must be able to:

■ handle a range of payment methods
  - personal cheques
  - credit cards

- debit cards
- cash
- gift vouchers

■ be accurate when totalling bills and giving change

■ provide an itemised bill for the client

■ issue receipts

■ record the transaction.

Payments in cash

The basic procedure will be as follows:

■ You will receive information from the therapist on the treatment the client has received. An itemised docket or bill is required. This may also include retail items. (Remember the retail payments will need to be recorded separately for auditing purposes.)

■ Total the bill and inform the client of the cost.

■ Key in the amount(s) into the till.

■ If appropriate, ask the client how they would like to pay.

■ When payment is in cash, accept the money and look carefully at the note(s) you have been given. There are special facilities for detecting forged notes. It is a good idea to place the note(s) on the till whilst you calculate the change.

■ Count out the change into the client's hand and ask them to confirm that it is correct.

■ Place the note(s) from the top of the till in the till drawer in the appropriate section and close it.

■ Give the client a receipt and thank them.

Payments by cheque

The procedure is as follows:

■ Before accepting a cheque, make sure the client has a cheque guarantee card. This card guarantees payment up to a certain amount, usually £50 or £100.

■ Check the card details are valid (see Figure 2.3).

■ Write the card number on the back of the cheque.

■ Make sure that the signature on the card matches the one on the cheque.

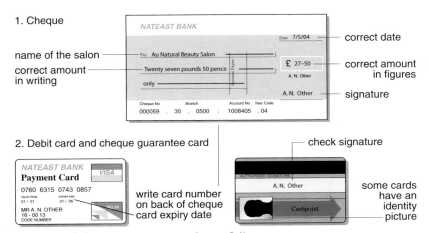

Figure 2.3 *Check cheques and cheque guarantee cards carefully*

When receiving payment by cheque follow the details shown in Figure 2.3. Do not rush, take time to check all the details carefully. Remember a cheque that is made out incorrectly may result in the bank delaying payment or refusing to pay the money into the salon account.

Look closely at the signature on the cheque and make sure it matches the signature on the client's cheque card.

Payments by credit card

The salon must have an agreement with companies such as **Visa** or **Mastercard** if they want to accept credit cards. A charge is made by the credit card company, usually a percentage of each transaction.

If a client wishes to pay by credit card the following procedure should be followed:

- Look closely at the card and check the hologram and bank name.
- Check the expiry date on the card. If it is out of date, do not accept it. Request some other form of payment.
- If the card is valid take a credit card voucher supplied by the credit card company (this is carbonised, giving three copies). Using the card machine, imprint the card details onto the voucher. This will include the card number, which must be clearly visible.
- Complete the details of the service and the amount charged using a ballpoint pen.
- Ask the client to check the details and sign.
- Check the signature against the card. Return the card and the top copy of the voucher to the client.
- Place the copies in the till, one for the credit card company and one for the salon.

A computerised terminal may be used for credit cards and debit cards. The procedure to follow is described below.

Payments using debit cards/credit cards

An electronic payment system such as **Maestro** or **Connect** is used by many people instead of cash or cheque. The system uses debit cards, which are issued by the bank. (These cards may also act as cheque guarantee cards.)

You may be familiar with this system from supermarkets and other shops where payment points or checkouts have this facility. If the salon has a debit/credit card terminal the procedure is as follows:

- The terminal is linked to a main computer which recognises the customer's card as it is swiped.
- The details of the transaction are keyed into the terminal and a printout authorising payment direct from the customer's account is produced.
- The customer checks and signs the authorisation printout.
- The signature is checked against the card and a copy of the transaction and the card is returned to the customer.
- PIN numbers are becoming more widely used instead of a signature.

Payment by gift voucher or discount voucher

Gift vouchers are **prepaid vouchers** that are treated in the same way as cash. Most vouchers are dated to be used within a certain time, usually six months or a year from the date of purchase. The vouchers should indicate the value clearly and will usually be sold as £1, £5 or £10 'notes'. Each voucher should show the name of the salon, a signature and a number that corresponds with an entry in a book recording the date it was sold. This will guard against possible fraud.

Discount vouchers are a way of promoting salon services and may be part of an advertising campaign in the local paper: '£3 off when you spend £20 or more on presentation of this voucher' or 'A free manicure with every full facial on presentation of this voucher before Saturday June 15'. These discount vouchers are a form of payment and must be collected for the salon records.

Dealing with invalid payments

In a busy environment such as the beauty therapy salon, mistakes can be made. These may not be noticed until the end of the day.

Discrepancies and invalid payments include:

- unsigned cheques
- incorrect date
- suspected fraudulent use of a payment card
- foreign currency (usually only small amounts in coins)
- out-of-date gift voucher
- incorrect adding up of a bill
- giving the wrong change
- pressing the wrong keys when entering amounts into the till.

These should be dealt with as soon as possible by contacting the client, if appropriate. If an error, such as accepting a cheque without a cheque guarantee card has occurred, the cheque may bounce. This happens if there are insufficient funds in the client's account and may lead to loss of the payment by the salon. The cheque can be presented to the bank again, but if there is no money in the client's account the salon must stand the loss.

Fortunately, illegal transactions are not common, but the receptionist must be aware of the possibility of a client using **forged** notes or a **stolen** credit card or cheque book.

If you have any doubt about the payment being made by a client, a senior member of staff should be called immediately. This must be done discreetly and without alarming the client.

The salon will usually have a **policy** on handling situations such as bad debts and fraudulent payments. Your job will be to take advice from the manager or senior therapist. Check what situations you have authority to deal with as they arise.

How to keep cash and other payments safe and secure
Money

- Money should not be left on the premises overnight.
- The till drawer should be left open to show that it is empty.
- An electric till should be installed. This ensures that takings are locked away, that there are receipts and a record of transactions on the till roll.
- The salon owner will decide who has access to the till security code or keys and who is responsible for cashing up at the end of the day. Any discrepancies should be dealt with immediately.

ACTIVITY

If, as part of your duties as a receptionist, you are required to 'cash up' at the end of the day, keep a copy of the dockets or takings sheet.

Write a brief explanation of how your particular system of recording works. Remember there are many different methods of keeping financial records.

Get your supervisor or assessor to check the accuracy of your records and ask them to sign to show that all financial transactions that you were responsible for were correct for the day.

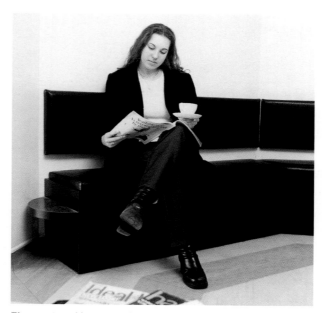

Figure 2.4 *Always make the client feel comfortable*

Chapter 3

PROMOTING PRODUCTS AND SERVICES TO CLIENTS

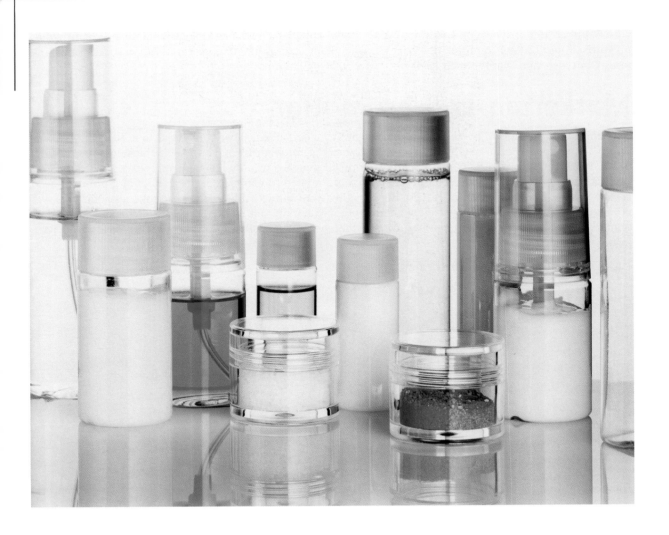

IN THIS CHAPTER YOU WILL LEARN ABOUT:

- Marketing and promotion
- Identifying the need for additional products and services
- Ethical selling
- Legislation
- Client feedback and how to deal with it

Introduction

In order for any salon business to survive and make a profit, customers must be encouraged to return. The responsibility for making this happen falls upon everyone within the establishment. Effective marketing and promotion by management will draw new clients into the salon, but all staff are responsible for providing the right circumstances to ensure their return custom. This involves professionalism, a comfortable environment, client care, good quality treatments and a friendly atmosphere. Once a client has become loyal to the salon, their interest in new or different treatments should be encouraged. The correct promotion of the salon's product range should complement the treatment without the client feeling pressurised into buying. Additional services and products sold by the therapist not only increase salon profits but also can improve their salary by accumulating commission.

Marketing and promotion

A definition of promotion is, 'the means by which we make known what we have to sell or what we want to buy'. A definition of marketing is, 'to create a demand for what we have to sell'. The salon may decide to glean information from new and existing clientele by means of a market research questionnaire. This can be placed on the reception desk, where clients are invited to complete it. New ideas and promotions can be based on the information gained. Encouraging new and existing clientele to take up additional products and services relies on effective advertising, promotion and marketing. Special events can be organised by the management team but it is the therapist's responsibility to take a willing and active part in the event to benefit all.

The reasons for a promotion may be to:

- announce a new product or service
- attract new clients
- announce a change to the business
- make a special offer
- invite enquiries
- announce the location of stockists
- educate new and existing clientele
- maintain sales
- challenge competition
- remind existing clientele.

There are four steps to effective promotion and marketing:

Advertising

Advertising can be described as paid for, non-personal communication in a mass medium such as newspapers, magazines, radio, television and billboards. Radio and television adverts may certainly feel out of the reach of a local salon, but local radio stations may be able to promote a special event more widely than an advert in the local paper and so should not be dismissed on cost alone.

Placing an advert in a newspaper or trade magazine is expensive, so careful choice of media is essential. Consider the readership of a trade journal, for example, as it will be clients you are seeking to attract. Leaflets or a mailshot can be a cheaper option but your target group should still be considered. A window display to promote a new service or product range can work if the salon's position encourages 'walk-in' trade. Organising a demonstration to local groups is an effective way of telling people what you have to offer.

ACTIVITY

Design a leaflet or mailshot advertising a special promotion for your salon.

Selling

This usually involves the therapist in 'face-to-face' communication with the client. Excellent communication skills are therefore essential for effective selling technique. A therapist may feel uncomfortable selling in this way but they are in a perfect position to do so. Ethical selling should be seen as helping the client to achieve their needs and expectations. More on ethical selling techniques later in this chapter. Effective communication techniques are discussed fully in chapter 5.

Questioning techniques using open-ended questions to obtain accurate information from the client is only one part of effective communication. Listening to the information and watching for non-verbal communication signs ensures that accurate and appropriate advice is given to match the client's needs and expectations to the appropriate product and service. Gain commitment from the client to the discussion by asking a closed question, for example, 'Would you like to try the moisturiser I have used today?'

Publicity

Publicity can be described as non-personal communication in a mass medium such as a newspaper that is not paid for. It can come in the form of a favourable editorial comment or news story. Word of mouth is possibly the best form of publicity. If a client has received good service in all aspects of their visit to the salon, they are likely to inform friends and relatives. This can generate significant extra trade.

Sales promotion

These are persuasive activities, that may involve displays, demonstrations, exhibitions, competitions, vouchers, gift tokens, free gifts and sampling. (See also chapter 6, Make-up planning and promoting activities.)

Sales promotion should give products and services a short period of added value and can be used to improve sales. Techniques used are:

- Introductory trial – a special reduced cost to encourage clients to try a new product or service. Frequently used when a salon is introducing a new service. After the trial period the price of the service returns to normal.
- Building customer loyalty – a reduced rate on treatments for a number of sessions or block bookings rather than payment for single sessions.
- Combined services – a reduced rate is offered on an additional service when booked with another. For example: book a facial and get a manicure half price.
- Sampling – samples of products are given to encourage clients to try new product ranges or a new one within an existing range. A useful promotion when linked with the products used within the treatment or as aftercare.

- Vouchers – this technique can include gift vouchers to be redeemed at a later date or money-off vouchers redeemable against services or products.

- Free gifts – to be used with caution but can encourage additional purchases. For example: 'If you buy a cleanser and toner you will receive a free trial-size moisturiser'.

- Competitions – when a salon or supplier donates a prize such as a product or treatment, either within the salon or at a related event, e.g. a health page in the local newspaper. This promotes additional interest in the salon or service.

- Trade incentives – often suppliers will offer special discounts and incentives in order to encourage salons to 'stock up'. Although these can result in an excellent return for the money spent by the salon, care should be taken in these situations. If the reduction by the supplier is given in order to sell stock in old packaging, for example, the salon may have difficulty selling the products to clients without reducing the price, so cancelling any benefits that may have been gained.

- Talks and demonstrations – given in offices, at women's clubs, on local radio or to newspapers, these are an effective way of promoting services and are often given in return for prizes of free treatments.

- Editorials – these take the form of unbiased reports on treatments or products. They are very effective as a means of publicity as it is thought that one page of editorial is worth twelve of advertising. It is, therefore, worth building up a good relationship with the local press.

Identifying the need for additional products and services

The need for promotion has two aspects. The salon's need as a business is firstly to survive and then to make a profit. The therapist's time is an expensive commodity and as such should be utilised properly. Staff will expect to be paid even when not performing treatments, so to ensure that each therapist is kept busy makes economic sense. Commission is often paid to therapists on products and services sold to clients to increase salary and encourage the therapist to promote these areas. It is thought that approximately one-third of a salon's profit should come from product sales.

Of course, the most important need to consider is that of the client. Whether they are a new or existing client, they should be considered in the same way.

Establish the client's needs and expectations

Communication is the key to establishing the client's needs and expectations. Discussion should be based around the client's perception of their requirement, but the therapist may need to educate if the client has unrealistic expectations. This is important if the therapist is to fulfil their client's needs accurately, sending them away happy and likely to return or even tell a friend.

Recommending the wrong service or product is short economy as the client is unlikely to return and may even recommend friends not to visit the salon.

The timing and location of the discussion are important too. The client may have walked into the salon without an appointment to make an enquiry. It is important to provide privacy for the discussion as the enquiry may involve a treatment of a private nature and the client may not wish to discuss this in a busy reception area.

For clients who have booked appointments, the consultation is the correct time to discuss the client's needs and expectations. A lot of emphasis is placed on the contraindication to treatment, but once these have been considered and it has been established that the treatment can safely go ahead, the emphasis should turn to providing the most suitable treatment for the client. (Consultation techniques are discussed in chapter 5.)

A regular client should not be overlooked in this regard. It is a mistake to assume that the client is still in need of the treatment or product prescribed on a previous visit. Regular analysis of the treatment area and asking questions that follow up on the aftercare advice and/or treatment provides the therapist with the relevant information to judge whether or not change is necessary.

Additional products and services could be:

- **New to the client** – during conversation the client may express an interest in a new or different product or service they have seen advertised. Additionally the therapist may suggest a new product or service when a problem or requirement presents itself. For example, the client announces that their daughter is getting married, an ideal time to promote 'The Wedding Service' offered by the salon.

- **Replace an existing** – the process of regular analysis of the client's condition allows another product or service to be highlighted by the therapist.

- **More of the same** – a repeat analysis and discussion may determine that the treatment and products recommended are still suitable. Do not change a product or service that a client is happy with and that is fulfilling their need.

- **Referral to another** – a service or product, highlighted by the therapist or client enquiry, may not be available from the salon or their usual therapist. Referral to another professional person to fulfil the client's needs may be necessary. This should be done without bias and professionalism must be maintained e.g. referral to a chiropodist after a pedicure.

The therapist's responsibilities

Everyone in the organisation has a responsibility to promote additional products and services but the therapist is in a prime position to do so. The therapist's responsibilities to the client are to:

- **Know what is available** – the therapist must have knowledge of the services and products that the establishment offers in order to promote them effectively. This may mean attending seminars, training days or reading promotional material from manufacturers.

- **Understand effects, benefits and features** – describe how the service or product will aid the client in fulfilling or correcting the requirement or problem established during discussion. The therapist must ensure the information given is correct in order for the advice to be accurate. Inaccurate advice results in a dissatisfied client and possible prosecution under the relevant legislation, e.g. The Trades Description Act 1972.

- **Know your limitations** – referral procedures are firmly established within an organisation regarding contraindications, but there are times when client's wishes are beyond the responsibility of the therapist. The therapist must be aware of their own limitations. For example, a client with severe acne may need referral to a doctor. The therapist must also be aware of the limitations of the products and treatments they are performing and not claim that a remedy is likely when impossible.

Ethical selling

Ethical selling relies on the professionalism of the therapist to only promote products and services that are going to benefit the client. This should concentrate on providing solutions to the client's problems and requirements and must not be based on the latest trends, the services the therapist prefers to perform or the amount of stock in the stockroom.

The therapist is in an ideal position to advise a client on the best suitable product or service.

Selling procedures

- **Create the desire** – in the form of promotions, displays, posters, demonstrations, talks, etc. All this should create an exciting visual salon image aimed at persuading the client into trying new or different products and services and enticing new clients into the salon.

- **Establish the need** – with good consultation, analysis and communication skills the therapist can determine the most suitable product and/or service.

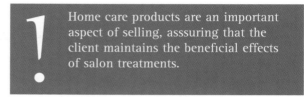

Home care products are an important aspect of selling, asssuring that the client maintains the beneficial effects of salon treatments.

- **Prescribe and educate** – the therapist should use their knowledge of the services and products on offer to fulfil the need established at the consultation. This is a time when the client can be educated to guide them away from misconceptions or unrealistic expectations.

- **Closing the sale** – to close the sale effectively the therapist must remember that they are the professionals and should have faith in their recommendations. Repeat the benefits the client will gain by taking up your recommendation. Offer a choice to overcome problems presented by the client as to why they cannot and give them the chance to try the products or service by suggesting they try introductory offers, samples or trial sizes. Place the client in the position of ownership with phrases such as, 'When you have the treatment your nail condition will improve'. Finally, ask, 'Would you like to book for that treatment?' or 'Would you like to try that product?'

Legislation

The following legislation relates to sales and promotion of products and services.

Any person who buys goods or services is protected by the law to ensure that:

- goods are not faulty
- goods are of good quality
- there is an accurate description of the goods or service
- the client is treated fairly and respectfully.

Legislation includes:

1. The Sale of Goods Act
2. The Supply of Goods Act
3. The Supply and Sale of Goods Act
4. The Consumer Protection Act
5. The Trades Description Acts
6. The Data Protection Act
7. Equal opportunities legislation
   - The Sex Discrimination Act
   - The Disability Discrimination Act
   - The Race Relations Acts

1 The Sale of Goods Act 1979

This was the first of the laws that required **goods** to be accurately described without misleading the customer. The law takes into account the:

- suitability of the goods for a particular purpose
- quality
- description.

2 The Supply of Goods and Services Act 1982

This went further than the 1979 Act to include **standards of service**, which should be:

- of reasonable quality
- described accurately
- fit for the intended purpose.

The Act also required that the service provided to a customer should be:

- carried out with reasonable skill and care
- within a reasonable time
- for a reasonable cost.

3 The Sale and Supply of Goods Act 1994

This amends the previous Acts by introducing guidelines on defining the **quality** of goods.

4 The Consumer Protection Act 1987

The European Community legislation provides consumers with protection when buying goods or services to ensure that products used on the client during treatment or retail products sold to the client are safe.

5 The Trades Description Acts 1968, 1972

The Act protects the client from misleading descriptions or claims relating to treatments and retail products. For example, to claim that a treatment is a miracle cure that will prevent skin from ageing is not likely to be true and is therefore regarded as misleading.

6 The Data Protection Act 1984

The increase in the use of computers by businesses to store information about their clients has brought about a need for legislation to protect clients' personal information.

The Data Protection Act requires the business to be registered and to comply with rules on storage and security of data. Companies should:

- only hold information that is relevant
- allow individuals access to information held on them
- prevent unauthorised access to information.

7 Equal opportunities

Equal opportunities relates to the rights of all individuals to respect, without discrimination on any grounds: race, language, colour, disability, sex or religion. When working with the general public the therapist has a duty to treat clients respectfully and equally regardless of colour, race, religion, cultural differences, gender or disability.

Some of the legislation relating to equality includes:

- The Race Relations Acts 1976, 2000
- The Sex Discrimination Act 1975
- The Disability Discrimination Act 1995

The Race Relations Act 1976, amended in 2000, relates to promoting good race relations between people in their communities and respecting each other's differences. The UK has a very diverse population and it is the aim of the legislation to encourage people to work together, to pool their energies and talents to achieve common goals.

The salon employer has a duty to treat all employees equally and to promote good race relations through the services offered to clients in meeting the needs of the ethnic mix of the community the salon serves. This includes:

- range of treatments for clients in the community
- retail products – make-up and skincare range for all skin colour and types
- promotional materials to include images relevant to the community.

Discrimination on the grounds that a person has a disability is unlawful. The employer and the therapists should make every effort to meet the needs of all clients who come to the salon for treatment, regardless of their disability. However, a small business may not have the resources to accommodate a client with physical disabilities, e.g. quite often the beauty salon is on an upper floor.

Beauty therapy has traditionally been a female profession with few male therapists or clients. Yet the trend for men to be more aware of skincare has resulted in an increase in the number of male clients to the salon, and the increase in male make-up and skincare consultants has brought male students into training. The Sex Discrimination Act ensures that both sexes are treated equally, e.g. equality in employment prospects and pay for both males and females.

The therapist and the law

The implications of the legislation for the therapist are clear. The customer or client has a right under the law to expect quality in respect of:

- the service they receive
- the products used during treatment
- the cosmetics or products that they purchase.

The therapist should be aware that not giving accurate information to the client, or claiming that a product or treatment can do something that it clearly does not, is misleading and the client can demand their money back. If incorrect information is given, a product could be regarded as unfit for the purpose intended or not accurately described. The client must be reassured that information given during the consultation process is confidential and secure.

Meeting clients' needs and expectations
Gaining feedback

The salon manager will need to be constantly aware of the clientele of the salon and whether they are satisfied with the services being offered. It is good practice to carry out surveys from time to time using questionnaires or comments cards. Anonymous feedback may give a more accurate response as some people are reluctant to make negative comments face-to-face.

Ways in which clients' comments can be collected:

- A suggestions box will encourage people to make comments.
- Comments cards can be left in the waiting area of reception. These cards could be like the ones you find at your table in some fast-food restaurants – simple and easy to complete.

- The therapist should make a point of asking the client at the end of the appointment whether they enjoyed the treatment and were satisfied with the result.
- The manager may use observation on a daily basis to gain information by checking the efficiency of appointment schedules, health and safety practice, client care or client satisfaction.
- Staff can contribute by listening to their clients and informing senior staff or the manager of any dissatisfaction or by making suggestions for improvement.
- Surveys or questionnaires can help to maintain and improve salon services as well as provide staff with valuable feedback on how they are doing within the team.

The manager will want to know that clients are being dealt with efficiently and that staff are meeting the targets of the business. Some clients with a negative attitude may use the opportunity to complain and criticise rather than make helpful suggestions. However, if there is a common thread running through the comments, it may indicate a need for action.

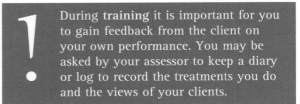

During **training** it is important for you to gain feedback from the client on your own performance. You may be asked by your assessor to keep a diary or log to record the treatments you do and the views of your clients.

The salon manager may also wish to gain client feedback before a staff appraisal.

Following up client feedback

It is always necessary to balance the needs of the client with what is viable for the business. To achieve this balance, feedback from both clients and staff is essential. However, it is no good requesting suggestions and comments unless the information gained is acted upon.

Urgent action will be required where matters of health and safety, security or client distress are encountered. Non-urgent matters may be used to develop an **improvement plan**.

Comments from clients that will require urgent attention may include:

- 'The carpet is worn on the steps and I nearly tripped.'
- 'The temperature control on the shower is broken, causing very hot water to come through.'
- 'The towels used for my treatment did not smell fresh.'
- 'The therapist was rude and abrupt when I phoned.'
- 'I was given the wrong change again today.'
- 'There is still no cleanser available for my skin type.'

It can be seen that these are matters of health and safety and service and must therefore be dealt with immediately.

The client may make comments on things that are desirable but not matters of urgency:

- 'I have read about a new face cream – are you going to stock it?'
- 'I wish you stayed open until 8.00 p.m. on Friday instead of Thursday.'
- 'I would rather have fresh coffee than instant.'

It is not always possible to act on every piece of client feedback. The salon manager will have to consider whether suggestions for improvement are sensible and whether the business can afford to implement them. There may be implications for:

- financial investment in the salon for new equipment, products or staff
- staff training
- refurbishment.

ACTIVITY

Design a short questionnaire that could be given to clients to gain information on how satisfied they are with their salon visits.

Use the following headings to help you:

- First impressions of the salon and staff

- Salon appearance/decor

- Hospitality and comfort

- Enjoyment of treatment(s)

- Value for money.

If possible, use your questionnaire to collect some views. You will need to type or word-process the questionnaire and plan how it is to be issued to the clients. Completed questionnaires will need to be collected and the results analysed. From the results you may be able to make recommendations for improvement to the service your salon offers.

> As many clients as possible should complete the questionnaire to ensure that sufficient information is collected.

Chapter 4

PERSONAL PERFORMANCE AND TEAMWORK

LEVEL
2

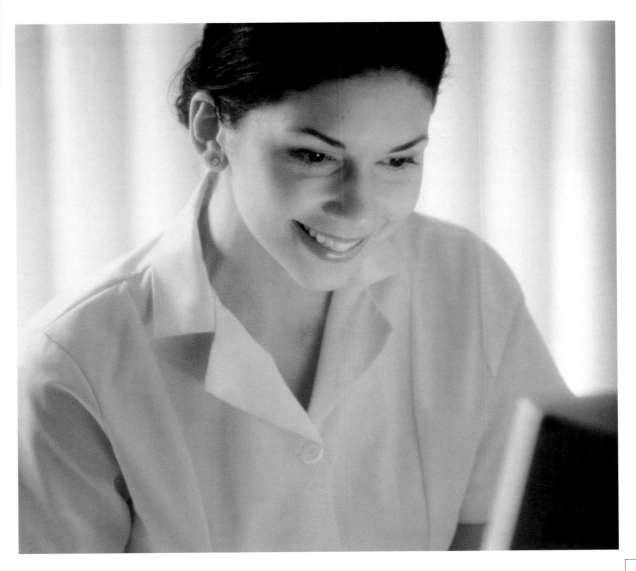

IN THIS CHAPTER YOU WILL LEARN ABOUT:

- Working in a team
- The different roles and responsibilities of staff in the salon
- Communicating with others
- Personal development
  - job description
  - appraisal
  - setting targets
  - reviewing personal progress and development

Introduction

The success of any business depends on the way in which the staff work together to meet the aims of the business. Working as part of a team helps to spread the workload, promote good relationships with colleagues and ensure that the business runs smoothly.

Knowing what your role and responsibilities are within the salon is important to ensure that tasks are satisfactorily completed and that you can constantly review how effective you are and plan for your future development.

Being part of a team

You will at some time have experienced being in a team. This might have been in sport (hockey, for example), in an orchestra or pop group, or as a member of the school play or local amateur dramatic society.

A team works to **agreed aims** or **goals**. A sports team aims to win a match, an orchestra or pop group aims to put together lots of different sounds from people playing many different instruments, a drama group aims to take different characters and put together a play or musical. This will involve a team of not only the actors but also people to do make-up, costumes and lighting.

Many aspects of life involve working together as a team. This is particularly important in the workplace. Whatever the business, be it in the manufacturing, retail or service industry, it will rely on a team or teams of people working together to meet the aims of the company.

A beauty therapy salon is in the **service sector** of business, with the broad aim of providing a range of beauty therapy treatments to its customers or clients. The salon owner will have a **business plan** in which the aims of the business are set out in more detail. The owner will require all the therapists to work together to achieve these aims.

Being a team member in a beauty salon

You must be able to:

- anticipate the needs of others and be willing to **provide help and support** when it is needed
- **communicate effectively** and share information
- **get on** with all members of the team

- **accept responsibility** from your supervisor and work within the limits of your authority
- resolve misunderstandings with colleagues.

Providing help and support

When someone is very busy they can become flustered and agitated. As a good team member you will recognise that this person is under pressure and needs help. This may be something as simple as checking the temperature of the wax or preparing a treatment room for the next client. Anticipating when a job needs to be done and keeping an eye on those tasks that need to be carried out throughout the day are important aspects of your role.

 Support staff in the salon are as important as the therapists themselves. The smooth running of the salon depends on their behind-the-scenes work.

Preparing treatment rooms or cubicles

Ensure that:

- equipment and materials from the previous client are cleared away
- the treatment couch is set up for the next client
- clean laundry is available
- products and equipment for the treatment are in place
- equipment is checked for safety and set up ready for the treatment
- the client's record card is available.

(See chapter 5 for further details.)

Care of clients and reception duties

The duties of the receptionist are described in more detail in chapter 2. However, in a busy salon everyone must play a part to ensure that the client is cared for.

Unplanned situations such as late arrival of clients, overbooking of clients or staff absence will require you to use your initiative by providing the therapists with assistance and by ensuring that waiting clients are served with coffee, have a magazine to read and are kept informed. Clients who arrive without an appointment should be accommodated if at all possible. Remember this can give you the opportunity to provide the treatment yourself and gain a new client.

Salon care

Ensure that the salon is clean, tidy and running smoothly. This will include seeing to the laundry, doing some cleaning, sterilising and hygiene procedures, dispensary or stockroom duties such as stock checks, dispensing or mixing treatment products.

Chapter 1 deals with aspects of health and safety and salon care and maintenance. It also explains the importance of everyone taking responsibility for health and safety in the salon.

Communicating effectively

Communication is always important, not only between clients and staff, but also between staff and management and between the therapists themselves. Most beauty therapists are good communicators because of the demands of the job. They are able, through effective communication, to develop a good relationship with clients, provide professional advice and be a good listener.

Good communication between staff will ensure that everyone is clear about the aims of the business and their individual part in achieving those aims, as well as their role as part of the team.

Team meetings

Team meetings are a very good way of ensuring that there is effective communication. If held on a regular basis, they can help to:

- encourage and motivate staff
- provide training opportunities
- allocate tasks in the salon through negotiation
- identify and help to resolve problems
- avoid misunderstandings, disagreements or mistrust within the team
- provide an opportunity for the exchange of ideas for the future development of the business.

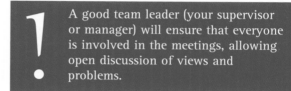

A good team leader (your supervisor or manager) will ensure that everyone is involved in the meetings, allowing open discussion of views and problems.

Methods of communicating in the salon

- Written
  - messages
  - fax
  - e-mail
  - memorandum (memo)
  - appointment book
  - stock book
  - salon policies, rules and regulations.
- Verbal
  - team meetings
  - telephone
  - oral instructions.
- Visual
  - training videos
  - demonstrations
  - body language.

Body language

Body language is a method of communicating. The wrong impression can be given easily by gestures, posture, facial expression and manner. A poor attitude will be reflected in your appearance. Be aware of yourself and how you appear to others. A glum, stern face with the body posture in a slouching position with round shoulders will give totally the wrong impression. The therapist needs to be aware of their looks and posture. A bright smiling face which is clean or well made-up reflects the skincare and appearance of the beauty industry they wish to promote. An alert body stance with good posture will give the impression of being ready to help the client and assist them with their appearance.

ACTIVITY

Put together a range of communication methods that you have used, for example a message, a fax or an extract from the appointment book.

Remember for the evidence to be valid for assessment it must relate to an activity that you have carried out. It must be signed and dated by your assessor before you can use it as evidence for your portfolio.

Getting on with the team

Maintaining good relationships within the salon makes for a happy working environment. Clients can sense an atmosphere of discontent and disharmony, and this may put them off coming back. Building good relationships will require you to be aware of others (their needs, temperament, moods) and will encourage you to treat them with respect.

Accepting responsibility

Accepting responsibility for your actions and how you may affect others is an important aspect of life at work. It is essential to maintain the aims of the business and to carry out your job effectively. An understanding of job roles and responsibilities within the business will help you to fit into the team by knowing what you are expected to do, who you should report to and who makes final decisions.

As an employee you should have a **job description** that outlines your work role and how you contribute to the overall work of the team. This needs to be reviewed as you gain experience.

ACTIVITY

There are many examples of teamwork. Working together in a group, discuss your involvement in a team and what responsibilities you had as part of that team. You might discuss your role in a previous job or in a sports team, for example.

The job role

The **job role** consists of the **duties** and **responsibilities** defined in the **job description**.

The job description

A job description will give details of your job, responsibilities and job title. A job description is necessary to enable you to define the limits of your authority: to ensure that you are aware of those things that are your responsibility, but also where your responsibility ends. Further details of your job, such as hours of work, pay and holidays, form part of your **contract of employment**.

Your job title will give you an indication of the level of your job (assistant, senior therapist etc.).

Name: _____

Job title: _____

Place of work: _____

General description of the job:

_____

_____

_____

_____

_____

Responsible to:
- ▪

Responsible for:
- ▪
- ▪
- ▪
- ▪

Main beauty therapy tasks (treatments):
- ▪
- ▪
- ▪
- ▪
- ▪

Other tasks (general salon duties):
- ▪
- ▪
- ▪
- ▪
- ▪
- ▪

Figure 4.1 *An example of a job description proforma*

Salon Owner
Part-time therapist with regular clients
Works in the salon on Thursdays and Fridays
Only member of staff trained in advanced epilation, so has clients from the hospital
Responsible for: running the business, checking takings/till, banking, paying the wages,
ordering stock, health and safety, staff appraisals, staff training

Manager/Senior Therapist
Full-time, six years' experience, works every day except Thursdays (unless the boss is away)
Does all treatments and has regular clients
Responsible for: the day-to-day running of the salon and supervising the staff, client records,
appointment book, allocating salon duties, stock checks, health and safety checks,
staff rotas and holidays, daily cashing up
Responsible to: Salon Owner

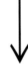

Beauty Therapist
Full-time, two years' experience
Building up her clientele, when not busy assists the Senior Therapist
Responsible for: daily hygiene practices and salon appearance, retail display, retail sales figures
Responsible to: Senior Therapist and Owner

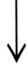

Assistant Beauty Therapist
Part-time, recently qualified to NVQ Level 2, taking NVQ level 3 course part-time at college
Manicurist and nail technician, waxing and make-up
Assists all the therapists by preparing treatment rooms, equipment and products
Responsible for: general cleaning duties including laundry, reception duties
Responsible to: Senior Therapist

Trainee Beauty Therapist
Full-time, attends college 1 day per week for NVQ level 1 and 2
Assists all staff in the salon, observes treatments as appropriate
Responsible for: greeting clients, providing coffee, general cleaning duties
Responsible to: all therapists with training from the Senior Therapist

Figure 4.2 *An example of a flow chart of staff roles and responsibilities*

Personal performance and teamwork

If you have already been in employment you will have had a job description and a contract of employment. Share your experience with someone in the group who may not have been in employment by discussing:

- your job title

- the job description

- the tasks you were expected to carry out

- who you were responsible to.

In your group use the proforma on page 54 to design a job description for a member of staff in a beauty therapy salon. To enable you to do this you will need to look at the staff in your salon or your work placement and make a flow chart of all the staff. Use the flow chart on page 55 to help you.

Appraisal and personal development

Throughout your time at school, college or work you will have been involved in **reviewing** and **checking** your performance and achievements. At school or college you may have experienced tutorials where you discuss your progress with your tutor and set targets for future learning, called an **action plan**. In employment, the tutorial is replaced by a **staff review** or **appraisal**, which looks at your performance at work.

'Where do I want to be?' is when you ask yourself what your future aims are. Setting out your aims is important in all aspects of your life, but particularly in relation to your career and future training needs.

'How am I going to get there?' is the point in an appraisal where you identify who can help you achieve your goals. During a staff appraisal the salon manager will discuss your strengths and weaknesses with you. You must be prepared to accept that they may have identified different strengths and weaknesses in relation to your performance in the salon. The manager may have different ideas for your future so it is important that an appraisal is a joint discussion with

Whether you are having a tutorial or an appraisal, it is useful to think about the following questions:

- **Where am I now?**

- **Where do I want to be?**

- **How am I going to get there?**

agreement on the goals and targets to be achieved. The question you need to ask is: who and what will I need to help me to achieve my goals and targets? It is essential to put the goals and targets in writing so that they can be reviewed regularly.

'How am I doing?' is the question you should ask as you aim to achieve your goals and targets. After an agreed period of time your manager will review your targets with you.

Appraisal is sometimes referred to as a **review cycle** because each time the targets are reviewed and the goals and targets are achieved, the process starts again with new or modified goals and targets.

During the appraisal interview the appraiser, who may be the manager or the person you are responsible to, will encourage you to plan your training and development needs.

An **action plan** is agreed, setting out your targets and what support you will need to achieve them. An action plan may include short-term targets – for example, to practise using the new waxing system so you are able to work on clients by next month – or long-term targets – to achieve the beauty therapy NVQ level 2 by July.

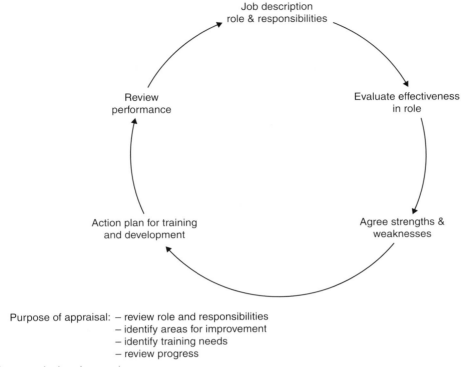

Purpose of appraisal: − review role and responsibilities
− identify areas for improvement
− identify training needs
− review progress

Figure 4.3 *An appraisal review cycle*

The date to review your targets will be agreed on the action plan and a copy retained by your appraiser. You will need to refer to the action plan to ensure that you stay on course to achieve your targets.

To enable you to plan for the future, whether in your career in beauty therapy or in your everyday life, you will need to set targets or goals. This will give you the encouragement and motivation to work hard to achieve these targets.

Managers in business use staff reviews or appraisals to evaluate the effectiveness of the whole team. During an appraisal, you and your manager (in an interview situation) review your progress and contribution to the performance of the salon against the targets of the business and your personal goals. As well as thinking about your past performance, you will also look to the future. This will involve setting targets for your personal development, including training.

> **!** Appraisal is not just about identifying problems and planning how to solve them. It needs to be a positive process providing you and the manager with the opportunity to discuss all aspects of your job role. Targets that you set together should be written down on an action plan. They must be achievable and completed within an agreed timescale.

Appraisal

Self-appraisal or appraisal with your manager will help you to manage yourself within your job role and to think about your future development.

You may find the questions listed above useful for appraisal. Begin with, 'Where am I now?'

To help you answer this question you will need to spend some time looking at your **strengths** and **weaknesses.** This is not always an easy thing to do as we are often more comfortable talking about our weaknesses rather than stressing our strengths. A useful exercise is to use the **SWOT** analysis. SWOT stands for Strengths, Weaknesses, Opportunities and Threats.

Doing a SWOT analysis

1. Begin by making a list of the broad areas of your job, such as assisting therapists with treatments and reception duties.
2. Then ask yourself, 'What do I do well and with confidence?' This will usually indicate your **strengths**.
3. Then ask yourself, 'What do I find difficult?' This will be things that you probably avoid doing or put off if you can – things that make you feel anxious. This will be an indication of your **weaknesses**.
4. **Opportunities** will need to be considered through discussion with your manager during your appraisal. These refer to the limitations when setting targets. So, if you identify a weakness such as using the new roller waxing system, this will require training. Therefore the opportunities for training will depend on the manager making the time available for you to go on a course or for someone to spend time with you in the salon for training.
5. The **threats** refer to the cost of such training and whether it would be cost-effective to take time for this particular training need when there may be other priorities, for example, training staff in the use of a new range of products.

strengths	**weaknesses**
– smart appearance	– not confident using electrical treatments
– good communication skills	– need to be quicker with treatments
– enjoy working with people	– find it difficult to choose products from the range available for individual clients
opportunities	**threats**
– attending course at college for NVQ level 3 in September	– employed part-time with little job security
– go to the trade shows in London to gain information about new products, new treatments and equipment	– work in a small salon with only 2 other therapists who are also part-time so do not get much time together

Figure 4.4 *An example of a SWOT analysis*

The SWOT analysis or any method of assessing your strengths and weaknesses will help you to monitor your progress and set your personal goals for the future.

Training and development

Beauty therapy is a fast-growing industry that requires the beauty therapist to be skilled in a wide range of treatments. The beauty therapist needs to keep up to date with new techniques, treatments and products, health and safety legislation and emerging technology.

Training needs of the staff will vary depending on their position, role and responsibilities within the salon. Training can include:

- nationally recognised qualifications such as NVQs or equivalent vocational qualifications (National Diploma)
- manufacturer's courses and information

- keeping informed of the latest technology and trends through trade journals and professional bodies
- in-house training to meet the needs of the salon, for example, using a new product range
- job shadowing, allowing less experienced staff, possibly trainees, to observe treatments being carried out by senior therapists
- management training for senior staff.

There is a constant flow of new products and techniques into the market. It is important that the therapist keeps up to date with what is happening in beauty therapy to enable them to offer new treatments and retail new products to their clients.

Trade magazines and newsletters from professional bodies should be available in your salon as they are particularly useful for learning about the latest research and development in skincare, cosmetics and treatments. Trade fairs offer the very latest in products and equipment with demonstrations leaflets and free samples available. The Internet can provide valuable information, although a great deal of it is from the USA and may not apply to the UK.

Chapter 5

PREPARATION FOR TREATMENTS AND CLIENT CARE

LEVELS
1+2

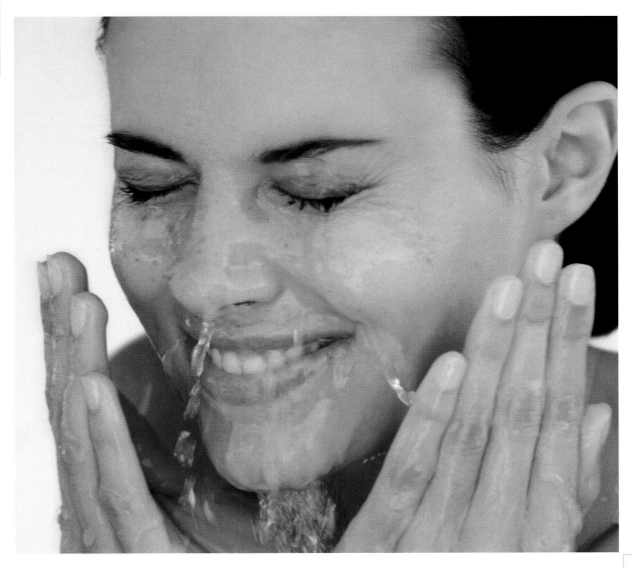

- Service to clients
- Service standards and codes of practice
- Approaching the client
- Recognising client feelings
- Dealing with complaints
- Client referral
- Communicating with clients
- Client consultation
- Preparing for treatment
  - preparing the treatment area
  - preparing the trolley
  - preparing tools and equipment
- Personal hygiene and appearance
- Salon rules and regulations, policies and procedures

Introduction

The customer is at the centre of every beauty therapy business. Therefore it is necessary for the business to provide service of the highest quality to its customers, generally referred to as clients. The experience the client receives during their visit to the salon will influence whether they will return for further treatments and become a valued client.

Service to the client

The way in which the staff approach their jobs will influence the success of the business. Consideration should be given to the following:

- technical skills of the staff to provide efficient and effective treatments
- salon environment, decor and ambience
- professionalism of the staff
- health, safety and security in the salon.

The technical skills of the staff rely on good training through recognised qualifications and ongoing skills updating and experience. Treatments should be of the highest quality and should meet the client's needs as closely as possible. All work should be carried out efficiently and be cost-effective.

The salon environment depends largely on the investment in the business by the salon owner(s) and the image they wish to project. Cleanliness is of utmost importance and this is reflected in the decor and care of fixtures, fittings and equipment of the salon.

The ambience of the salon will be very important to the client. Clients will wish to feel relaxed and comfortable in a peaceful and unhurried atmosphere.

The professionalism of the staff is important as it is they who contribute to the image of the salon and the quality of the treatments. Codes of practice provided by any one of the professional beauty therapy organisations give guidelines on the practice and procedures for treating the client. The salon will also set standards of appearance and behaviour for the therapists to follow, which will take the form of salon rules and regulations. The therapist must aim to represent the salon in a positive way and follow standards of behaviour that comply with the organisation's service standards.

The responsibility for health, safety and security in the salon should be shared by all staff to ensure that clients are never put at risk (see chapter 1).

The following activity is designed to help you to consider how you would ensure that your client has a positive experience when they attend the salon.

ACTIVITY

Using the following list of negative impressions to help you, write a list of positive impressions you should be giving your client.

Negative impressions   *Positive impressions*

- no information available for your client
  (price list, product information)

- your client is ignored as they arrive at the salon

- telephone is left ringing

- promises you make to do something for
  the client are forgotten

- surroundings are dirty or untidy (magazines
  are old and torn, the plants are dusty and
  dying due to lack of care)

- client is left waiting without an explanation

- you forget to give a message from a client
  to one of the staff

You may be able to think of others:

Service standards
Salon rules and regulations

The client's perceptions of you and the salon are very important. The image you project should follow the salon policy on standards of appearance and client care. The salon may have a manual or a notice in the staff room that outlines salon practice and procedures and rules and regulations. New members of staff will normally receive information on salon practice during their induction.

The professional way in which the salon staff approach their job will influence the success of the business. There are accepted standards of behaviour for the therapist outlined in the codes of practice supplied by the professional organisations. These guidelines may be adapted by a business to provide their own service standards.

The standards set by your salon or training organisation provide you with rules and regulations relating to:

- hygiene
- professional practice and behaviour
- dress
- treatments.

Hygiene

During your training you will be constantly reminded of the importance of hygiene and the need to carry out thorough hygiene procedures. The nature of beauty therapy requires close contact with the client and it carries the risk of cross infection. Clients have a right to expect high standards of hygiene throughout the treatment, making cleanliness a priority for the salon. (For personal hygiene, see page 81.)

There are new strains of viruses that are resistant to simple cleansing methods. This makes strict working practices a necessity (see chapter 1 for health and safety procedures).

- Cleaning equipment, **work surfaces** and **implements** should be part of your working routine. Ways of storing specialist equipment and safety checks are outlined in chapter 1.
- Fresh laundered **towels** and **bed linen** must be available at all times. Therefore, attending to laundry will be an important part of your salon duties.
- **Washing hands** is the simplest but one of the most effective hygiene procedures. It must become second nature to you to protect yourself from infection and also your clients and all those within the salon environment. Use **bactericidal hand wash** from a dispenser and have the water as hot as possible, followed by thorough drying with a disposable hand towel.
- **Cover cuts** or **abrasions** on your hands or the area to be treated on the client with a waterproof plaster.
- **Wear rubber gloves** for treatments where there is any possibility of coming into contact with blood or body fluids (depilatory waxing, particularly underarm and bikini line waxing where blood spots during treatment are common). There is some concern about the possibility of passing on the HIV virus or hepatitis through some treatments such as electrical epilation, ear-piercing or where the skin can become broken. Studies have given contradicting information as to the risks, however procedures must minimise risk of cross infection from any source.
- **Sterilise** small implements using an autoclave or sterilising fluid.
- **Disposable items** such as paper towels, spatulas, tissues and cotton wool must be used where possible and disposed of immediately after use in a covered waste bin.

Professional practice and behaviour

The approach to the client is dealt with later in this chapter, however acceptable standards of behaviour whilst in the working environment will include:

- speaking politely without the use of slang or bad language
- courtesy and regard for others
- no smoking, eating or chewing
- appropriate topics of conversation within the salon.

Behaviour is learnt from others and what may be acceptable for one person or within some work or social environments is not always appropriate for the beauty therapist.

ACTIVITY

Observe the way in which senior therapists who are experienced in working with clients in the salon behave. Use the headings on page 64 to check appropriate behaviour.

Dress

Salon dress or uniform should project an image of cleanliness and professionalism. White uniforms are the standard dress for beauty therapists, with individual salons using coloured trim or badges as distinguishing features to promote the salon image. Smart shoes (not sandals due to the possibility of injury to the therapist's feet from equipment) with low heels should be worn.

ACTIVITY

Look through beauty therapy trade magazines or write to salon wear manufacturers for a brochure and select a uniform for your salon. Briefly describe the reasons for your choice.

Treatments

The therapist must keep up to date with professional practice and has a duty to find out about new treatments. Treatments are becoming more advanced, with lasers and microcurrents being used to meet the demands of the client.

Professional qualifications, training courses, trade shows and trade magazines will keep the therapist up to date and ensure that treatments are performed to the highest possible standard. **Litigation** (legal action) resulting from alleged negligence by the therapist is becoming more common. It is therefore essential that the therapist is qualified and competent to practice.

Professional codes of practice

The **codes of practice** provided by the professional beauty therapy organisations lay down standards for their members including:

- **codes of ethics** – rules that aim to protect clients from improper practice. New members are usually required to sign an agreement that they will abide by the code of ethics
- **professional codes of practice**, which keep the therapist up to date with methods of treatment and procedures for beauty therapy such as hygiene practices, new treatments and findings from research.

Failure to comply with your professional organisation's codes of ethics and practice can lead to expulsion from the organisation. Students of beauty therapy can apply for student membership and receive valuable information about events and new products and treatments.

ACTIVITY

What are the rules for your salon on dress and appearance? Refer to chapter 1 to check your appearance.

Ask to see the salon's service standards and make a checklist for your staff noticeboard on salon rules and regulations. This should be well presented so that it is easy to read. Word process your checklist if possible.

Contact one of the professional organisations and ask for information on their codes of practice.

Approach to the client

The way in which you approach the client is important. Client care is an essential part of the beauty therapist's role from the moment a client makes an enquiry to the end of the treatment. You will be required to:

- listen carefully
- observe the client

- make appropriate conversation with the client
- offer advice
- provide one-to-one attention throughout the treatment.

It is important that the therapist is aware of the client's feelings and makes the effort to build good relationships by:

- practising good communication skills
- empathising
- caring
- taking responsibility
- showing courtesy and respect.

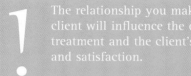

! The relationship you make with your client will influence the quality of the treatment and the client's enjoyment and satisfaction.

Practising good communication skills

- Listen carefully to the client and others.
- Question appropriately and in a sensitive manner.
- Write clearly using memos, reports, messages, etc.
- Use non-verbal body language and facial expression.
- Make appropriate conversation with the client.

Empathising

Put yourself in your client's place. Everything you do should be seen from the client's point of view. The client may sometimes feel confused or anxious about their visit to the salon. It could be the first time they have had a treatment and they will naturally feel apprehensive about what it will involve. They may feel embarrassed about having to remove clothing or be concerned about whether the treatment will be uncomfortable.

You must make every effort to explain fully what will be involved, and avoid any embarrassment to the client by ensuring privacy and adequate covering to maintain their modesty. The following activity will help you to think about your feelings in a range of situations.

ACTIVITY

How do you feel when:

- you make a phone call and are left on hold for a long time with no explanation?
- you are kept waiting with no explanation or apology?
- a shop assistant ignores you when you are trying to buy something?
- someone is serving you while they have a conversation with someone else?
- someone looks angry and speaks aggressively to you?
- you arrive for an appointment to find that it has been changed to another time?
- someone promises to do something for you but forgets?
- people are giggling in front of you as if they are laughing at you?
- you try to explain something but the person does not seem to be listening?

You may be able to think of other situations.

Have you ever felt uncomfortable or embarrassed?

Choose two situations and write down or discuss with a partner how the person should have behaved to make you feel more comfortable.

Caring

This is a genuine feeling of wanting to help others by:

- being able to recognise when someone needs assistance
- showing a willingness to help clients and others (remember the client will observe how the staff work together)
- showing genuine concern for the well-being of the client
- ensuring that the client is not put at risk
- recognising when clients have special needs and offer assistance.

Taking responsibility

You will need to:

- make decisions or solve problems that affect your client, quickly and within the limits of your authority
- refer your client to a doctor or another therapist as necessary, without delaying or inconveniencing them
- avoid passing on problems to others because you cannot be bothered to handle the situation
- take ownership of a problem and resolve it in the best way you can.

Showing courtesy and respect

Being polite and showing respect for others is essential in all aspects of life. You should:

- be aware of others
- show tolerance for differing views and behaviour (different cultures, religions and backgrounds will influence behaviour)
- not judge others or view them as inferior because they may appear to be different to you
- recognise that being tolerant and having respect for others does not mean that you have to compromise your own standards and beliefs.

Dealing with a client and recognising feelings

We all have days when we feel irritable, upset, confused or anxious. This is part of human nature. What is important is that you can recognise these feelings in yourself and in others and learn how to handle them. **Facial expressions** and **body language** can give a good indication of a person's mood or attitude.

Facial expressions

Facial expressions can show:

- sadness
- anger
- thinking
- confusion
- disgust
- anxiety.

Body language

The way in which you respond to the client when you recognise expression of feelings can affect the whole experience for the client and may influence whether they return to the salon for treatment in the future. Equally, the way in which you handle your own feelings by overcoming such things as anger, frustration and unhappiness, for example by presenting a professional image, will influence how successful you will be as a beauty therapist. You will be expected to display a calm and efficient manner at all times.

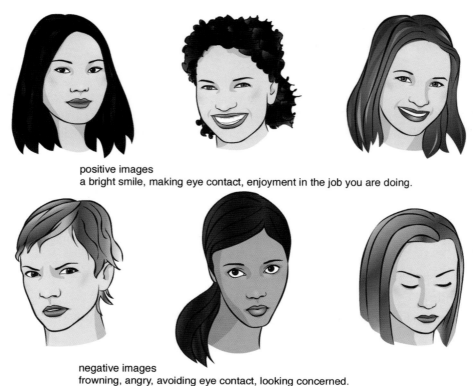

positive images
a bright smile, making eye contact, enjoyment in the job you are doing.

negative images
frowning, angry, avoiding eye contact, looking concerned.

Figure 5.1 *Facial expressions give away a lot about your mood*

Clients who are confused

It may be that the client has not visited the salon before or is having a new treatment. They may feel unsure and anxious about what to expect. You must recognise these feelings and give the client reassurance by explaining fully what the treatment involves and what they might expect to feel, making sure that they are comfortable and answering any questions they might have before you start. To enable you to reassure your client you must be confident in what you are doing and knowledgeable about the treatment. The manner in which you reassure your client should not be patronising, but should aim to give them confidence in you and the salon.

ACTIVITY

Describe a situation when you have felt confused and unsure about what to do. This may have been your first day at college or when you have had to travel somewhere on your own for the first time.

- How did it feel?

- What would have made it easier for you to cope and feel more confident?

Challenging behaviour

The client may, in certain situations, display anger or aggression. This could be due to a range of reasons such as:

- dissatisfaction with the treatment
- poor communication where a situation has arisen because things were not clearly explained
- the wrong attitude of a member of staff
- the client may have personal problems that make them feel stressed
- the client may have been kept waiting with no explanation.

Remember the client has a right to question what you are doing even though it can feel threatening for you. You must respond in a positive manner, without challenging the client or displaying anger. If at any time you feel that things are getting out of hand and beyond your control, excuse yourself and see a senior member of staff. This lapse in time can sometimes defuse the situation, allowing space for the client to calm down and for you to regain your composure.

Client complaints

It is inevitable that there will be occasions when the client will make a complaint. These may include:

- dissatisfaction with a salon treatment (a depilatory wax not completely removing leg hairs, for example)
- being kept waiting
- an appointment mix-up.

A more serious complaint would involve damage to the client's clothing or injury to the client. Complaints may be made as they happen, verbally to the therapist or the client may request to see the manager. Alternatively clients may complain in writing after the incident. The salon may have a policy on the way in which a complaint should be handled. If so, this must be followed at all times.

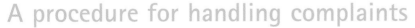

! Any complaint must be taken seriously and rectified immediately.

A procedure for handling complaints

1. Listen attentively to what the client has to say, preferably in a private area. You may need to deal with the client's emotions first if they are angry or distressed. Acknowledge that they are upset and make them feel valued by showing genuine concern.
2. Decide whether it is within the limits of your authority to deal with the complaint following the salon's policy, or whether you should pass it on to a more senior member of staff.
3. A serious complaint carries a threat of litigation and must be referred to the manager, who will make decisions on appropriate recompense or compensation. If the client wishes to take legal action there will need to be a formal record of events with witness statements and physical evidence of the complaint. Fortunately almost all complaints are fairly minor and can be handled by offering free treatment or by refunding the cost of the treatment.

The client's rights are protected by the legislation relating to the consumer. Details of these Acts can be found in chapter 3.

Client referral

It may be necessary to refer clients to other services within the salon or to recommend that they seek advice from other professionals, such as their GP or a chiropodist. A client may give details during the consultation of contraindications that prevent them from having treatment. You may need to advise the client to see a doctor.

For example, during a pedicure a client may ask you to remove hard skin on her toes. On examination you find the client has calluses and a corn, which you are not qualified to treat. The salon may work closely with a chiropodist, in which case you could refer the client by giving them a business card so that they can make contact themselves.

A procedure for referral

The salon should have a policy on referral to ensure that staff are aware of the procedure:

1. A full consultation to check for contraindications must be given prior to every treatment.

2. The therapist must be able to recognise infectious skin conditions, skin diseases and other disorders and establish what constitutes a contraindication to treatment.

3. Clients should be directed clearly towards medical advice where necessary.

4. Referral must be handled in a sensitive manner and on no account must a diagnosis be made by the therapist.

5. A letter from the client's doctor giving permission for a specific salon treatment may be necessary. This must be attached to the client's record card.

ACTIVITY

Think about how you would handle the following situations.

Case study 1
A client arrives at the salon reception where several other clients are waiting. She very loudly announces her dissatisfaction with a recent leg wax treatment. She mentions the therapist by name and complains about her directly. She asks you to make a comment on how good you think she is as a beauty therapist.

Case study 2
During a consultation, when you ask your client for information on her general health, she begins to give details of recent major surgery and becomes very upset.

Lines of communication

Communication can be seen as an essential part of the therapist's role and is vital for the efficient running of the salon. So, the way in which you communicate with your clients, colleagues and manager will affect the atmosphere and efficiency of the salon.

It is important to follow the agreed methods and lines of communication within the salon. Look at the lines of communication chart on page 55.

Many of the problems that arise in the workplace are caused by poor or inappropriate communication. For example, interrupting therapists with trivial matters when they are treating clients is not good practice. Neither is holding on to an important piece of information that may require urgent attention.

Systems must be in place to allow effective communication between salon staff and may include:

- messages using a whiteboard
- pigeon-holes for paper messages and information

- staff meetings
- minutes or notes from meetings
- newsletters.

Making conversation with your client

One of the most daunting tasks when training to be a beauty therapist is meeting clients and knowing what to talk about. Clients can be any age, but young therapists may find it difficult to relate to the older person.

Conversation with the client is an essential part of the service offered and is part of:

- making the client feel welcome
- gaining important information during the consultation
- receiving feedback during and after the treatment to ensure that the client is comfortable and satisfied.

Some clients see the opportunity to unwind and talk about their problems as part of the treatment, whilst others prefer to be quiet without unnecessary talking. It is your job to assess the client's needs and provide conversation or peace and quiet as appropriate.

Starting a conversation

- Find out your client's name from the appointments book or ask the receptionist. Find out what treatment the client is booked for.
- Greet the client by using their title and surname. First names are too familiar for a first meeting and should only be used if the client specifically asks you to (or you know them personally).
- If the client comes to you regularly, you should try to recall things from her previous visit to start the conversation. For example:
  - 'How did you get on with the night cream you bought last time?'
  - 'What dress did you decide to wear last Friday night?'
- The client record card can provide you with information that may help you to start the conversation. For example:
  - 'I see you have been using the new product range, Mrs James, how are you liking it?'
  - 'Has your allergy settled down, Mrs Andrews?'

The British are renowned for discussing the weather, perhaps because it is one of the easiest ways of breaking the ice! It will invariably lead to other topics of conversation.

We so often ask the question. 'How are you?' without expecting a detailed reply. Most people just say, 'I'm fine.' Changing the question slightly will make it seem like a more genuine enquiry. This can lead to conversation and provide valuable information for the consultation. Try: 'It's nice to see you looking so well, did you have a good holiday?' or 'I am sorry you had to cancel your appointment last week. Are you feeling better?'

You will need to have some background information or to remember things about your client to ask these sorts of questions. If you have not met the client before, you could use general topics from the newspaper or television. Remember that you must not discuss other clients or gossip. In chapter 2, communication skills in relation to client reception are discussed.

Client consultation

Consultation requires the therapist to listen carefully and use questioning in a sensitive manner to illicit the important information required before the client's treatment. Information is recorded on a client record card or computer database. Client consultation for individual treatments can be found at the beginning of each relevant chapter. Client consultation must be part of every treatment to check for contraindications and to establish the needs of the client before carrying out a treatment.

Confidentiality

It is important that you observe strict rules on confidentiality when dealing with clients. Your discussions with the client should be discreet and, when appropriate, take place in private. You must never repeat what your client has discussed with you in confidence. In some circumstances it may be necessary for you to seek advice, making it necessary to discuss client details with your supervisor. This would be acceptable in a professional context, but you would need to ensure that it was carried out in a professional manner to maintain client confidence.

Junior staff should be instructed on the importance of confidentiality and follow salon rules on approach to clients and appropriate topics of conversation.

Client records

Client records are personal to the individual and should be kept in a locked filing cabinet. If stored on computer, you will need to comply with the Data Protection Act (see page 26) to ensure that personal details remain confidential at all times.

Consultation, treatment planning and treatment records are essential. These are discussed in more detail below.

At the start of every treatment, time must be allowed for client consultation. You should assess whether the treatment is suitable for the client and then prepare a plan of what the treatment involves. Sometimes a client will be offered a separate consultation to establish whether or not a particular condition can be treated in the salon.

To enable you to gain sufficient information during the consultation you will need to follow three stages:

1. **Questioning**.
2. **Visual check** – look closely at the area you will be treating and the overall appearance of your client.
3. **Manual examination** – touching the skin is important as it enables you to feel the texture and elasticity.

Questioning the client

Begin by explaining to the client what the treatment involves. This will help them to relax and gain confidence in you and what the treatment has to offer.

Questioning the client about requirements and expectations

Making sure that the client has realistic expectations of the treatment and the products is an important part of consultation. The client may have misinformed views on what can be achieved or how they should be caring for themselves. It may be that they have experienced pressure selling with overenthusiastic cosmetic sales assistants claiming that a product will do far more than is actually possible, or they may have read exaggerated articles in women's magazines. It is the job of the therapist to produce actual results by either improving the client's home care regime or changing their views on the benefits of good salon care.

Where client's expectations are not achievable you should politely make alternative suggestions and give as much explanation as possible.

It is against the law to make false claims (The Trades Description Act 1968 and 1972). Truthful and realistic outcomes are what matter if you are to keep your clients. Work together to change bad habits, to keep clients motivated and to keep them informed in best practice.

Question the client on home care routine

The way in which the client cares for themselves between salon treatments is important information that is gathered during the consultation. It will give an indication of how committed the client is to skincare and health regimes, whether they spend time and money on themselves and recognise the importance of visits to the beauty salon.

Question the client about their lifestyle

Selecting appropriate treatment for the client may be dependent on their needs at a particular time. This can be influenced by such things as eating habits, smoking and alcohol intake, exercise and sleeping patterns, a busy life and whether they are happy and contented.

Question the client about previous salon treatments

These will be shown on the record card if the client visits your salon regularly. This is one of the reasons why record cards should be completed fully after every treatment and filed correctly for future reference. Any problems, such as adverse reactions to a treatment, can be recorded, enabling you to establish appropriate treatment quickly and efficiently. If the client has had treatment at other salons it will be more difficult to gain information other than what the client tells you. You can, however, expect the client to be more relaxed if they have experienced salon treatments before.

Question the client about their general health

You should also ask about any medication they may be taking. Medical referral procedure should be followed when conditions are present that the therapist does not recognise as contraindications. The therapist must under no circumstances diagnose or make comment on any condition the client might present at the consultation.

Very often the relationship is such that the client may discuss a problem with the therapist rather than a member of her family. This is a difficult situation, which must always be handled sensitively.

Examples of the sort of conditions you may come across relate to things like skin lesions, lumps or swelling or where a client is taking medication that causes skin irritation or rash. Under all such circumstances the client should contact their doctor and provide a letter advising you that it is safe to provide the treatment. This will also apply to long-term health problems.

Most conditions, however, are temporary and you can advise the client to wait until the condition has cleared up before having treatment. On no account should the therapist make direct contact with the client's doctor by telephone or letter. The responsibility lies with the client, although you may wish to write down for her some details of the treatments or products you would be using.

Many conditions are localised: a verruca on the foot would not prevent you from doing a manicure or facial on the client, for example.

Discuss your recommendations for treatment

Use your skill and experience to ensure that the treatment relates to the individual needs of each client. The choice of product for treating the skin will depend on the client's skin type and the choice of depilatory wax method will depend on the client's hair growth. Explain your reasoning and provide an opportunity for the client to ask questions.

Use questions to clarify

It is important to ensure that details recorded on the record card are accurate and that the client is aware of what you have written. Give them the opportunity to read the details and to sign the card. This information is confidential and should be stored in a locked filing cabinet or secure computer for access

FACIAL TREATMENT CARD

Name:

ADDRESS:

TEL: Work:
Home:

MEDICAL HISTORY:

MEDICATION:

DOB:

SKIN ASSESSMENT

	date	date	date		date	date	date		date	date	date
SEBORRHOEA				OPEN PORES				MILLIA			
COMEDONES				ACNE				SCARS			
SENSITIVE				DRY				DEHYDRATED			
MATURE				FLAKY				LOSS OF FIRMNESS			
SKIN COLOUR				DILATED CAPILLARIES				PIGMENTATION			
SUPERFLUOUS HAIR				SKIN BLEMISHES				LINES/AGEING			
OTHER											

Client Signature: Date:

TREATMENT

Date	Products used	Advised for home use	Products purchased
1			
2			
3			
4			
5			
6			

Reassess the skin carefully after six treatments to judge changes in skin condition, success of home product use and make changes in salon and home routines as required.

7				
8				
9				
10				
11				
12				
TREATMENT PROGRESS:				
Client comments:				
HOME CARE CHECKLIST				
Client Signature:	Date:		Therapist Signature:	Date:
CLIENT COMMENTS:				

Figure 5.2 *An example of a client consultation card*

only by the beauty therapy staff. Alternatively, information may be stored on a computer database. This is governed by the Data Protection Act.

Questioning techniques

- Ask appropriate questions that are not intrusive. It is not necessary to pry into your client's private affairs. It should only be necessary to ask general questions that allow the client to tell you as much or as little as they want to.
- Ask questions in a tactful manner.
- Display empathy and understanding when questioning your client.
- Use open questions as much as possible to gain information.
- Only question to gain the minimum appropriate information.

Open and closed questions

With an open question, the client can give you a detailed answer. The answer to a closed question is either yes or no. Examples of open and closed questions that may be used in consultation are:

- Open question: 'Can you tell me about the skincare routine you follow at home?'
- Closed question: 'Do you cleanse your skin at home?'
- Open question: 'If you are taking any medication will you explain what condition it is for?'
- Closed question: 'Are you taking any medication?'

A visual check

The therapist should be prepared to look for signs of infection first and foremost, and then observe any abnormalities in the area. While diagnosis of any condition is against the therapists' code of practice, you may need to make certain judgements about a skin lesion or unusual swelling, for example. The client will invariably be able to explain the condition and, providing you can establish that it is not a contraindication or that the treatment will not aggravate it in any way, you would be able to start the treatment.

Your assessment of the client will depend on a visual check of the condition of the area you are treating. This will enable you to select appropriate products and treatment. For example, you must establish the client's skin type before beginning a facial.

Observing the client as they arrive at the salon can help with your assessment, by giving you an indication of their temperament and attitude. If you are doing make-up for the first time, it can be useful to look at the client's clothes, the colours they wear and how they do their own make-up.

You should observe your client's body language to see if they are relaxed or uncomfortable.

Manual examination

Assess the client by touching the area to be treated to feel the skin's texture or the warmth of the skin. When waxing, establish the length and coarseness of the hair to be removed by touch.

It may be necessary to palpate the skin to feel muscle tone or to assess the elasticity of the skin. The therapist must be confident when touching the client and always have freshly washed hands.

Manner and attitude

A professional manner will require you to speak clearly, ask only appropriate questions, listen carefully to what the client has to say, and show respect. The way in which the consultation is carried out will give the client confidence and trust in your ability. Be prepared to give the client time to ask questions. It is important to build the relationship with your client and make them feel relaxed.

The treatment plan

The information gained throughout the consultation is used to establish the best course of action to meet the needs of the client. This is called a treatment plan.

Each treatment requires specific information and the detail appears in the relevant chapter of this book. However, the general information that needs to be recorded includes:

- client's name, address and telephone number (e-mail address if appropriate)
- type of treatment and products
- area to be treated
- contraindications – notes on any medical referral
- any known contra-actions
- client's home care routine and any relevant information on lifestyle
- aftercare advice given and products purchased
- course of treatments – number and advanced payments
- outcome of treatment – results and effects
- client's comments and signature
- therapist's recommendations and signature.

The treatment plan should be ongoing and record progress over a period of time. Looking back over past records and seeing improvements can be very encouraging for the client.

Informing the client of costs and time taken for treatment

The client will want to know how long they will spend in the salon for treatment and how much it will cost. An up-to-date price list must be available in the salon. Should there be a change to the published prices, the client must be informed during the consultation. This will avoid any embarrassment when the client comes to pay. It is not good practice to spring extra cost on the client when you have completed the treatment.

The client should be given an estimated time for the treatment to be completed. This allows them to make arrangements and for you to keep to your appointments schedule. The therapist must be aware of time so that treatments are cost-effective. For example, taking an hour to do a treatment that would usually be done in 45 minutes is not making the best use of time and your manager may question how efficient you are being. If, however, you are able to sell further treatments or products, this would be regarded favourably by your manager, providing your next client is not kept waiting.

Courses of treatment paid for in advance offer financial benefits to the salon. A special offer for the client of one free treatment or a free skincare product can be an added incentive to attend the salon regularly.

Selling

Beauty therapists must recognise that an important part of their role is to sell. This may be selling treatments, retail products or promotional packages for example. Therapists should be selling and promoting new treatments as they are introduced to the salon. They should also ensure that the client is aware that some salon services require a course of treatments. The application of individual false eyelashes will, for example, require the client to return for the lashes to be replaced periodically, or the application of nail extensions will require maintenance.

The client must be made aware of this during the initial consultation and it should be noted on the treatment plan. It is wise to offer courses of treatments as a whole package. This allows the salon to offer discounts and other incentives to the client. The client then understands exactly what it will cost both in monetary terms and in time. You should also include any products required for home use in the total package.

Home care

The client must be encouraged to undertake a home care routine. The importance of this routine must be stressed if the treatment plan outcome is to be achieved. The client needs to be aware of what to do, what to use and when to use it. The use of a home care plan, which can be tailored to meet the individual requirements of the client, can assist in changing old routines and improving the skin condition. By including products that the client will need to purchase with the cost of the course of treatments, a weekly cost could be given to the client, which will cover all their needs.

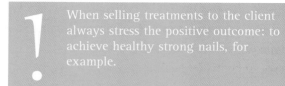

When selling treatments to the client always stress the positive outcome: to achieve healthy strong nails, for example.

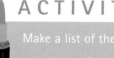

ACTIVITY

Make a list of the skills you will require to carry out a consultation and treatment plan, for example:

- accuracy in writing down information
- empathy.

Preparing for treatments

Preparation before starting any treatment is essential to ensure that hygiene and safety procedures have been carried out. A treatment area must never show signs of the previous client, for example crumpled bed paper, used towels, used products left on the trolley.

Time must be allowed between treatments to:

- prepare the treatment area
- allow the therapist to check their appearance.

Preparing the treatment area

The appointment book will indicate what treatment(s) the client has requested. This may change after consultation with the client but the therapist can usually decide what clean laundry will be needed and how the couch, trolley and equipment can be set up.

It is the responsibility of the therapist to ensure:

- the health and safety of the client
- the visit to the salon is enjoyable for the client
- the surroundings are clean and tidy
- the environment is warm and well ventilated.

The health and safety of the client

- Be well prepared for the treatment by ensuring products are available and equipment is in good working order.
- Check your appearance.
- Check that hygiene procedures are fully carried out – wash your hands.
- Check for contraindications.

- Check the client's record card for details of previous treatments.
- Always apply skin tests for treatments that require them, e.g. lash tint, and enter results on the client's record card.
- Be prepared to adapt the treatment to meet the client's needs.
- Observe the skin during treatment for any adverse reactions.
- Check for any contra-actions during and after treatment and be able to treat them appropriately.
- Ensure that the finished treatment meets the client's needs.
- Enter treatment details on the record card.
- Provide aftercare advice.

The visit to the salon is enjoyable for the client

- Check the ambience of the treatment room – heating, ventilation, lighting, pleasant smell (perfumed candles), soft music as appropriate.
- Work to appointment schedules and recommended treatment times as closely as possible.
- Communicate with the client using a friendly but not too familiar manner.
- Ensure the client's belongings are secure and be particularly careful if the client has to remove jewellery for treatment.
- Check the client's expectations from the treatment.
- Maintain the client's modesty throughout the treatment.
- Be aware of the client's body language or facial expression to ascertain whether they are relaxed and enjoying the treatment, or in the case of something like a leg wax where relaxation is difficult, check that the treatment is not causing too much discomfort.
- Always ask the client if they are comfortable throughout the treatment.
- Provide home care advice and where appropriate offer a leaflet detailing procedures for home care.
- Discuss products used and offer samples and/or retail cosmetics.
- Offer further appointments and include offers such as: a free product with every facial, two for one, introduce a new client get a free treatment, etc.

Clean and tidy surroundings

- The floors in the treatment area must be cleaned daily and anything split wiped up immediately to avoid slipping.
- All work surfaces must be wiped down with a disinfectant solution.
- Cupboards should be neat and tidy, free from spillages and dust
- Waste products must be handled with care and disposed of immediately.
- The waste bin must have a liner and be disposed of into a main bin after each client.
- Clean linen must be used for each client. This will require efficient laundry procedures.
- Disposable paper products should be used wherever possible.
- Magazines should be arranged neatly (they should be up to date and in good condition).
- Used coffee cups must be cleared away and washed.
- Food must never be consumed in treatment areas.
- The salon should be a no smoking area.

Before the start of treatment

- Wipe the trolley with disinfectant and cover with disposable paper.
- Tidy bottles and containers on the trolley. Wipe bottle tops and ensure lids and tops are secure.

- Prepare products and materials for the next client by checking the appointment page for treatment required, i.e. ensure wax is heated to the correct temperature, prepare make-up pallet, prepare manicure trolley, etc.
- Prepare couch with clean towels and disposable paper.
- Prepare disposable gloves if used.
- Ensure there are sufficient disposable materials – bed paper, tissues and cotton wool.
- Wash hands thoroughly.
- Collect sterilised tools, e.g. tweezers, cuticle implements, etc. and place in disinfectant until required.

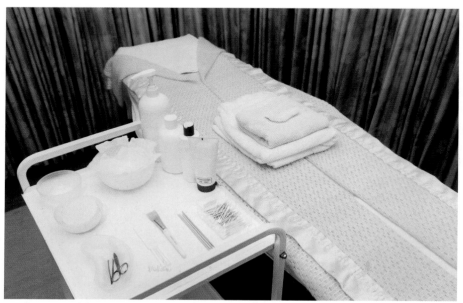

Figure 5.3 *A couch prepared for a facial treatment*

Preparing the trolley

Product trolleys, manicure trolleys and equipment trolleys must be wiped over with disinfectant and covered with disposable paper. Dust and spillages on trolleys can harbour infection and will give a very poor impression to the client. Bottle tops should be wiped, containers will need washing and a supply of dry and damp cotton wool and tissues will be required.

Preparing tools and equipment

Any item that is used on the client's skin has the potential to carry infection. Wherever possible such items should be disposable and thrown away after use, or be easily washed and sterilised or disinfected. Small tools and equipment such as tweezers should be wiped over or washed as appropriate and placed on the trolley in a jar containing disinfectant. Disposable items such as eyeshadow applicators should be placed in the bin to be thrown away.

Facial sponges and cosmetic brushes can very easily harbour infection when they are left unwashed after use. The damp, warm conditions encourage growth of micro-organisms. Sponges can smell sour if left dirty or placed in plastic bags. While the use of sponges can be economical, saving on cotton wool, the chances of passing on infection is greatly increased.

Sponges and cosmetic brushes must be thoroughly washed in hot soapy water, rinsed in disinfectant solution (such as Milton), allowed to dry naturally and stored in an ultraviolet sterilisation unit or in an airtight container.

Check your appearance and hygiene

High standards of personal hygiene are essential to guard against cross infection and to project a good image of the salon. There are basic procedures that must be followed by the therapist:

- **Hair** must be clean, styled and away from the face. Constantly pushing the hair back during treatments is unhygienic and unprofessional.
- **Jewellery** should be kept to the minimum, particularly rings and bracelets which may come into contact with electrical equipment or the client.
- **Shoes** must be comfortable and appropriate for long hours of standing. Sloppy sandals or boots are not acceptable. Stockings or tights must be clean each day and free from unsightly snags or ladders. Keep a spare pair at work just in case.
- **Salon wear** will usually be a uniform and may be a full-length overall or top, usually white or a pale shade, worn with trousers or skirts. Whatever choice of salon dress, it is important to have at least two overalls to allow for daily washing. Salon dress should not be worn outside the salon where it may pick up undesirable smells and become soiled.
- **Hands** must be well cared for, smooth with short manicured nails and no nail polish. Dirt can become trapped under the nail and nail polish can mask this, risking the spread of infection. Any cuts or sores on the hands must be covered with a surgical dressing to avoid cross infection.
- **Fresh breath** is essential because of the close proximity to the client. Cigarettes and spicy foods containing garlic and onions can taint the breath. They may be offensive to the client and should, therefore, be avoided. Brushing the teeth morning and night and after food removes particles of food and plaque that can cause bad breath. Bad breath (**halitosis**) may be the result of stomach disorders. Brushing the teeth or using a mouthwash while at work will help to avoid unpleasant mouth odour.
- **Body odour** (BO) is unacceptable and can be avoided by a daily shower or bath. Deodorants can help to maintain freshness, but remember they cannot cover up poor personal hygiene. BO is caused by perspiration becoming stale on the body or clothing. Underwear must be changed daily and more often during the menstrual cycle when extra care must be taken to avoid unpleasant odour.

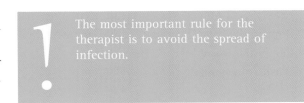

The most important rule for the therapist is to avoid the spread of infection.

- **Day make-up** must be worn at all times when coming into contact with clients. It should be immaculate with particular attention to skincare. It is often the best way of selling cosmetics to a client. The client will expect to see the therapist practise what she preaches!

Thorough **washing of the hands** is essential before treating the client, after carrying out treatment and at any time during the day when the hands have come into contact with a possible source of infection, for example after visiting the toilet or carrying out cleaning tasks in the salon.

Washing hands thoroughly

- Use hot water and a good liquid detergent in a dispenser, preferably antiseptic, to wash hands. (Bars of soap can harbour germs.)
- Disposable towels should be available for drying and disposed of immediately in a closed bin.
- Wash hands before starting any treatment and immediately afterwards.
- Washing hands throughout the day is also important, especially after visiting the toilet, before eating food and following cleaning jobs.

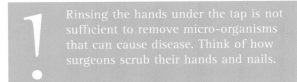

Rinsing the hands under the tap is not sufficient to remove micro-organisms that can cause disease. Think of how surgeons scrub their hands and nails.

During treatment

- Personal hygiene is essential for the therapist when working in confined areas and in such close proximity to the client. Check personal hygiene and appearance regularly throughout the day.
- Prepare the area to be treated as appropriate (see individual treatments for preparation of the area to be treated).
- Wash hands before and after treatment or at any time it is necessary to break away from the treatment, e.g. a sneeze, answering the telephone.
- Always place tops back on containers immediately after use to prevent micro-organisms contaminating the product.
- Wipe up any spillages immediately.
- Tidy the treatment area and the trolley.

> ! You will come into close contact with your clients. Bad breath from smoking or spicy foods can be very offensive. Good personal hygiene is of the utmost importance to avoid unpleasant body odour.

After treatment

- Discuss the results of the treatment with the client and ensure that it is completed to the client's wishes.
- Provide aftercare advice.
- Dispose of all waste materials, any contaminated tissues, etc., in a plastic bin liner and tie securely.
- Clean equipment, particularly depilatory wax heaters, immediately after use. The heaters can become unsightly and harbour germs if they are not kept free from wax.
- Make-up pallets should be cleaned and stored until required.
- Nail polish tops must be wiped before replacing the cap. This ensures that the tops do not stick, making opening difficult, and that the solvent does not evaporate, making the polish thick (for further examples of procedures for clearing up after treatments see individual treatment procedures).
- Prepare the couch/manicure table, etc., with clean linen ready for the next client.
- Empty the waste bin.
- Wash your hands.

ACTIVITY

Use the following checklist to assess your appearance on a regular basis.

Personal hygiene and appearance checklist

- Is your salon uniform spotless and neatly ironed?
- Is your hair clean and in a style that prevents your hair falling over your face during treatment?
- Are you wearing comfortable, low-heeled shoes that are clean and not scuffed?
- If you are wearing tights or stockings, are they changed every day and free from holes or ladders?
- Are you wearing jewellery that may come into contact with equipment or the client, e.g. rings and bangles?
- Have you brushed your teeth today?
- Did you take a bath or shower before starting work today?
- Are you wearing day make-up?
- Does your make-up look professionally and carefully applied?
- Did you wash your hands using hot soapy water and disposable towels to dry them, before and after treating your client?

Think ahead

The key to good preparation is to think ahead.

- What do I need to carry out the treatment?
- Will my client be comfortable?
- Is the treatment area clean, tidy and hygienic?
- Have I accounted for likely hazards that may put me or my client at risk?
- Is my appearance immaculate and professional?

> **!** The preparation for specific treatments will be dealt with at the beginning of the relevant chapter.

Salon rules and regulations

Health and Safety legislation demands that employers set out **policies** on safe working practice. This will usually take the form of salon rules and regulations that are posted on noticeboards in staff areas or as part of the employee's contract of employment.

Generally speaking the policies will follow the **codes of ethics** supplied by the various professional beauty therapy organisations as well as current legislation described in chapter 3.

Rules will cover such things as:

- salon care and maintenance
- hygiene procedures
- fire precautions
- emergency procedures
- salon dress
- approach to clients
- safe working practices.

A code of ethics deals with the behaviour of the therapist towards clients, other beauty therapists and allied professionals through:

- referring clients as necessary to other professionals such as chiropodists
- upholding standards of treatment and not making false claims
- having loyalty to and respect for other beauty therapists by not criticising their work or 'poaching' their clients
- not gossiping or betraying the confidence of the clients.

A code of ethics will also ensure that the quality of treatment is maintained, stipulating that:

- each client has a consultation to establish any contraindications and to find out requirements for treatment
- written permission is obtained from the client's doctor for certain treatments where the client's medication or condition requires it
- the therapist is competent and keeps up to date with the latest treatments
- the therapist does not make false claims and does not attempt to treat medical conditions.

A code of ethics will also ensure standards of health and safety are maintained by requiring that:

- practices and procedures are implemented and monitored
- staff are trained in safety procedures.

Salon policies and procedures

ACTIVITY

Use the following checklist to check your own working practices to ensure that you follow salon policies and procedures that are in place to reduce risks to health and safety.

To work safely you must:

- dispose of different types of waste in the correct way
- check all products are in date and equipment is safe
- position yourself so that you do not have to overstretch or bend
- position your trolley so it is within easy reach
- not trail electrical cables across the floor
- check all electrical equipment and ensure that electrician safety tests are up to date
- position your client to make sure that they are safe and comfortable
- make sure the lighting is suitable for the treatment to be performed
- ensure that staff are competent to carry out treatments through adequate training
- ensure staff are up to date with new treatments and working practices through training and following the manufacturer's instructions for the use of products and equipment.

To work hygienically you must:

- wash your hands thoroughly before starting the treatment
- keep your work area and work surface clean and tidy throughout the treatment
- wipe bottle tops and secure tops/lids on products
- use disposable paper couch covers and clean towels for each client
- throw away all disposable items after each client and set up the treatment area with clean towels and couch paper before starting the next treatment
- empty the treatment room bin after each client
- check all equipment is sterilised or disinfected as appropriate for each client.

Chapter 6

MAKE-UP

LEVEL 2

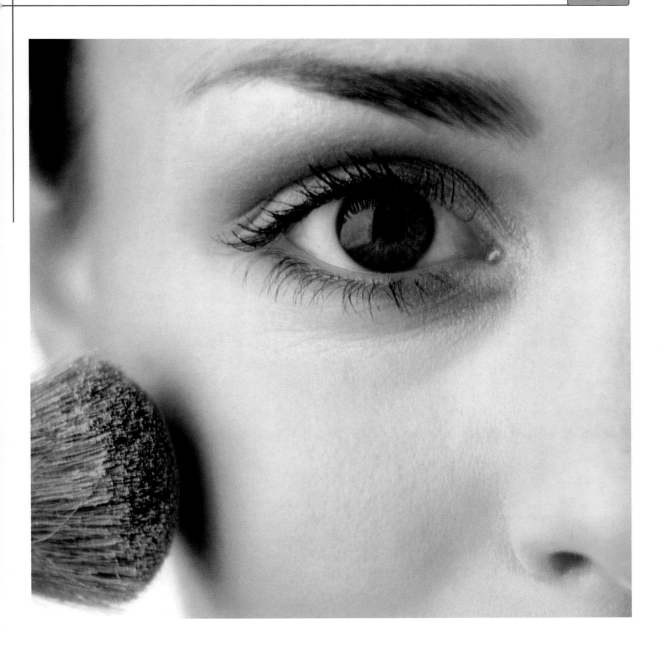

IN THIS CHAPTER YOU WILL LEARN ABOUT:

- Tools and equipment
- Preparation
  - treatment area
  - skin
- Make-up products and how to select them
- Application of make-up
- False eyelash application
- Planning and promoting make-up activities

It is essential that you have a clear understanding of the skin: function, structure, disorders, disease and damage. Please refer to chapter 14, Related Anatomy and Physiology, for full details.

To obtain a perfect make-up finish, knowledge of the skin is essential. The beauty therapist must be able to make an accurate assessment of the client's skin in order to select the correct cleansing and make-up products, as well as the right application technique. Learning about skin disease and disorders is important, as the presence of a condition can determine whether a treatment should be performed.

Prepare the work area and the client for the application of make-up

The use and effect of a professionally applied make-up should not be underestimated. Make-up is an important part of a facial but it is also becoming increasingly popular as a salon service in its own right. Many salons include make-up lessons as part of their menu of services. It is also a response to the growing demand for professional make-up application for weddings and portrait photography.

Make-up is used to 'say something' about the wearer. Therefore, it is vital to undertake a thorough consultation with the client to ascertain their needs and desires. A consultation also provides an opportunity to advise the client of achievable outcomes. All findings from the consultation should be recorded on the client's treatment plan (see page 74).

Make-up can be used not only to improve and enhance, but also to correct minor imperfections and to balance the features. Within most hospitals there are facilities available for cosmetic camouflage. Specialised make-up products and methods of application are used effectively to camouflage pigmentation abnormalities and skin disorders.

Specialised techniques are also used for photographic work, fashion and catwalk shows, stage, television and for creating special effects within television and film.

This chapter, however, is dedicated to basic make-up product selection and application. Once these principles have been mastered, they will form the foundation for the further development of these skills. The art of make-up application is acquired through practice and experimentation with colour and different techniques.

Personal preparation

It is important to instil confidence in your client and, as discussed in chapter 5, you must ensure your appearance is appropriate. A client will expect you to be professional both in appearance and

 Remember to wash your hands before commencing make-up and to ensure that the client can see you doing this.

manner. It is particularly important to wear make-up. This should not be heavy but will indicate that you take care with your appearance.

Tools and equipment
Lighting

One of the most important requirements for make-up application is good lighting. Ideally this should be **natural daylight,** however this is not always possible. You will need a good quality lamp, one that is capable of simulating natural daylight and that does not flood the face with bright white light. It should also be adjustable to accommodate client positioning.

Fluorescent lights should be avoided, as should fixed lighting, which may cast shadows on the face. It is important to ascertain the conditions in which the make-up will be worn and to adapt accordingly, for example you will have to consider the effects of artificial light on evening make-up.

Brushes

A good set of brushes will last for many years. You will soon find them familiar tools, ones that can be easily selected to meet the special needs of particular make-up techniques. Professional brushes should be long handled and made from **sable** or **soft bristle.**

You will require a large-headed powder brush, a blusher brush, a contour brush and a selection of eyeshadow brushes. These should include a sponge-tipped applicator, an angled brush head, a dome-shaped brush head and a wider brush, which

!

Refer to chapter 1 for information on sterilising equipment.

Contour brushes
These are used to apply highlighter shades and other corrective products. The longest contour brush is usually for powder blusher application.

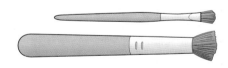

Lip brush
This is used for applying lip colour with accuracy

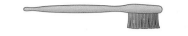

Eyebrow brush
This is an essential brush and should always be used. Eyebrows should be brushed as part of the general make-up procedure to give a groomed appearance. This brush should also be used when shaping the brows.

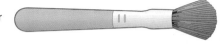

The **powder brush** is the largest brush. It is used to dust off excess powder following application. By brushing upwards and downwards, a velvety finish is given to the skin.

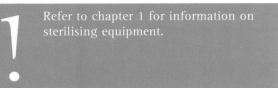

An **eyeliner brush** is very fine and can be used to apply eyeliner with accuracy. It can also be used for intricate detailed corrective make-up.

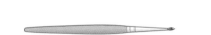

Eyeshadow brushes
These are used to apply and blend eyeshadows.They are usually square-ended or tapered.

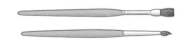

Figure 6.1 *Different types of make-up brushes*

is useful for blending. You will find that most professional brushes will have the suggested function identified on the handle. You may disregard these if you wish and use whichever suits the need of the application. A combined brush/comb is required for grooming the brows and for separating the eyelashes. A fine brush is essential for eyeliner application and a lip brush is vital for applying cosmetics to the lips with precision. You will also require a selection of sponges and facial wedges. Eyelash curlers are another essential item as they enhance the eyes considerably.

You should also have a mirror available to show the client the finished make-up or to talk the client through each stage of a make-up lesson.

> ! Remember to check for contraindications.

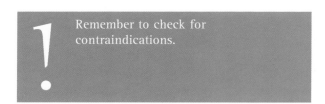

Eyelash curlers
Used before mascara application to curl lashes.

natural sponge

synthetic sponge

latex wedge

Figure 6.2 *Sponges, wedges and eyelash curlers*

Preparation of the treatment area

It is important to ensure the trolley and work station are prepared prior to the client's arrival. Your work station should be equipped with:

- cleansing, toning and moisturising mediums – a selection should be available to accommodate the findings of the skin analysis
- corrective products – green tinted moisturiser, concealer products
- foundations – a selection of shades
- contour cosmetics – highlighters, shaders, blushers
- eyeshadows – a selection of colours with both matt and pearlised finish
- mascaras – block-type with disposable wands
- false lashes – individual and strip lashes
- brow cosmetics
- lip cosmetics.

In addition you will need:

- cotton wool and cotton-wool buds
- tissues
- spatulas
- a selection of small bowls
- clean headbands
- mirror
- a covered waste bin
- client treatment plan or record card.

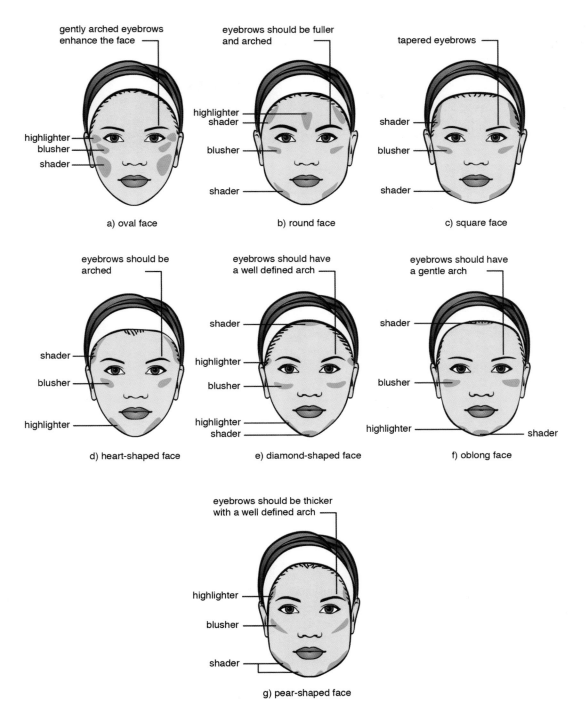

Figure 6.3 *Highlighter, blusher and shader are used in corrective make-up*

All tools and equipment should be sterilised in the appropriate way (see page 21) and should not be brought to the trolley until you are ready to use them.

The client should be comfortably positioned on the couch or in the make-up chair. The client should be in an **elevated** position and should not be lying flat for make-up application. It is important that the effects of gravity on the facial features are considered. The hair and clothes should be protected. The therapist can be either seated or standing, depending on the working height of the couch or chair. At least 30–45 minutes should be allowed for make-up application in the treatment schedule.

Preparation of the skin

The skin must be clean and free from grease, stale make-up and cleansing products. Once the skin is cleansed, a suitable moisturiser should be applied to the face and neck. (See chapter 7 for more detail on cleansing and moisturising.)

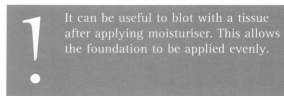

It can be useful to blot with a tissue after applying moisturiser. This allows the foundation to be applied evenly.

Foundations

The right foundation is the basis of a successful make-up. Although it is not essential, it does provide the ideal surface to receive other cosmetics. A good foundation will even out the complexion, correct any imperfections and act as a barrier between the skin and any atmospheric pollution. Many foundations contain sunscreens to protect the skin from the damaging effects of ultraviolet light.

Selecting the right foundation

Factors to consider:

- skin type
- coverage
- skin colour
- lifestyle
- occasion
- expense
- age.

Types of foundation

Foundations are available in many forms, the most common types being **creams, compacts, liquids, cakes, gels** and **mousses.**

Type of Foundation	Method of Application
Creams – originally cream foundations were colour-free, oil-in-water emulsions known as vanishing creams. Modern foundations are tinted and are usually oil-in-water emulsions containing mineral oil and ceresin wax. Colours range from the palest tones through to rich dark brown, thus providing a foundation colour to suit all skin colours. The cream may be coloured by the use of inorganic pigments such as iron oxides. The inclusion of titanium dioxide in the formulation produces a more opaque cream, increasing the covering power.	The foundation is removed from the container using a spatula and a small amount is placed on the back of the therapist's hand or onto a palette. It can then be applied with fingertips using a light effleurage movement, producing an even film over the skin.
Compact foundation – this type of product is a mixture of cream foundation and face powder, which produces a foundation with a matt finish. The products are gaining in popularity, as they dispense with the need for separate foundation and powder.	These products are usually applied with a facial wedge or sponge. A small amount of the product is placed onto a palette. The foundation is then applied using the sponge to one area of the face at a time and blended.

(Continued)

Type of Foundation	Method of Application
Liquid – these contain similar ingredients to creams, but with a higher proportion of water. Some liquids are oil-free, containing clay to thicken and hold the pigment in an alcohol or water base.	Liquid foundations should be gently agitated prior to use to disperse the pigments evenly through the formulation. The product may then be applied into the palm of the non-working hand of the therapist or onto a palette. Fingertip application is better for this product as moistened sponges can remove rather than apply. It is important to let this product dry before proceeding to the next stage.
Cake – cake foundations are usually emulsions containing mineral oils, wax, powder and pigments that are dried. The product is then powdered and compressed into cake form. Cake foundations give dense cover and can be used for correcting or concealing blemishes. This formulation is also used for **concealers**.	Cake foundations should be applied with a moistened sponge, slowly building up to the required finish.
Gels – these foundations produce a glossy film, often used to produce a tanned look. Gels have very little covering power and are therefore unsuitable for less than perfect skins.	Care should be taken with their application. Do not dot all over the face as this can lead to irregular patches and staining. The gel sets quite quickly on application, leaving a concentration of colour. Instead, a small amount should be dotted on one area at a time and blended in before applying elsewhere.
Mousses – these foundations are sheer, light textured foam, usually in pump dispensers. They can be used on all skin types and are most effective when a light, natural look is required, i.e. day/bridal make-up.	Mousses can be applied with fingertips for a light finish or with a sponge for a more intense colour. It is preferable to layer the applications rather than apply a large amount as it can be difficult to work with.

Skin type and foundation

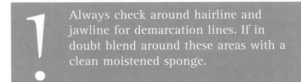

It is vital, when selecting a foundation, that the client's skin type is considered. If the wrong product is selected, the completed make-up may be poor and the effect may not be long-lasting. Moisturisers, whilst an essential element of the process, will only have a temporary effect. The skin will revert to type as the day progresses. If the right product is selected and it is applied correctly, foundation should last throughout the day, should not change colour or need to be reapplied.

Always check around hairline and jawline for demarcation lines. If in doubt blend around these areas with a clean moistened sponge.

Skin Type	Choice of Foundation
Dry	Cream or Moisturising Liquid
Mature	Cream or Moisturising Liquid
Sensitive	Hypo-allergenic liquid or cream
Combination	Liquid or compact
Oily	Liquid, water based, oil-free
Blemished/Acne	Oil-free liquid, which is medicated

When selecting a foundation, you should aim to match the colour as closely to the natural skin colour as possible. If the colour is not selected with great care, the result may be an unattractive mask-like appearance. This is a particular problem when selecting foundations for black skins. Foundation is not always necessary on darker skins, if the colour is even. Instead, a light dusting of translucent powder should be used to take off any excess shine and to provide a good base for the rest of the make-up application. If foundation is used, then it should be selected on the basis of complementing the lightest tones of the skin. Foundation should always be tested on the face, **NOT** the back of the hand. The skin on the hand is very different in both colour and texture and will not show the true effect of the product.

> **!** There may be an erythema present after cleansing, particularly on clients with a sensitive skin condition. This condition may be temporary and must be considered when making your foundation selection.

Colour suggestions

Skin Tones	Foundation Tones
Fair/pale, translucent skins	Light ivory, porcelain, apricot and peach tones
Medium skin	Beige and honey tones for medium light skin
	Warm apricots and olive for medium dark skin
Dark skin	Beige, bronze and olive tones
Vascular complexions	Always use green corrective products to tone down redness
	Use beige and olive tones
Sallow skin	Pink, beige or tawny tones
Pigmented skin	Areas of pigmentation should be covered with camouflage cream before foundation is used

Hints

1. Choose a foundation to suit skin type and colour.
2. Choose a foundation as near to the natural skin colour as possible.
3. On dark skins select a product nearest to the lightest skin tone.
4. To reduce a florid skin apply green corrective cream before the foundation.
5. To brighten a sallow skin apply lilac corrective cream.
6. Apply foundation with a dampened make-up sponge or fingertips.
7. Apply foundation to small areas at a time and blend well.
8. If the under-eye area is very lined, mix a little moisturiser with the foundation and blend in up to the base of the lashes.

Face powders

Face powders can be either translucent (loose) or highly pigmented (usually compressed). They work in very different ways.

Translucent powder

Translucent powder is extra fine and filtered. It allows light to diffuse through without changing the underlying skin colour. The foundation should always be followed by application of loose powder. Translucent powder is designed to set the make-up but not to change the colour. Translucent powders enhance the foundation and tone down shine.

Compressed powder

Compressed powders offer dense coverage and, therefore, are restricted to corrective work or for make-up 'touch-ups'. The use of traditional compressed powder has decreased. This is due in part to the introduction of refined compressed foundations that offer good coverage with a velvety finish all from one product.

The main constituent of powder is **talc**, which gives slip, translucency and covering power. Metallic particles may be added to give a pearly look. They should be used with caution. They can make the skin look moist, especially when photographed, as the metallic particles reflect light. This type of powder is particularly effective for evening wear and could easily be added to adapt day make-up for evening.

> A good face powder should be easy to apply, smooth on the skin and allow the colour of the foundation to be seen, without changing the base colour. Some powders can be worn without a base and can be used to give a glow to the skin, particularly on black or dark skins.

Corrective effects of face powders

Translucent

Usually colourless and will not alter the desired effect of the make-up.

Green

As with tinted moisturisers, this coloured powder can be used under normal face powder to tone down a florid or red skin. It should be used sparingly, especially on the nose and cheek areas.

Lilac/pale pink

This can liven sallow skins. It should be used under normal face powder.

White/pearly powder

It may be used as a highlighter to enhance facial features.

Face powder application

A small amount of loose powder should be taken from the container using a clean spatula. The powder should be placed onto a tissue in the therapist's hand. A clean, sterile powder puff or ball of cotton wool should be dipped into the powder and the excess tapped off. A light twisting motion should be used to apply the product. A large headed powder brush should then be employed to dust away the excess powder from the face. This should be done with light upward and downward movements and will create a velvety finish to the skin.

> Always apply a light dusting of powder to the lips and eyelids. This will help the eye and lip cosmetics adhere to the area.

1. Always use loose powder.
2. **Never** apply powder that is darker than the foundation.
3. Apply sparingly if the skin is excessively dry or if the under-eye area is wrinkled.
4. If there is a lot of facial hair, powder should be avoided.

Contour cosmetics

Contour cosmetics comprise three main types: blusher or rouge, highlighter and shader. They can be used to accentuate and diminish features or to add colour and warmth. Shading and highlighting can be done effectively on light or darker skins. However, shading will be less prominent on darker skins while highlighting will be more obvious.

The use of highlighters and shaders can help to transform day make-up into evening make-up by accentuating features and creating interest in the face. Remember evening make-up will need to be stronger to allow for the effect of artificial lighting.

Blusher or rouge

Blusher and rouge have the same function. Blusher is the modern name for rouge. It is designed to add colour to the cheek area, simulating a 'natural' cheek colour or adding warmth. It can be in cream or powder form and the colours available vary from very pale pinks through to brick reds and dark browns. Powder blusher is applied over foundation and after the powder has been applied. Cream blusher is usually applied after the foundation but before the powder.

Application

A small amount of powder blusher should be taken up onto a blusher brush. The excess should be tapped off over the back of the hand. The application should proceed using an inverted triangle as a template shape. Application should start from below the centre of the eye, working up to the top of the ear. The application should not start beyond the centre of the client's eye. Without reloading the brush, small strokes gradually fanning out back up the cheekbone should be applied.

Do not exceed application beyond the centre of the client's eye. This can make the application look unnatural and can lead to the cheek having a 'clown-like' appearance.

Highlighters

Highlighters are used to enhance positive features. They are usually light colours: beiges and pinks through to white. Some may have pearlised or iridescent finishes and they can be cream or powder based. They are commonly used to accentuate the eyelids, under the eyebrow or across the cheekbones. Less common but equally effective is the application of highlighter to the cupid's bow on the lips to accentuate the pout. On darker skins, highlighting can be used to great effect. Areas of the face can be brought into prominence and interesting planes given to the features. Highlighting is particularly effective when used to slim and straighten the centre of the nose and give definition to the cheekbones.

lighter matte shadow
creates width

highlighter

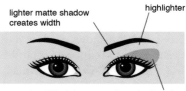

should be taken upwards and outwards
from the outer corner of the eye

a) close-set

deeper colour provides depth to the
inner corner of the eye

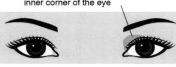

b) wide-set

lift eyeshadow and eyeliner applicaton
beyond outer corner of eye

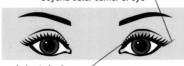

darkest shadow
colour to the centre of eyelid

c) round or prominent

highlighter

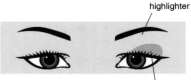

blended shadow working from applying
darker colour over the lid area and blended

d) overhanging lids

dark shadow applied above
natural socket line

highlighter

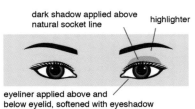

eyeliner applied above and
below eyelid, softened with eyeshadow

e) small or deep-set

highlighter

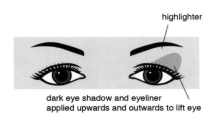

dark eye shadow and eyeliner
applied upwards and outwards to lift eye

f) downward slanting

darken the socket line extending above
natural socket line, blended into highlighter

highlighter

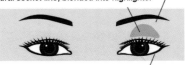

eyeliner applied to lower lash line
and softened with eyeshadow

g) narrow

shading above the natural
socket line gives depth
to the eyelids

lighter matte eyeshadow
blended across the eye
socket gives depth and
fullness to the eyes

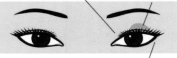

eyeliner and eyeshadow applied to
the lower lash line widens and enlarges

h) oriental

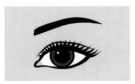

proportioned lid and brow

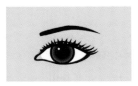

small lid, small brow

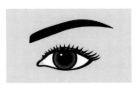

small lid, large brow

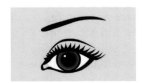

large lid, small brow

Figure 6.4 *Corrective eye make-up*

Shaders

Shaders, as a range of corrective products, have been replaced with blushers and foundations. The **concept** of shading, however, is still very important. The effect of shading is to reduce or diminish a particular facial feature. Dark pink, tawny or brown shades are used and always have a matt finish. Shading is usually only used on darker skins to give depth to a rounded face around the lower cheek area. The wide colour range of foundations and blushers provides alternatives to a traditional shading product. Two foundations of contrasting colour can provide a natural shading effect.

Hints

1. All cream products should be applied **before** the powder. Powder products should be applied **after** the powder.
2. Blusher should always be kept high on the face and never applied to the centre plains of the cheeks.
3. Do not apply blusher too near to the nose or eyes.
4. The effect of contour products should be subtle and natural.
5. Check the application on completion to ensure it is symmetrical. Balance can also be achieved by applying a touch of colour at the temples.
6. Blend contour cosmetics carefully to ensure there is no demarcation line.

Concealers

These are specially formulated to disguise minor imperfections and blemishes. They are cream based and are available in a range of flesh tones. These products are usually applied with a brush, cotton wool bud or fingertips, and normally before the foundation is applied.

Hints

1. The use of a white concealer cream is particularly effective in disguising dark circles under the eyes.
2. Clients with high colouring or broken capillaries (couperose skin) could have a green tinted cream applied to the area. This reduces the redness.
3. Minor blemishes can be masked with concealer or lighter foundation using a brush.

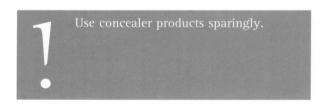

Use concealer products sparingly.

Eyeshadow

The eyeshadow is one of the most important aspects of a good make-up. The shape of the eyes can be flattered or altered with an expert application of eyeshadow products. The choice of eyeshadow available now is overwhelming and care must be taken to discuss with the client their preferences and needs. If the make-up is for a special occasion, find out more about the function and explore the colour of the outfit to be worn. Ascertain the type of function – a different effect will be required for a wedding, party or a job interview. The application techniques for the products already covered are largely the same, whichever type of function the client will be attending. The eye make-up application, however, will differ. The main function of eyeshadow is to accentuate the eyes and to make them look brighter. On a darker skin the eyes will need to be given added definition by emphasising the eyelashes as well as the eyelids. Eyeshadows are available in **powder**, **cream**, **gel** and **liquid** forms. They may have a matt finish, may contain metallic particles or have an iridescent effect.

Type of Eyeshadow	Method of Application
Powder eyeshadow – this is the type most commonly used. They are usually presented in a compressed cake, loose in a pot or in stick form. They are formulated in a similar way to cake products, but with stronger colour pigments added. Powder eyeshadow is very popular, but its staying power is limited unless foundation is used. Loose powders can irritate the eye, particularly if powdered metals are contained in the products. Clients with contact lenses should use compressed powders to prevent particles of powder entering the eye. A range of products has been designed to suit the needs of contact lens wearers and this could be a consideration when selecting a suitable retail range in the salon.	A small amount of colour should be taken onto a sterilised eyeshadow brush. The excess should be tapped off over the back of the hand. The product should be applied to the closed eye according to the desired effect. A clean tissue should be placed under the eye to catch any loose particles and to prevent the therapist's hand coming into contact with the prepared 'canvas'.
Cream eyeshadow – cream eyeshadows are not as popular as the powder varieties. Their staying power is quite poor and it is difficult to prevent creasing in the socket line. If the client does prefer cream eyeshadow, it is important to apply a light dusting of powder over the eyeshadow to help it to set.	Cream eyeshadows can be applied with the fingertips or with a moistened sponge-tipped applicator. A light dusting of powder should be applied to facilitate setting.
Gel or liquid eyeshadow – this type of eyeshadow has seen an increase in popularity. The effect created can enhance the eyes and the same product can also be used on the lips. They tend to give gloss rather than depth of colour. Several coats may be required to give adequate coverage.	These products can be applied with fingertips or with a small eyeshadow brush.

Corrective eye make-up
Hints

1. Cream eyeshadow must be applied before face powder.
2. Gel and powder eyeshadow are applied after powder.
3. Ascertain the function or effect required and explore colour themes.
4. Do not apply highlighter to loose, crêpey (thin, wrinkled) lids.
5. Introduce a small amount of blue to the base of the lashes. This will brighten the whites of the eyes.
6. Take care to avoid contact between the client's face and your hand by placing a tissue underneath the hand.
7. Where there are dark circles under the eyes, concealer may be applied to lighten the area.

Eyeliner

Eyeliner is available in **liquid**, **pencil** or **cake** formulations. It is probably the most difficult cosmetic to apply, but once the technique is mastered it can add real definition to the eye. It can be used to encircle the eyelids or on the outer edges of the lids only. The softer, non-setting formulations such as cake or pencil can be smudged using a sponge-tipped applicator or a cotton-wool bud. This gives a softer definition to the eyelid.

Make-up

97

Liquid

This is used to give a definite line. Liquid liners are applied with a very fine brush for accuracy.

Pencil

Pencil liners should be sharpened before use on each new client. They can be applied in a hard line and then blended to soften the line depending upon the desired effect. Kohl also is available in pencil form and is soft and waxy in texture. It can be quite difficult to control because of its composition and the effect of the body heat on the waxes.

Cake

Cake liner is applied with a wet fine brush. It is similar to eyeshadows in composition and can be smudged once dry for a softer effect.

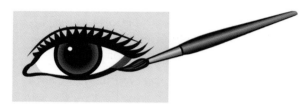

Figure 6.5 *Application of eyeliner*

Mascara

Mascara is used to give definition to the eyes by thickening and darkening the lashes. There are two types of mascara: **cake** and **liquid**.

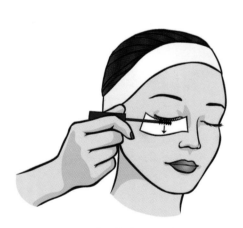

apply with downward strokes

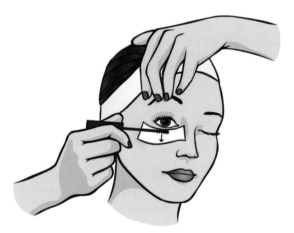

apply with upward strokes

Figure 6.6 *Applying mascara*

Cake

This is applied with a moistened disposable brush. Cake mascaras are made from waxes and pigments in a soap base. The moisture from the brush creates the formation of an emulsion on the surface of the cake. The brush takes the emulsion up and it can be applied to the lashes.

Liquid

Liquid mascaras are available with a wide range of functions: waterproof, smudgeproof, hypo-allergenic, lash-lengthening, thickening, protein enriched. Colour pigments and resins are contained in a base

Always wipe over the lashes with a mild tonic solution before starting the make-up. This will ensure the lashes are completely grease-free.

of water or alcohol and water with castor oil to prevent the mascara from becoming brittle. Filaments of rayon or nylon can be used to build and 'extend' lashes. Mascaras that contain such filaments should not be used on contact lens wearers as the filaments can irritate the eye. These mascaras come with their own applicator wand within the product and should not be used in the salon as there is a risk of cross infection.

Application

1. Curl the lashes prior to mascara application if required.
2. Apply to lower lashes first, thus enabling the client to look upwards without fear of marking the brow area with damp mascara.
3. Place a tissue under the lower lashes.
4. Lift the skin of the eyelids from underneath the brow when applying to the upper lashes.
5. Build up in fine coats, allowing each one to dry.
6. Separate using an eyelash comb if necessary.

> **!** Always use individual disposable applicator wands for each client to prevent cross infection.

Hints

1. If the client's eyes water, gently blot the corner of the eye with a soft tissue.
2. Don't apply to lower lashes if the skin is crêpey.
3. Ensure the client is advised of the type of product used and the method or product to be used for removal. This is especially important for waterproof products.
4. Application of a light dusting of powder will help to thicken the lashes and increase adhesion of the mascara.

False eyelashes

These are used for fashion, photographic and catwalk make-ups. They are particularly useful for enhancing short or sparse lashes. They are made from natural hair or nylon and there are two types:

- temporary
- semi-permanent.

Temporary

These are preshaped lashes on a flexible strip, which are applied to the edge of the eyelid. A special latex-based adhesive is used to adhere the lashes to the skin.

Semi-permanent

Available as individual or clusters of three or four flared lashes held together by a fine knot. These are applied to the natural lash using a special adhesive.

> **!** The client should always be patch-tested prior to application of semi-permanent lashes as the adhesive may irritate the skin.

Contraindications

- Sensitive or sensitised eyes.
- Reaction to patch test of bonding adhesive (semi-permanent lashes).
- Swollen or inflamed lids.
- Eye infections.

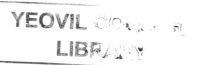

Procedure for applying temporary lashes

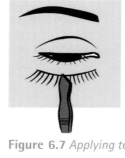
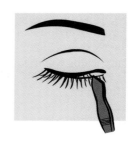

1. Apply small amount of adhesive to a spatula.
2. Using tweezers, gently pick up the strip of eyelashes. Care should be taken to pick up from the centre of the lash side.
3. Stroke the base of the strip through the adhesive so there is a fine line of adhesive along its length.

Figure 6.7 *Applying temporary eyelashes*

4. Lift the brow area to gently pull back the lid. This allows close application to base of the natural lashes.
5. Line tweezers with the centre of the eyelid and gently press strip into place on the closed eye.
6. Secure the inner and outer corners of the strip.
7. Repeat for the other eye.
8. Using a clean mascara brush, blend the false and natural lashes together.

At least 10 minutes should be allowed for the application of temporary lashes in the treatment schedule.

Procedure for removing temporary lashes

1. Hold the eyelid taut and gently pull the lashes away from the outer edge.
2. Remove adhesive from strip.
3. Wipe over natural lashes with mild toner.

Procedure for applying semi-permanent lashes

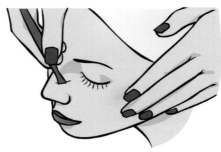

1. Ensure natural lashes are clean and free from any oil, which may prevent the adhesive from sticking.
2. Using tweezers, carefully remove lashes individually from the pack and arrange on a tissue. The lashes should be facing away from you.
3. Apply a small amount of adhesive onto a spatula.

Figure 6.8 *Applying semi-permanent lashes*

4. Raise the client's head slightly.
5. Pick up a lash and dip the knotted end into the adhesive.
6. Ask the client to lower their eyes, but **not** to close them.
7. Lift the brow area to release the fold of skin from the base of the natural lashes.
8. Place the false lash over a natural lash. Stroke gently along its length and locate according to desired outcome.

 Always grab the flare, not an individual hair, as this will cause distension to the knot and spoil the lash.

9. Work alternately between each eye to ensure balance.

Allow at least 20 minutes for the application of semi-permanent lashes in the treatment schedule.

Procedure for removing semi-permanent lashes

1. Place dampened cotton-wool pads beneath the eyes.
2. Using special solvent or oily eye make-up remover, apply to false lash with a cotton bud.
3. Wait a few seconds and gently ease the lash off.
4. Wipe over with mild toner.

 Recommend that the client returns to the salon for removal of lashes. Avoid oily products around the eyes as the oil will loosen the adhesive!

A C T I V I T Y

Research trends in eyebrow and eye enhancement over the last four decades. Consider particularly brow shapes and eye definition. Use diagrams and cuttings to support your findings.

Eyebrow pencils

These are available in a range of hair colours: grey, brown and black.

They should be applied in light feathery strokes, not in hard defined lines. They are used to add definition to the eyebrow area and can also be used in corrective work to balance or to infill missing brows.

Take special care when using black eyebrow pencil to avoid dark, unnatural brow lines.

Application

1. The brows should be brushed into shape before applying the pencil.
2. When applying, aim to create the appearance of natural hair growth by using light feathery strokes and brushing through after application to soften the effect.

Hints

1. A light application of a softer shade of eyeshadow can be used to good effect, if definition rather than correction is required.
2. Brush through brows after cosmetic application to soften effect.

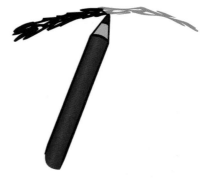

apply in light, feathery strokes

Figure 6.9 *Using an eyebrow pencil*

Lip cosmetics

Lip cosmetics are available in **pots**, **sticks** and **pencils**. They are each used to define, enhance and balance the lip shape. The main ingredients of lip products are oils, fats and waxes.

Lipstick

This has a high percentage of wax, which gives it its stiffened form. Lipsticks will vary in terms of their staying power and the choice of product will depend upon the finished effect required. When selecting lipstick for a darker skin, consideration should be given to the natural colour tones of the lips. It may be necessary to even the lip tone using a foundation or corrective product prior to application. A number of products claim to stay on all day. These products can be very drying and can also stain the lips. Softening ingredients such as petroleum jelly or mineral oil are also included in varying amounts depending on the formulation.

Gloss

This is usually formulated with a high grease content. Gloss can be clear or pigmented and is not durable. It should not be used on large lips as it will accentuate them. The introduction of a gel-based gloss has brought increased durability. This product may also be used on the eyes.

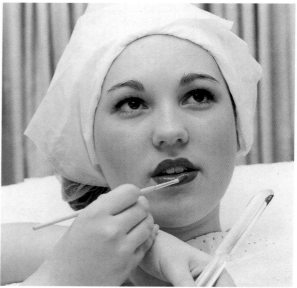
Figure 6.10 *Applying lipstick with a brush*

Pencil

This is used for outlining the lips. Pencils are difficult to sterilise and therefore must be sharpened prior to every use. They are formulated with a high proportion of hard waxes. Pencils are good for corrective lip work because they can be used to balance and even alter the alignment of the lips.

Application

1. If using a pencil, outline the line of the lip evenly.
2. If using lipstick, gently scrape a small amount of the chosen colour onto a clean palette or spatula and, using a clean, sterilised lip brush, apply a clear outline to the lips. Then fill in the lips evenly with colour.
3. Outline the lips from the sides to the centre with the lips slightly apart to allow application into the corners of the mouth.
4. Protect the make-up by using a tissue on the client's chin to support the hand.
5. Blot after the first application and reapply. This prolongs the duration of the application.

Hints

1. Apply lip gloss over the lip colour for fashion or evening wear.
2. Avoid using blueish tones on sallow skin.
3. For uneven lip tones, even out using foundation or concealer prior to applying lip colour.
4. Avoid overuse of lip gloss on large lips.

> ! It is particularly important to keep accurate records of the selected make-up products and application method. These details must be entered on the client's treatment plan or record card.
>
> The skin can take up to 48 hours to settle following a facial. This can affect the smooth application of make-up as the skin can be blotchy following a facial treatment. A simple cleanse is all that is needed prior to make-up.

General procedure for make-up application

Make-up is usually applied in a routine order. This order allows the effect to be created gradually. The application of foundation can be likened to the artist whitewashing the canvas prior to painting. It evens out the tone and creates one even 'canvas' to work on. The blusher creates the planes and the eyes and lips can be defined using eye and lip cosmetics to complete the total look.

1. Prepare client for make-up by gently cleansing the skin.
2. Check for contraindications.
3. Remove make-up brushes and sponges from the steriliser.
4. Conduct consultation with the client.
5. Select a foundation to suit the client's skin colour and type (see page 90).
6. Apply concealer if required.
7. Using a dampened cosmetic sponge, apply the foundation to the face. Take care to blend the hairline and avoid demarcation lines.
8. Place a small amount of loose powder onto a tissue. Using a dry piece of cotton wool or a sterilised powder puff, take up a small amount of powder. Lightly twist the powder into the foundation. Do not rub.
9. Select a large powder brush and sweep away any excess powder. Use upward and downward strokes to ensure that the fine facial hairs are lifted away from the skin. If you select a cream blusher this should be applied prior to the powder.
10. Apply blusher (see page 94).
11. Apply eyeshadows (see page 97).
12. Apply eyeliner (see page 98).
13. Apply mascara using disposable sterilised wands (see page 98).
14. Apply lipliner (see page 102).
15. Take a small amount of the selected lipstick onto a spatula and apply using a sterilised lip brush, blot and reapply.
16. Check overall effect for balance.
17. Remove hair covering and tidy client's hair.
18. Show client the finished result.
19. Allow the client to comment and make any adjustments if necessary.

Plan and promote make-up activities

A popular role for the therapist is one of offering make-up lessons. Clients who like the finished effect following make-up in the salon will often want to recreate the effect. This is also an opportunity for the therapist to sell items from the make-up product range. Normally a make-up lesson would take 45 minutes.

There are a variety of make-up applications a therapist may be required to offer. These include

- day make-up
- evening make-up
- bridal make-up
- photographic make-up
- catwalk and fashion show make-up.

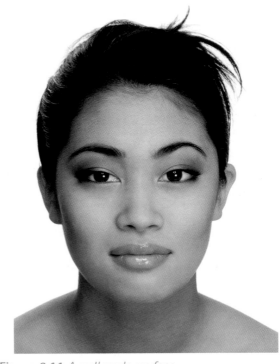

Figure 6.11 *A well made-up face*

Make-up artistry is also becoming increasingly popular as a career. For example, a person who has developed specialist make-up skills may work for a photographer, on film and promotional shoots, for fashion magazines or for a cosmetic company. Working for cosmetic companies will usually require the make-up artist to promote the product range through demonstrations.

Whatever the occasion, the effects of lighting on make-up must be considered.

<table>
<tr><td>!</td><td>It is important to discuss the client's wishes when providing a make-up. Listen carefully to what the client is saying. You can gain valuable information about their perceptions on what the make-up will look like. This is really important for brides and clients having make-up for the first time. The client may not feel confident about wearing make-up. You must be sensitive to their opinions.</td></tr>
</table>

Day make-up

Make-up for daywear should be well blended and natural looking. Lightweight products should be used in neutral, subtle shades. Some special occasions require a more defined make-up, which has to look good in daylight.

Evening make-up

Evening make-up will be well defined using bolder/deeper colours. Shading and highlighting can also be used to accentuate facial features. Lip gloss, pearlised products, false lashes and eyeliner can all be used to create a dramatic evening effect. The effect of artificial lighting must be considered when planning the desired effect.

Lighting

Natural light or daylight is a pure light. It clearly shows the colour and texture of make-up. It is also a reflected source of light from windows, walls and any light surface.

Artificial light can distort the effect of colour. There are several forms of artificial light.

The **fluorescent** light is usually delivered through strip lighting, which is tubes of blue-white light that remove the warmth in make-up colour. This type of lighting usually has diffusers, which soften the light and spread the light source. This has the effect of removing shadow. However, there is a special type of fluorescent light that is designed to recreate daylight. This gives out a warm white light. It is essential for make-up/treatment rooms to have a good source of daylight and special 'daylight' (warm white) lighting.

Filament lamps are the standard household light bulbs, which give off a yellow light. This deepens the red colours and flattens blue tones.

The make-up lesson

The make-up lesson should be conducted in a private well-lit treatment area, with the client seated facing a large mirror. Remember it is important to keep each stage separate and to discuss them thoroughly with the client. A record card in the form of a make-up chart should be kept, clearly detailing the products and colours used and the effects achieved.

This is also an opportunity to stress the importance of preparation of the skin before the application of make-up. For example, the use of cleansing and moisturising products and their application.

<table>
<tr><td>!</td><td>A make-up artist is not always concerned about skin preparation as they do not want the skin to be over-stimulated or warm, which could affect the colour of the make-up.

Models/actors will arrive for make-up having cleansed their own skin.</td></tr>
</table>

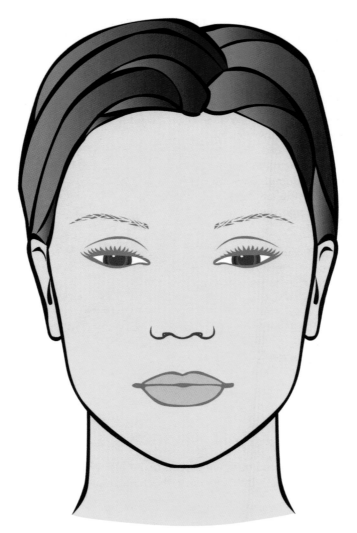

Figure 6.12 *Make-up chart*

It is important to explain to the client the importance of handling the skin carefully without over-stimulating it. General hygiene should also be discussed, as well as the cleaning of brushes and sponges, the use of disposable applicators and mascara wands, care of the make-up application and touch-up tips such as using a dampened pad of cotton wool to freshen the make-up.

Choosing make-up products

Return to Chapter 3, where the range of salon make-up products is discussed.

The make-up artist may include a broad range of colours and products and include materials from the theatrical make-up product range. Specialist make-up manufacturers

A C T I V I T Y

Contact two make-up manufacturers and review the range of products and colours. You will want to build up your own make-up range for use on clients.

Remember it is unprofessional to use your personal make-up on clients for hygiene reasons. Make-up for clients should be kept separate in a vanity case.

Bridal make-up

Bridal make-up should be carefully planned and rehearsed prior to the big day! It is important to have several sessions with the bride to allow you to understand her needs and ideas. It is important that the bride has scheduled appointments for facial treatments leading up to the wedding, allowing sufficient time for the skin to settle and for the make-up to be practised. It is important that the bride feels confident with the look.

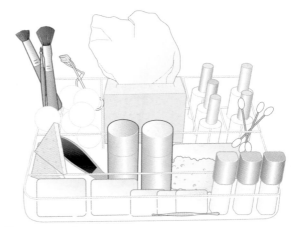

On the big day the make-up is usually applied before the hair is finally dressed. Once the hairstyle has been finished the final touches to the make-up can be made.

It is important that the colour scheme of the bridesmaids, flowers, etc. are considered and reflected in the make-up where possible, particularly in the nail polish colour and the lipstick.

Figure 6.13 *Demonstration kit*

Photographic make-up

The effects created for make-up to be photographed can really allow the creative talents to come to the fore! The use of strong lighting, filters, diffusers and reflectors can create some wonderful effects on the image.

Highlighting and shading should be used when creating make-up to be photographed. A light foundation, which is suitable to cover the skin and mask imperfections, should be used. This will allow the defining effect of highlighting and shading to be seen to the best effect. Make-up must be blended well as the camera will pick out any imperfections.

The lighting used in photography can create a lot of heat! It is important to set the make-up with light translucent powder and to keep reapplying it throughout the shoot.

Be wary of using pearlised products for black-and-white imagery as it can cause 'kickback'. This is where the metallic particles in the make-up are reflected, causing the skin to look shiny. Matte products are preferable for black-and-white photographs.

Airbrushing is now commonly used on finished photographs, which can simply erase any flaws or imperfections that appear on the finished image!

Catwalk and fashion show make-up

This can be an excellent way to promote your salon. Working collaboratively with a fashion house or local businesses provides good promotional opportunities. Make-up for such events is usually based on the same application principles used in photographic and evening make-up. Emphasis should be placed on defining eyes and lips and the principles of highlighting and shading should be applied. In some cases, however, you may be required to work to a specific brief, particularly when working with fashion designers who may require a specific look.

Remember models may have several costume changes and will require make-up to be touched up or refreshed. A fine spray of water will help to set the make-up and freshen the look.

Using make-up demonstrations to promote your business

A demonstrator is usually also a salesperson! By demonstrating the range of products available and their application, the demonstrator is creating opportunities for selling the products. If you are representing the salon you should take price lists and details of any promotions or special offers and free samples if available. Take product display stands with the full range on view. This will allow members of the audience to browse before and after the demonstration. For demonstrations to be cost-effective the aim must be to encourage members of the audience to come to your salon for treatment. This particular role requires confidence and a good understanding of the products being demonstrated and the range of treatments available in the salon. This is where a well-designed price list or promotional offer is essential, something the client will keep to share with a neighbour or member of the family. A thin, poorly designed leaflet will not give a good impression.

ACTIVITY

Design a promotional leaflet for a demonstration you are going to do at the town hall as part of a fashion show.

Use a word processor and include the salon name and a design that best represents your salon. Evaluate your leaflet by asking another therapist for their views.

It is important to ascertain the type of audience. This will allow you to target the demonstration with the particular client group in mind. It is important to have knowledge of the venue beforehand. Visit the venue and check where you will work to ensure all the audience can see. You will need to check whether there is a hot-water supply and suitable lighting. It is also important to consider disposal of waste products such as facial tissues and cotton wool. Pack a small bin liner into your demonstration kit.

The demonstration kit

The demonstration kit should comprise a clean, well-organised box or holdall containing:

- small lightweight bottles or jars of cleanser, toner and moisturiser
- small box of facial tissues

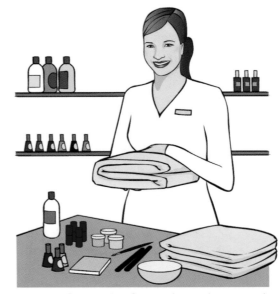

Figure 6.14 *Preparation for a make-up demonstration*

Make-up

107

- antibacterial wipes
- cotton buds/cotton-wool rounds/sterilised brushes and sponges
- range of cosmetics with a good selection of colours
- container of water (in case there is no water supply)
- tweezers
- small disposable bag for waste.

Demonstrating

Standing in front of an audience, particularly for the first time, can cause a great deal of anxiety. It is important to prepare well and to do your homework on the products and the client group you are addressing. Remember to smile and to introduce yourself clearly. When you select a demonstration model from the audience it is usually a good idea to choose someone who appears not to wear cosmetics. You will then be able to demonstrate a greater effect to the audience.

It is important at each stage to discuss what you are doing and why. It is also important to impart any hints or tips the audience may find useful. By stating your intention as the demonstration commences you will be able to review how successful you have been in meeting the stated aims at the end of the event.

! It is also essential to be able to manage your time well. There will be a limited amount of time to demonstrate the products, usually on a previously unseen client who has volunteered to be the 'model' from the audience.

Spending too long can become boring to the audience. They are interested in the finished result, not a lengthy explanation. Limit the time spent on cleansing and preparing the skin.

! Be organised – carefully plan what you will need by rehearsing the demonstration in your head. Prepare for a range of possible clients, e.g. age, skin colour, by ensuring you take a good selecton of colours and products.

! Remember to thank your 'model' and present her with a gift. An item from the demonstrated range would show your appreciation!

Evaluating the event

Demonstrations, particularly outside the salon, can be time-consuming. It is important for business to ensure that it is cost-effective. Gaining feedback from the audience about what they enjoyed or disliked about the demonstration will help with future planning of such an event.

Accurate figures on the take-up of any promotion will give an indication of how worthwhile it was in promoting the salon and creating further business.

A tally of the products sold at the event will show any profit from retail sales.

ACTIVITY

Collect pictures and photographs from magazines and other sources that have interesting make-up designs. Examine your cuttings and analyse technique. Look carefully at use of colour and continuation, and contrast of theme. Examine the use of accessories and backdrops. Put the pictures into a scrapbook and keep adding to it for future reference. This will become one of your most precious resources!

Experiment with different make-up colours and application techniques and produce a series of photographs. Include evidence of corrective work. These will be useful for your portfolio of evidence and will also be of value to demonstrate your abilities to prospective employers.

Chapter 7

FACIAL TREATMENTS LEVELS 1+2

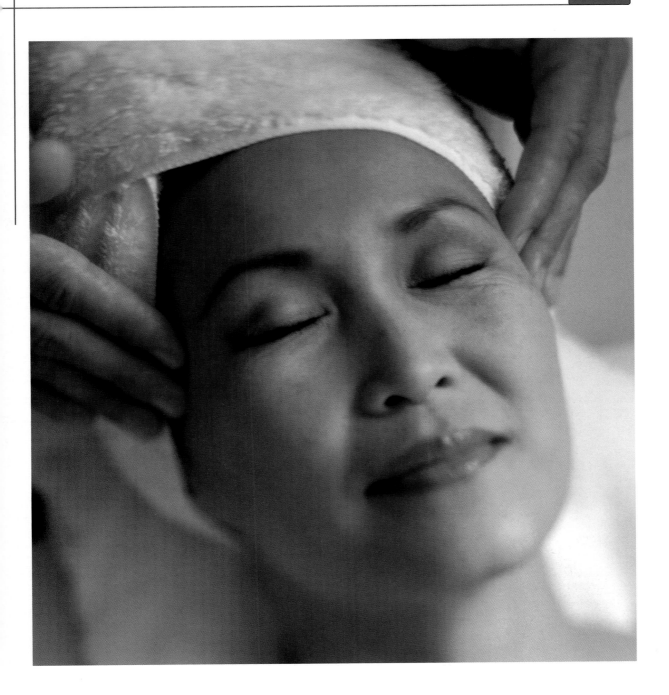

IN THIS CHAPTER YOU WILL LEARN ABOUT:

- Assessing and analysing client skin type
- Specialist and everyday skin products
- Preparing the client and treatment area
- Cleansing
- Massaging the client's face, neck and shoulders
- Face masks
- Advising on facial aftercare
- Ultraviolet light and the skin

Looking at skin

Accurate inspection of the skin is vital in assessing the client's needs and for the identification of contraindications. The following are contraindications specific to facial treatments. They are separated into those requiring medical referral and those that restrict treatment within the localised area. Refer to chapter 14 for a full list of skin diseases and disorders.

Contraindications requiring medical referral:

- bacterial, e.g. impetigo
- viral, e.g. herpes simplex
- fungal, e.g. tinea
- conjunctivitis.

Contraindications that restrict treatment:

- recent scar tissue
- eczema
- allergies
- cuts
- abrasions
- bruising
- vitiligo
- sties.

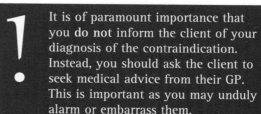

It is essential that you have a clear understanding of the structure and function of the skin, bones and muscles of the head, face and neck, and composition and function of blood and lymph. Please refer to chapter 14, Related Anatomy and Physiology, for full details.

It is of paramount importance that you **do not** inform the client of your diagnosis of the contraindication. Instead, you should ask the client to seek medical advice from their GP. This is important as you may unduly alarm or embarrass them.

You need to understand the structure and function of the skin and the actions of the facial, neck and shoulder muscles.

The key to improving the condition of the client's skin is the correct analysis.

To carry out a skin analysis you will need:

- good lighting or additional illumination
- magnifying lamp.

You must be prepared to look at the skin with care and talk to the client about their current skincare regime. Ask them to tell you about their perceptions of their skin.

It is important to find out what skin type the client believes they have. This information will provide you with clues to any anomalies you may notice during your inspection. It will also help you to make your own decision. If you are assisting the senior therapist you should discuss anything you are unsure of.

> **!** The client has come to you as a professional, an expert. Therefore, do not rely on or be misled by the client's own diagnosis of their skin.

Client groups

Beauty treatments are becoming increasingly popular with both female and male clients. There is a wide variation in both skin characteristics and skin types. It is important to understand and recognise these differences when analysing skin and planning treatments.

Skin characteristics

The skin functions in basically the same way irrespective of type or colour. The colour of skin is determined by pigmentation caused by the amount of melanin present. Melanin is constantly produced to maintain the skin's natural colour. There are, however, important differences in the skin characteristics of people from different ethnic groups.

'White' skin

This describes those who originate from East and West Europe, North America, Canada, South Australia and New Zealand. This group is sometimes referred to as **Caucasian**. This skin has very little defence to ultraviolet light and burns easily. The group has problems with spots and blemishes, particularly through puberty, but may also have a tendency towards sensitivity and dryness during their twenties and thirties. The delicate nature of the skin means that premature signs of ageing occur in the early thirties. The pale tones of the skin are usually accompanied by fair, red or mid-brown hair.

'Yellow-toned' skin

This describes the yellowish tones of people originating from Southern Europe, South and Central America, parts of Asia, the Far East and the Middle East. This group has a tendency to skin displaying a mild oiliness, a consequence of which is a delay in the skin's ageing process. There is also more sudoriferous activity. The signs of ageing will generally start during the late thirties and early forties. This skin is prone to hyper-pigmentation and, therefore, any blemishes on this type of skin should be treated with care. Relatively minor skin damage – sometimes even expressing comedones (blackheads) – can lead to hyper-pigmentation. Hair colour is usually mid- or dark-brown to black.

'Black' skins

This describes a range of dark skins that may vary in tone from light to dark with a wide variety of undertones. There is generally more sebaceous and sudoriferous activity in this group. The skin does not display signs of the ageing process until the forties are reached. The first sign can be greying of the hair. It is easy to mistake the sheen on dark skins as excessive oiliness. The sebaceous glands

> **!** A lack of pigmentation, usually in irregular patches, is known as **vitiligo**. Dark irregular patches of pigmentation is known as **chloasma**. Corrective make-up techniques can be used to disguise both conditions.

are larger, however, the darker the skin and more reflection of light occurs. This reflected light can be mistakenly diagnosed as too much oil. Another common mistake, particularly on dark Asian skins, is the identification of comedones on the centre 'T' panel. Close and careful examination will actually show the presence of dark facial hair around the nose and forehead, not comedones. It should be noted that black skins easily form keloid scars (an over-thickening of the skin) when damaged and caution should be exercised. Dermatosis papulosa nigra is a condition found on the cheeks and across the nose on the skin of both males and females of African origin. Black raised spots of varying sizes can be seen.

General differences

1. Skin cancer is rare in darker skins as the pigmentation filters ultraviolet radiation.

2. The epidermis on dark skins is thicker.

3. Acne is rare in darker skins, despite having more sebaceous glands.

4. Paler skins are more prone to product-related allergies.

> **!** The condition of any skin will be affected by climatic changes and extremes of temperature.

5. Dark-skinned people have a greater heat tolerance due to the increased number of sudoriferous glands.

6. Paler-skinned people have a greater tolerance to extremes of cold.

7. Black skin desquamates (naturally sheds surface cells) easily compared to white skins.

Skin types

There are five main skin types:

1. oily
2. dry
3. combination
4. mature
5. young.

Oily skin

The skin is usually coarse in texture and appears shiny, particularly around the nose, chin and forehead. Comedones and open pores will be present. The coarse texture is due to pores which have been stretched by a previous blockage.

The skin will appear coarse and grainy. It will be moist and the epidermis will appear thick. It will be sallow and have a yellowish hue.

The cause of oily skin is an over-secretion of sebum, caused by hormonal imbalance, for example through the effects of puberty.

Dry skin

Dry skin appears taut, fine lines may be evident and there may be flaky patches. There is a tendency for dilated capillaries; these are the permanent dilation of tiny capillary blood vessels. Blood has leaked from the capillaries leaving a spidery appearance across the cheekbones and around the nose (sometimes referred to as couperose tissue).

The skin will be fine in texture, sensitive and finely lined but will have a coarse surface. It is unlikely that the skin will have any comedones or open pores.

The causes of dry skin are:

- not enough sebum, with low fluid content in the upper layers of the skin
- excessive use of soaps and degreasing agents such as astringents
- exposure to sunlight without due care and attention
- extremes of temperature
- central heating, which will also have a drying effect.

Combination skin

The face has a central panel commonly referred to as the 'T' zone, which includes the forehead, nose and chin. In this skin type these areas will appear oily and congested, whilst the rest of the skin may be dry. This is one of the most common skin types.

Mature skin

This condition describes skin that has started the ageing process. It lacks natural oil (sebum) and moisture. Character lines and wrinkles begin to form around the muscles of facial expression. There is some loss of underlying muscle tone and the subcutaneous (fatty) layer is shrinking.

Young skin

Beauty treatments are becoming increasingly popular with a younger clientele. Young skin can present a variety of characteristics. Typically it is firm to the touch, even in texture and colour with few blemishes. However, some young clients may have seborrhoeic conditions caused by the onset of puberty. This is readily identified by oily skin with enlarged pores and comedones.

Skin conditions

You will also need to recognise and differentiate between skin types and skin conditions. The following are skin conditions that you should be able to identify (see chapter 14 for details):

- sensitive
- comedone
- milia
- dehydrated
- broken capillaries
- pustules
- papules
- open pores
- hyper-pigmentation
- dermatosis
- papulosa nigra
- pseudo-folliculitus
- keloids
- in-growing hair
- seborrhoea.

Sensitive

Sensitive skin is thin; it can become blotchy and is quickly irritated. It may be recognised by its high colour and warmth. There may be fine dilated capillaries around the cheeks and nose.

Comedone

A comedone is a term given to a blackhead. Comedones are formed when sebum is trapped within a pore; keratinised cells at the top of the pore multiply and block off the exit from the sebaceous gland. The surface of the blocked pore becomes black due to oxidation (a chemical reaction when exposed to air). When there is a build-up of sebum it may cause the gland to erupt, which will allow sebum into the lower levels of the skin. When this occurs it leads into the formation of a papule. If it becomes infected it will become a pustule.

Milia

Milia is the name given to sebum trapped within a blind duct. It is common on dry skin types, particularly around the eye and cheek area. It appears as a white pearly nodule and is a clear indication of a tendency towards dryness in that localised area. If the milia is not established it may be possible to disperse with gentle massage. If, however, it is a hardened mass then it will be necessary to remove it using a sterile lance on pre-warmed skin. The top of the milia is split using the sterile lance and the milia is lifted out. The skin is then left to heal. Milia should never be expressed in the way that other spots and blemishes may be. It would cause the client a great deal of discomfort and may lead to permanent damage of the skin.

Dehydrated

Dehydrated skin lacks moisture and appears dull. It may become itchy and tight. It may also have a smooth sheen but must not be confused with oily skin. Any skin type can become dehydrated and it would be considered a temporary condition.

Seborrhoea

Seborrhoeic conditions are caused by overactive sebaceous glands, creating too much sebum on a skin that is already naturally oily.

It is a common condition in young people and is particularly associated with the onset of puberty. It may also be the start of acne if it is left untreated. The sebaceous secretions are increased and the skin becomes grainy with enlarged pores and comedones. The pores can become blocked with the sebaceous secretions. As the hormones settle down the condition subsides.

The danger triangle

The danger triangle covers an area from the centre of the eyebrows at its tip spreading outwards to the lower lip at its base. The client should be advised not to express spots around this area. Important blood vessels lie directly under the area and if the skin is damaged they may be prone to bacterial infection. This may cause a condition known as **deep cavernous thrombosis**.

Ageing and the skin

The general characteristics of ageing usually occur around the age of 40 or with the onset of the menopause. Skin ages at different rates depending upon several factors. These may include ethnic group, hereditary or health-related factors and the treatment it has received. Incorrect cleansing, harsh treatment, overexposure to ultraviolet light, smoking and extremes of temperature all play a part in the ageing process. Despite the best possible skincare regime, the underlying muscle structure tends to lose its tone and inevitably a softening of the features occurs.

The softening of the skin and decrease in muscle tone creates character lines, particularly around the muscles of expression. There is a loss of elasticity in the skin and the expression lines become permanent. This effect is caused by the breakdown of collagen and elastin fibres within the dermis. It is the bundles of collagen that make the young skin supple and smooth.

The formation of wrinkles occurs along the lines of facial expression. This is why wrinkles are often referred to as character lines! The regular contraction of the muscle forms the lines and, while the skin can stretch easily, it cannot contract in the same way as muscles. Thus as the skin loses its elasticity the lines become more and more etched.

A combination of these factors clearly indicates the onset of the ageing process. The appearance of the skin reflects the underlying changes.

The physical and physiological signs of ageing

The following features are signs of ageing skin:

1. Circulation slows down, therefore waste is not removed as efficiently.
2. The elasticity of the skin decreases and character lines are formed.
3. There is an accelerated growth of fine lanugo or baby hair, particularly on the cheek and upper lip.
4. There is a decrease of skin permeability leading to gradual dehydration.
5. There is an increase in hyper-pigmentation, for example chloasma.
6. The skin becomes noticeably thinner, especially around the eyes.
7. The capillary network can be more easily ruptured due to the inelasticity of the skin.
8. There is a decrease in sebum production.
9. There is a decrease in the activity of the sudoriferous glands.
10. The basal cell metabolic rate slows down.
11. There are open pores present.

Analysing skin

It is essential that time is given for a full consultation and skin analysis. Take care not to make a superficial diagnosis, but to ask appropriate questions, to look at the skin closely (preferably using a magnifying lamp) and to touch the skin to judge texture, temperature and muscle tone.

> Refer to chapter 5, pages 71–78, for a full explanation of client consultation and treatment planning.

A common error is to examine the skin, but fail to talk to the client about their skincare routine and their own perceptions of their skin. Correct analysis is like an investigation, which will require good detective work to find the clues and piece them together. It is important to gather as much information as possible. The client may be using inappropriate products, which are stripping the skin's protective acid mantle. This leaves the skin feeling taut, shiny, prone to infection and bacterial invasion. Clients may feel that their skin is oily because of the effect of using these products and will mistakenly use a product for oily skin, which will be too harsh and will exacerbate the problem.

> The longer the client uses inappropriate products, the more the body attempts to restore the acid mantle through increased secretions. This may lead to even more shine!

The group who are most likely to fall into this trap are those going through puberty. Companies still tend to target this vulnerable group with products so harsh they can upset the delicate skin balance at an early age. Incorrect selection of products can also sensitise areas. If the product is too strong it can induce vascular response, which can result in the underlying capillaries stretching or dilating. In some cases the capillaries may rupture.

Look out for clients who use sunbeds or those who have recently been exposed to sunlight. They will display signs of dehydrated skin, but remember this is likely to be a temporary state. A note should be made on the record card and subsequent changes recorded. The range of false or self-tanning products, while harmless, can affect an effective

> **!** The therapist must take care when analysing darker skins, as imperfections readily visible on a lighter skin may not be immediately noticeable.

diagnosis. It is possible, weeks after application, when the skin colour has normalised, to have open pores still stained with the product. The clear liquid-type products are more likely to do this than the cream formulations. It may require a series of exfoliating treatments to remove the problem. Clients should be advised of the correct application of such products.

It is important not to rush the skin analysis and you should allow at least 5 minutes for a thorough analysis in the treatment schedule.

Establishing the correct skin category, in terms of skin type and condition, has implications for the effectiveness of the recommended treatment. If you are in an assisting role, seek clarification from the senior therapist of any aspect you are unsure about.

> **!** It is important that you treat the current condition of the skin. It is vitally important that you conduct a thorough analysis each time the client visits and note all changes.

The systems for recording findings will differ from one salon to another. It is usual for salons to design their own system of record cards based on their 'house style'. Salons also use treatment plans. A treatment plan is a record of the proposed schedule of treatment and the therapist's recommendations. Plans may be one double-sided form or two separate ones (see page 74).

Remember a treatment plan should include:

- client's full name
- client's usual skincare routine
- result of skin analysis
- contraindications
- recommended treatments and products – including costs and duration
- outcomes of treatment
- contra-actions
- aftercare advice given
- client's signature
- record of client feedback.

A record card should include:

- client's full name
- client's address and telephone number(s) (and e-mail address)
- date of birth
- medical history.

> It is important to record your findings neatly; other therapists may need to refer to the records.

ACTIVITY

1. Design a treatment plan and record card that encompasses all of the listed characteristics in the 'house' style that best suits your salon environment (an example can be found on page 74). Where possible use a word processor to achieve a professional finish.

2. List five important questions to ask your client during an initial consultation.

Selling in the salon

Beauty therapy trainees have always found selling within the salon environment a difficult concept to grasp! They are usually very able when it comes to putting together a suitable treatment plan but for some reason find selling products very difficult. If you can sell a service (a treatment) then logically you should be able to sell a product. More emphasis is now placed on retailing in training

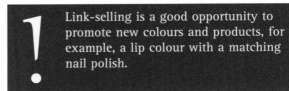

> ! Link-selling is a good opportunity to promote new colours and products, for example, a lip colour with a matching nail polish.

situations and you will be expected to retail alongside the recommended treatment. Retailing is now part of the therapist's role and it is a very important one. It benefits the clients in that they are purchasing products from a professional range that the therapist has recommended. Beauty therapists usually receive commission on products sold, so this is a good way of increasing your salary!

The advice you have given to the client about the products you have used and the recommended aftercare must be clearly recorded on the record card or treatment plan. This should be discussed within the privacy of the treatment room so that the client is clear about the items required at the reception or sales area (see page 77).

Find the gap in the client's product range and fill it rather than insisting they purchase all the products. If the product is more appropriate for them, they will purchase more.

Stock

It is important that you know your way around the stockroom! The shelving should be adjustable and easy to clean. Shelving should be labelled and popular lines should be stored at eye level.

It is important to keep a note of how particular products are selling and then to inform the salon supervisor, manager or whoever has responsibility for ordering stock. A stock check must be carried out regularly to ensure that product ranges are complete and available for treatments.

Displays

The reception area is one of the most important areas in the salon. It is here that the client will be greeted and sit either before or after treatment. Facial product leaflets should be available for the client to read. There should be attractive displays that highlight treatments and product range. The displays should be changed every few weeks to maintain client interest and to demonstrate that the salon is keeping abreast of new treatments and products. A well-thought-out display area will attract clients and increase salon profitability.

> ! Tips for displays:
> - keep them dust-free
> - have a theme
> - reflect the season, e.g. Christmas
> - have testers/samples available
> - restock often
> - do not have gaps!

Facial treatments

Products

You must be familiar with the range of available products in order to make the correct selection for each individual client. You need to know which products are required for each treatment.

Cleansers

A good cleansing medium should:

- remove make-up, dirt and grime effectively
- be suitable for the client's needs
- be easily applied and easily removed.

There are several types of cleansing preparation available: creams, milks, lotions, soapless cleansers and bars.

Creams

These are ideal for mature skin conditions and for dry skin types. They are designed to dissolve the pigmented waxes that are found in make-up products. They are usually water in oil emulsions and therefore do not soak into the skin. They have a cooling effect on the skin and are easily removed.

Milks

These are available in various consistencies. Most milks are liquid and are made from oil in a water emulsion. They are not very effective in removing a heavy make-up and are mainly used for superficial cleansing.

Lotions

Cleansing lotions are particularly useful on congested or oily skin. They leave very little residual oil on the skin after removal. However, they can be very strong so it is important that you know the product and that the skin has been accurately analysed.

Soapless cleansers (facial wash) and cleansing bars

These products are becoming the popular choice. They have changed the concept of cleansing, particularly in relation to the male market. Many clients will inform you that they prefer to use soap and water because they do not feel that their skin has been properly cleansed otherwise. This range of products now allows clients to use a more gentle complexion soap with water. Cleansing bars are made from soft soap but have a carefully balanced pH, which does not leave the skin feeling tight and shiny. They leave the skin at the correct pH balance and are particularly effective on seborrhoeic and acned skins. Soapless cleansers are made from laurel sulphates and soap bars contain potassium palmitate.

Toners

Toner is used at the conclusion of the cleansing treatment and prepares the skin for make-up application. It removes any product remaining on the skin after cleansing or face mask removal. Toners dissolve surface oil and have an antibacterial effect. They may also have a refreshing effect, depending upon the type selected. Toner refines the pore size as it evaporates, leaving the skin prepared for an application of moisturiser.

Toners are made from infusions of herbs and flowers, such as witch hazel, orange flower water, rose water, and small amounts of glycerine in distilled water. Other ingredients could include zinc sulphate and potassium sulphate. Toners also contain varying amounts of alcohol, which determines their strength.

As with cleansing products, there is a wide range to choose from.

Skin tonics

This range includes astringent solutions, which can be very strong. The amount of alcohol present and the active ingredient, for example witch hazel, will determine which tonic you select for a particular client's skin. If more than 20 per cent alcohol is present, use should be restricted to oily skin types. An astringent removes the surface oil and can disturb the skin's pH balance. It would therefore be contraindicated on blemished or sensitive conditions as it could be an irritant. Witch hazel has astringent properties and also should be used with caution.

Skin fresheners and bracers

These have a much gentler effect. The action is a refreshing but mild one and these products are suitable for dehydrated, dry, delicate and mature skin conditions. They contain only small amounts of alcohol and do not remove oil as efficiently as their stronger counterparts. A dilution of orange flower water or rose water is an example.

Eye make-up remover

These specially designed products need to have certain characteristics. They must not be heavy in texture, highly perfumed or excessively creamy, but must be effective in removing densely pigmented waterproof products. They are based on a mineral oil such as liquid paraffin or soft waxes such as paraffin wax.

ACTIVITY

1. What are the main differences between a skin tonic and a skin freshener?

2. What are the qualities required of an eye make-up remover?

3. What is the acid mantle?

Exfoliants

Exfoliants aid desquamation (the skin's natural shedding of surface cells). They smooth the surface of the skin, prepare the skin for further treatment and stimulate the blood and lymphatic flow, thereby aiding the elimination and absorption of waste products. All skin types benefit from using exfoliating products.

They fall into two categories: pore grains or facial scrubs and peeling creams.

Pore grains or facial scrubs

These are made up of detergent and small grains of almond shell, oatmeal and pumice or ground fruit kernels. They have a detergent cleansing action and when gently massaged over the skin remove surface adhesions, leaving the skin soft and smooth. Their regular use should be restricted to those with an oily skin and only limited usage for those wishing to refine and tone.

Peeling creams

These are based on clay and other natural biological ingredients. They are applied to the skin and allowed to dry. They can then be lifted off the skin or gently rolled using friction to slough off dead cells. These are effective on all skin types, particularly those conditions that require gentle treatment.

Exfoliation treatments

Brush cleanse is an intensive cleansing treatment. It has an exfoliating effect by loosening surface adhesions and increases blood circulation, creating warmth. It can also be used to remove specialised exfoliating face masks. The machine comprises a series of brushes which, when attached to the motor-driven applicator, rotate at varying speeds dependent upon need and purpose. There is a variety of brush heads available:

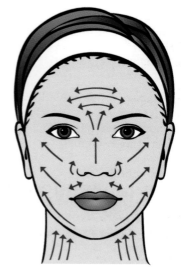

- soft complexion brushes – these are used for general cleansing purposes
- sponge heads – these are usually used with a foaming cleansing product and are a gentler alternative to the brushes
- bristle brush heads – these are used for a more stimulating effect and are good for working on male clients
- pumice block – this is used for peeling and refining a coarse skin texture.

Preparation of the skin

The skin should be cleansed to remove make-up and surface oil. A suitable medium should then be applied. The choice of medium will depend on need. You can choose from a variety of liquid detergent-based cleansing products to cleansing creams.

Figure 7.1 *A brush cleanse treatment*

Safety precautions

- It is important to ensure that a uniform pressure is applied.
- Do not over-wet the brush head as you will spray the cleansing product everywhere!
- Use a dampened cotton-wool pad or sponge to protect the eyes and mouth.
- Choose the brush head and medium with care.
- Avoid dragging the skin.
- Avoid over-stimulation of the skin.
- Ensure the brush heads are clean and sterilised before and after use.

Contraindications

This treatment would be contraindicated for those with a sensitive skin condition or loose crêpey skin.

ACTIVITY

1. What is exfoliation?
2. State two precautions to take when using exfoliants.

Massage mediums

Massage can be carried out using a variety of mediums. Most, however, will be based on either a cream or an oil formulation, which may have added ingredients to suit the individual needs of the client's skin. Mediums contain mineral oils, beeswax or paraffin wax and a large percentage of distilled water.

Moisturisers

Moisturisers comprise an oil and water emulsion. They can be presented in either a cream or liquid form.

They readily evaporate from the skin leaving a fine film of **emollient**. An emollient is a substance that softens the skin by increasing its water content and keeps it soft by slowing moisture loss. The gentle evaporation produces a cooling sensation, which temporarily refines the pores and leaves the skin feeling soft and supple. The moisturiser leaves an aqueous film on the skin, which is ready for make-up to be applied.

Moisturisers also supplement the skin's water content by attracting water from the atmosphere by the means of a **humectant** (water-attracting) product. Humectant materials are glycerol, sorbitol and glycol.

All skin types require the use of a moisturiser. Moisturisers prolong the appearance of make-up; they prepare the skin for the application of foundation by smoothing the surface. They also protect the skin from the pigments in the make-up. Moisturiser should always be worn even if make-up is not; it will protect the skin from the elements and pollutants in the atmosphere.

> ! Always check the content of products, particularly toners. Manufacturers are now legally required to list product ingredients.

The choice of moisturiser will depend on skin type.

Specialist skin products
Eye creams, gels and lotions

These specialist products are used to temporarily minimise the appearance of crow's-feet and character lines; they may also have a temporary tightening effect. The creams are formulated in the same way as moisturisers. They contain cocoa butter and vegetable oils. Petroleum jelly and high wax content are avoided as they can cause puffiness around the delicate eye area. Eye gels often contain astringents such as witch hazel. They have a cooling and firming effect on the delicate tissue surrounding the eyes. Lotions are similar to gels. They are usually applied onto a dampened pad of cotton wool and placed over the eyes. They produce a soothing, refreshing effect on the eyes.

Acne products

There are certain products that are now recognised as irritants to acne. These are products that contain petroleum jelly, lanolin and some vegetable oils. There are specifically designed lotions, which are spirit-based in a chemical formulation to prevent infections. The use of soapless cleansers facial wash and cleansing bars, as described earlier in this chapter are particularly effective on acned skins.

Neck creams

Neck creams are rich moisturising creams that may contain other active ingredients such as collagen. The action of these rich formulations is primarily to soften, tighten and tone the skin.

Lip balms

These are a range of specifically designed products for softening and protecting the lips. They form a protective film and prevent moisture loss. They are formulated from varying mixtures of oils and waxes and may contain colour pigments.

Night creams

Night creams are emollients and are generally heavier and thicker than other skin creams. They are usually formulated from a range of products including animal fats, vegetable oils, cocoa butter, olive and almond oils and beeswax. The action of a night cream is to soften and hydrate the skin. Most products contain a humectant.

ACTIVITY

1. State three reasons why using a moisturiser is important.

2. List two qualities of an eye gel, cream or lotion.

Preparation for treatment
Reception

The visual appearance of the salon and the manner in which the client is greeted are of vital importance. It is essential that there is a professional atmosphere at all times, in which the client feels comfortable and uninhibited. If the atmosphere at the reception is professional, it will instil confidence in the client.

> **!** Every person who walks through the door is a potential client for not only one, but many of the salon services. Know your services and products!

Personal appearance

The client is coming to you for a range of treatments and services that will help to maintain or improve a particular condition or meet a specific need. You are therefore perceived to be a professional, an exponent of your craft. It is important that your image projects your expertise! Your appearance will indicate to others how much care and pride you take in your role. Clients will judge you on your image, and the beauty business is one in which the correct image and appearance are paramount. You may be very confident and knowledgeable in the services and products offered, but if your image is not appropriate it sends the wrong message to the client. See chapter 5, which deals with personal appearance in more detail.

> **!** You only have one chance to make a first impression!

Preparation of treatment area

Safe and hygienic practices within a salon environment are crucial to prevent cross infection. Tools, materials and equipment must be sterilised before and after each client. Linen should also be changed after each client. The recognition of contraindications is of vital importance to prevent cross infection.

It is essential to create a calm and relaxing environment for the client. The salon furnishings and equipment should be appropriate and fit for the purpose.

It is likely that the client will be apprehensive, particularly if it is their first visit. It is important to avoid delays and you should have everything prepared and ready for the client's arrival. It will also increase salon efficiency if you work within the time parameters for each treatment. The recommended maximum service time for a facial is 60 minutes. However, specialist facials may require a layer, following manufacturer's instructions. You should check your column in the appointment book before commencing work and refer to salon records of previous visits where appropriate. If it is a new client, you should have all necessary paperwork ready for completion. You should also check the range of products available to ensure you can offer a range of options to suit the individual need and recommendations following initial consultation.

Trolley

Remember, visual impressions count! The trolley should be clean and tidy and contain all the products needed to carry out the required service or treatment. You will also require a magnifying light.

You should have on your trolley:

- cotton wool – dry and dampened – to remove cleansing products and for applying products such as toners
- tissues – to blot the skin and to remove cleansing products
- a selection of bowls – for holding dry cotton wool and dampened cotton wool
- spatulas – to remove creams and products from containers, to mix face mask formulation
- a selection of skincare products – always remember to replace lids, use spatulas to remove products or in the case of liquid products pour into the palm of your hand
- face mask brush – to apply formulation (do not remove from steriliser until ready to be used)
- facial sponges – to remove product, to remove face mask formulation
- a covered waste receptacle.

You should also have ready and prepared:

- record card or treatment plan
- protective headband
- towels
- hand mirror.

Facials are performed on the client in a reclining or semi-reclining position. The treatment chair or couch should be capable of adapting to meet the requirements of the treatment. The height of the couch is important both for client comfort and for the beauty therapist. Back problems are common amongst therapists and, therefore, it is important to prevent such problems by correct positioning. The beauty therapist normally works from behind the client and may be seated or standing to carry out the treatment. There should be pillows and covering available for the client during treatment to provide warmth and to promote relaxation. If you are working in a cubicle, it should have screening, which will ensure complete privacy from the rest of the salon.

You should have a steamer and brush cleanse unit available.

The client

The client should be given very clear instructions about what to do. Hair and clothing should be protected. You should ask the client to remove their outer clothing and you should offer them a robe or towel to protect their modesty. It would be expected that privacy would be a paramount consideration. You should ask the client to remove all necklaces and earrings.

Once the client is settled on the chair or couch ask them to remove or slip down any straps that will inhibit the facial treatment.

The client's head should be slightly elevated and their hair should be protected using a headband or other suitable covering. Finally, wash your hands – you are now ready to commence treatment.

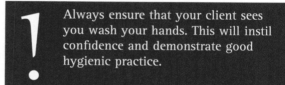

Always ensure that your client sees you wash your hands. This will instil confidence and demonstrate good hygienic practice.

ACTIVITY

Compare facial record cards with a fellow student. Design a record card for your own use. (Refer to chapter 4.)

The facial
Cleansing

Cleansing usually comprises two stages. The first stage is to superficially remove surface oil and make-up. The second stage is to thoroughly deep-cleanse the skin. The analysis of the skin type will be carried out after the superficial cleanse. You may be expected to conduct cleansing in a routine that has been adopted as the house style in your salon or training institute. Inevitably, the routine will be based upon common principles and practices.

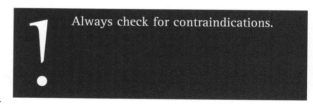

Always check for contraindications.

Procedure for a superficial cleanse

This is always carried out, whether the client is wearing make-up or not.

1. Ask the client to close their eyes and select a suitable cleansing product.
2. Apply the selected product using small gentle circular movements. Avoid exerting too much pressure over the eye. Apply to upper lid, lashes and under the eye.
3. If the client is wearing mascara, place a dampened pad of cotton wool under the lashes and apply eye make-up remover with either fingers or cotton bud until the mascara has dissolved.
4. Remove the loosened make-up and cleanser using dampened cotton-wool pads. Ensure you support the skin as you work.
5. Select a suitable product for the lip area. Apply using gentle circular movements.
6. Remove the loosened lip cosmetic and cleanser with dampened cotton wool. Blot the lips using a tissue.
7. Select a suitable product for the face and neck. Apply the selected product using light upward movements on the cheeks, forehead and neck. Work the product into the folds around the nose and chin.

a) small, circular movements

damp cotton wool pad under the lashes when removing mascara

b) removing cream and cosmetics

three downward strokes, one across brow, one under eye

c) small, light movements

wipe in direction of arrows

Figure 7.2 a b c *Steps in a superficial cleanse*

8. Remove the cleanser product by initially blotting with soft facial tissues. Tissues are used for their absorbency when using greasy or oil-based products. Dampened cotton wool may be used to remove water-soluble debris from the skin. The skin is clean when the cotton wool shows no soiling.

> ! Always cleanse the lip and eye areas first. This will ensure these areas are thoroughly cleansed and will prevent the spreading of densely pigmented make-up over the face and neck.

9. Apply a light application of mild toner using dampened cotton-wool pads.

10. Blot the skin using a facial tissue. Place a hole in the centre for the nose and blot. Then fold the tissue down onto the neck and blot again.

11. You should allow at least 5 minutes in the treatment schedule for superficial cleansing.

Deep cleanse

The analysis of the skin should take place before commencing the deep cleanse. Analysis should be carried out at each visit and you should not simply accept the previous diagnosis (see page 115).

The aim of the deep cleanse is to:

■ soften and loosen comedones and other skin blockages

■ increase circulation

■ remove any remaining make-up preparation

■ increase desquamation.

It is important that you adapt movements and pressure according to client need. Each movement should be repeated at least six times unless otherwise stated.

Procedure for a deep cleanse

(See figure 7.3)

Select a suitable cleansing product.

1. Place hands at the base of the neck. Work upwards over the platysma muscle to the jaw (mandible bone), using a light, flowing movement. Sweep across the mandible. Apply a light sweeping stroke down either side of the neck following the sterno-mastoid muscles.

2. Using a light sweeping movement work along the mandible from one side to the other.

3. Starting at the chin use small circular movements, moving slowly up to the sides of the nose. Glide along the cheeks (zygomatic muscle and zygomatic bone) without exerting pressure, and back to the chin.

4. Slide hands along each cheekbone and up to the forehead. Gently slide the hands down over the nose and back along the cheeks.

5. Using small circular movements work around the base of the nose.

6. Slide the fingers down the top and sides of the nose using alternating strokes.

7. Using large circular movements work across the forehead, slide across the cheekbones and back up to the forehead.

8. Using the pads of the fingers perform a scissor or zigzag movement across the forehead, working from one side to the other.

9. Stroke around each eye using the ring finger and gently perform a lifting movement, three times under each eyebrow.

Always conclude a facial routine by applying slight pressure at the temples, which indicates the end of the routine.

Remove the cleansing product by blotting the surface with tissues then using dampened cotton-wool pads. It is vitally important to ensure all trace of cleanser is removed. You should check around the hairline, under the jaw and in the folds of the skin. You may then apply toner.

You should allow at least 10 minutes for deep cleansing in the treatment schedule.

> **!** Always work the chosen cleansing medium between both hands to warm the product and to provide slip.

Extractions
Comedones

Comedones will have been loosened following a deep cleanse and extraction of skin blockages can take place at this point. The skin should be warmed using either hot dampened cotton-wool pads, a steamer or heated towels.

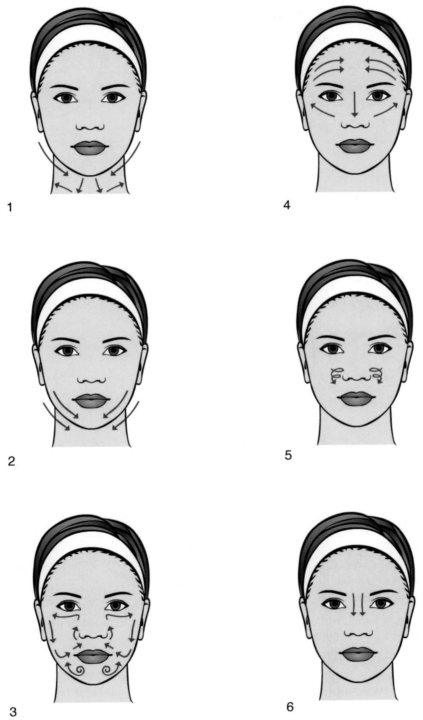

Figure 7.3 *Steps 1 to 6 in a deep cleanse (Continued)*

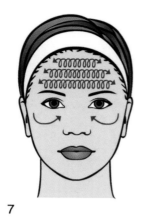

7

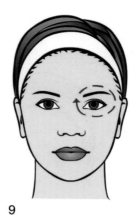

9

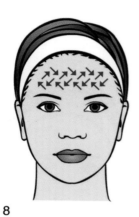

8

Figure 7.3 *Steps 7 to 9 steps in a deep cleanse*

Steaming

The steamer should be filled in accordance with manufacturer's instructions. It is usual to fill the steamer using distilled water. This prevents the element furring up with limescale, which can cause the unit to spit boiling water.

The duration of treatment will vary between 3 and 20 minutes. Positioning of the unit will depend upon skin type:

- 25 cm (10 in) for oily skin
- 30 cm (12 in) for normal skin
- 40 cm (15 in) for dry skin.

If the client has dilated capillaries or very sensitive skin you should avoid stimulating the circulation and, therefore, steaming would not be indicated.

Most steamers have an ozone facility within the unit. The use of ozone is particularly beneficial to those who have a blemished skin. It is drying and has an antibacterial effect. There are restrictions governing the use of ozone, however, and it is important that you check with your local health authority before offering the facility. The ozone option is not required for warming the skin.

You must make all the precautionary safety checks before using a steaming unit.

- Ensure that the unit is not overfilled.
- Make sure that it is on a safe, solid base.

- Place the unit at the correct distance for the skin type.
- There should be no trailing wires or flexes.
- Check that the vapour is evenly emitted before directing towards the client.

Heated towels

A towel can be soaked in hot water, wrung out and wrapped around the face, leaving a space for the nostrils to enable the client to breathe.

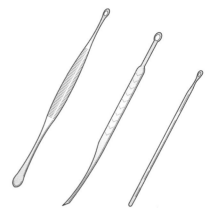

When steaming has been completed, the skin should be blotted. Extractions should be carried out using fingers covered with tissue or a comedone extractor. If the fingers are used, a rolling pressing motion should be used until the comedone is expressed. If a comedone remover is used then gentle even pressure should be applied over the blockage. You should work with caution to prevent exerting too much pressure, which may cause bruising.

Figure 7.4 *Types of comedone extractor*

Milia

Milia should also be removed following steaming. However, they should never be expressed by exerting pressure. They are usually formed into a hard pearly lump when they have become established. Following steaming the milia is gently exposed using a sterile lance. The lump can be lifted out. Great care must be taken to prevent infection.

ACTIVITY

1. State the differences between a superficial cleanse and a deep cleanse.

2. What precautions should be taken when carrying out extractions?

Facial massage
The benefits of massage

1. Cell division in the epidermis is optimised, resulting in an improvement in the appearance of the skin.
2. As the epidermis is being replaced frequently, the skin feels soft and smooth.
3. Skin colour is improved due to the increase in local blood circulation.
4. The collagen and elastin fibres maintain their elasticity, improving skin tone.
5. Skin texture is improved by the increased health of the epidermis and dermis.
6. Puffiness around the eyes is reduced due to the removal of excess tissue fluid.
7. Fine lines are reduced by the increased activity of the epidermis.
8. Dark circles around the eyes are reduced by the increase in blood circulation and waste removal.
9. Removal of waste products from muscle tissue prevents fatigue and gives a subsequent improvement in muscle tone.

Facial treatments

10. Continued good lymph drainage combats the signs of ageing, resulting in the client looking young for longer.

11. Acned or spotty skins are improved as there is a reduction in the risk of infection, so fewer spots result.

12. Skin healing is improved so scarring is less likely and there may be an improvement in scars already present.

13. If spots or other infections occur, the healing process will be quicker.

14. Skin appendages benefit, in other words, hair and nails grow stronger and more quickly.

All good facial treatments should be aimed at improving the skin tone and texture, firming the underlying muscles and tissue structure. A good facial massage will cleanse, tone and refine the skin, strengthen the muscles and relax the client. The stimulation of the circulation will increase cell regeneration and maintain the correct oil and fluid balance of the skin. By understanding the classification of massage movements and their effects, the therapist can tailor a massage to suit the need of the individual client.

The facial massage is based around four types of movements – **effleurage**, **petrissage**, **tapotement** and **vibrations**. Each of these movements has a specific purpose. You may be expected to learn a routine that has been designed as the salon or training institute's house style. Whatever routine is adopted, it will be based on these four massage movements.

Effleurage

Massage always starts with effleurage. This is a series of light, continuous stroking movements that are designed to relax the client and are used to link up other movements and manipulations within the routine.

Effects of effleurage:

- increases blood circulation
- increases lymphatic drainage
- aids desquamation
- promotes relaxation.

Petrissage

Petrissage is a series of compression movements that include kneading, knuckling, lifting, rolling and pinching. The movements are intermittent and deeper than those employed in effleurage. They are used over soft tissue.

Effects of petrissage:

- increases blood circulation
- improves lymphatic drainage
- improves muscle tone
- increases mitosis (the process by which cells reproduce)
- aids desquamation.

Tapotement

Tapotement movements are applied in a light, quick, stimulating manner. They include movements such as slapping and tapping. They should be applied in a continuous rhythmic series of strokes.

Effects of tapotement:

- stimulates the nerve endings
- increases blood circulation
- improves lymphatic drainage
- tones the skin.

Vibration

Vibrations are applied by producing a quick contraction and relaxation of the therapist's arm muscles. The client experiences a light trembling sensation.

Effects of vibrations:

- relaxing
- stimulates the nerve endings.

The overall effects of facial massage are:

- increases blood and lymphatic circulation
- increases mitosis
- improves skin texture
- promotes relaxation.

The repetition of movements will depend upon the needs of the individual client. The routine should take between 15 and 20 minutes of the recommended 60 minutes' duration for a facial. The selection of a suitable massage medium will depend upon client need, but will usually be a cream or oil-based product.

Procedure for a facial massage

1. Place fingers on the pectoral muscle at the base of the sternum. Slide across and around the shoulder (deltoid muscle). Turn the hands and slide back along the trapezius muscle to the neck.
2. Slide the fingers to the deltoid and use circular thumb-kneading along the trapezius to the top of the spine. Slide back and repeat.
3. Place the fingers on trapezius, at deltoid, and proceed with deep circular finger kneading.
4. Place the fingers at the back of the neck and vibrate up the back of the neck.
5. Circular kneading along platysma and sterno-mastoid.
6. Cup hands one above the other, place on the sternum, slide up the left side of the neck, across the jawline and down the right side.
7. Bend the fingers and, using the knuckles, knuckle up and down the neck area.
8. Place the thumbs on the centre of the chin. With first fingers placed under the jaw, slide the thumbs firmly down the platysma, bring the first fingers onto the chin, slide along the jawline to the ear, change and slide down to the chin.
9. Place the thumbs one above the other on the chin and proceed with circular kneading along the jawline to the ear and back. Reverse the circling and knead to the other ear.
10. Place the thumbs at the corners of the mouth and lift the mouth with a flicking upward movement.
11. Clasp the fingers under the chin, turn hands, unclasp and slide the hands up the face towards the forehead.
12. Place the hands on the forehead at the temples and stroke upwards from the eyebrow to the hairline from left to right.
13. Using the ring finger draw a figure of eight around the eyes.
14. Repeat movement 11.
15. Circular kneading from the chin to the nose to the temples.
16. With thumbs on the cheeks, carry out deep circular kneading to the cheek area.
17. From left to right, tap along the jawline.
18. Cup the hands and lift the masseter muscle on each side of the face and release.
19. Using thumb and forefinger, proceed with a deep rolling pinching movement to the cheek area.
20. Place the pads of the fingers on the mandible and proceed to work towards the ear, using a lifting movement.

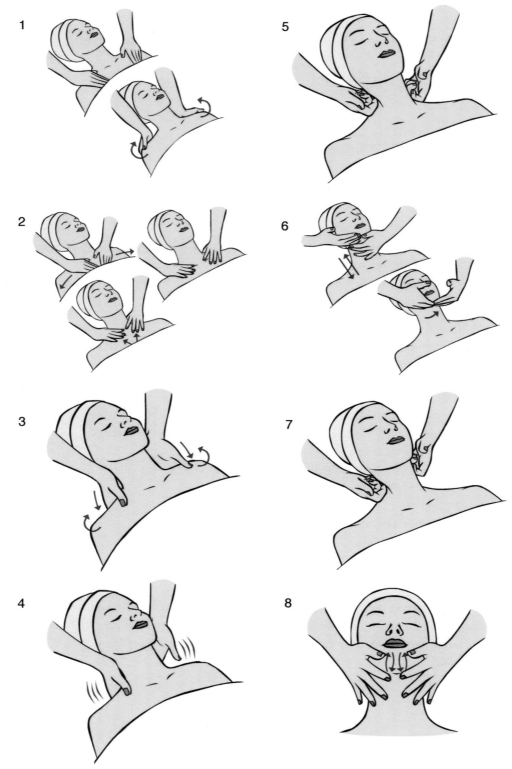

Figure 7.5 *Steps in a facial massage*

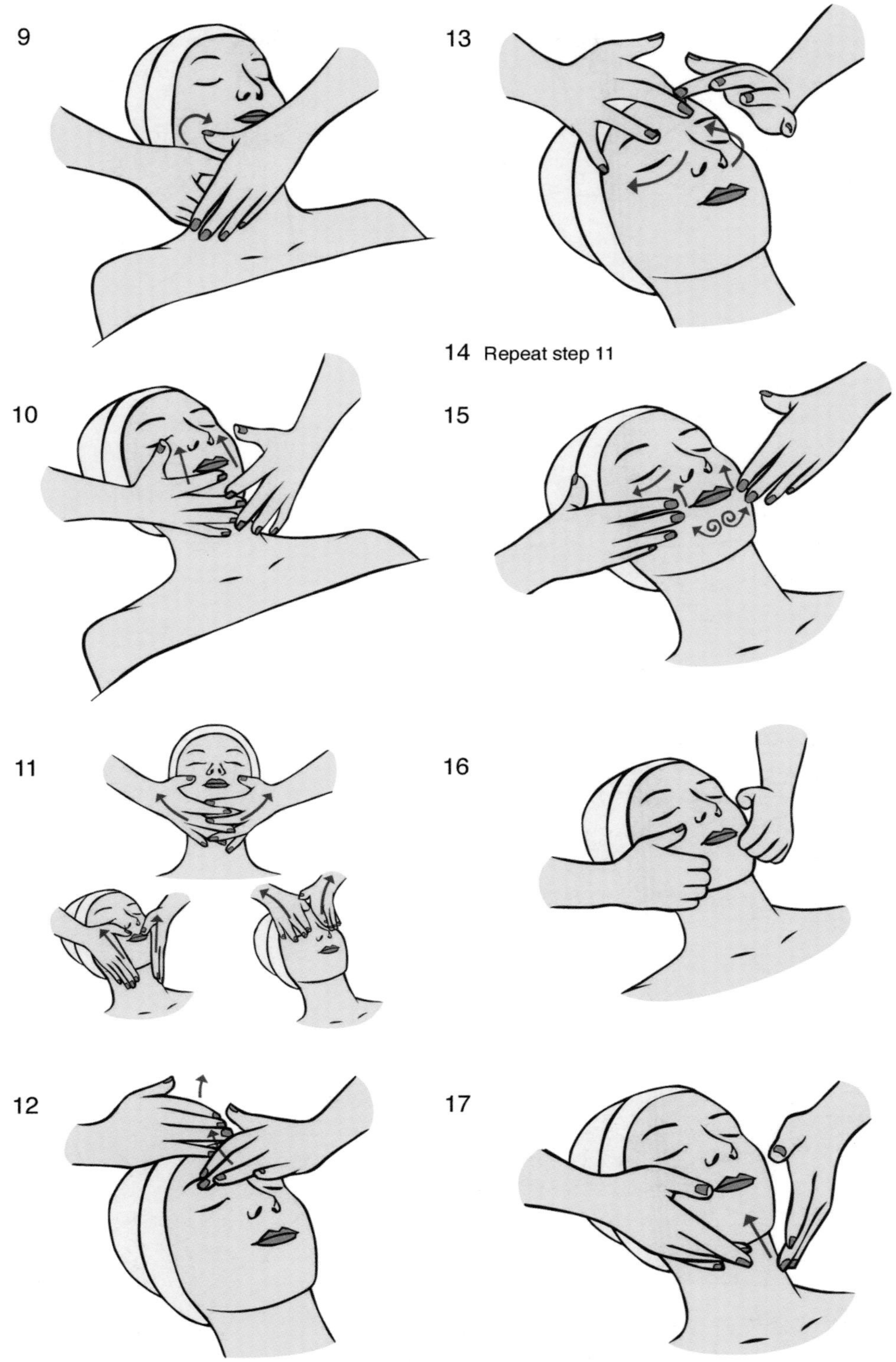

9

10

11

12

13

14 Repeat step 11

15

16

17

Figure 7.5 *Steps in a facial massage (Continued)*

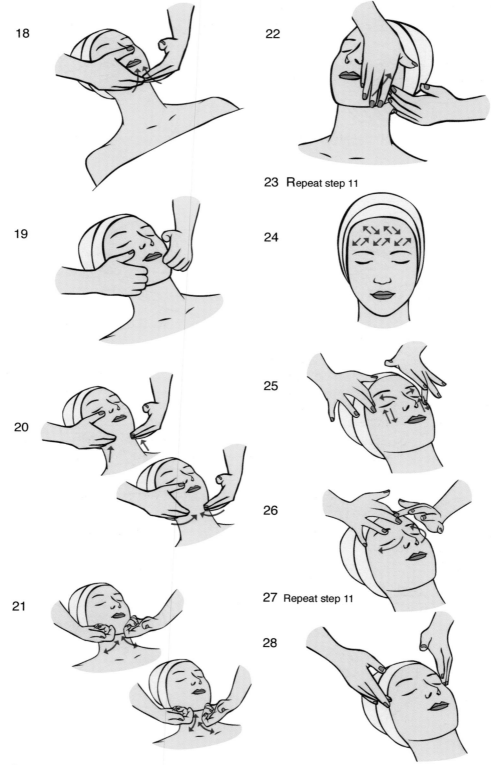

18

19

20

21

22

23 Repeat step 11

24

25

26

27 Repeat step 11

28

Figure 7.5 *Steps in a facial massage*

21. Knuckle along the jawline and on the cheek area.

22. Using the palm of the hand, slap along the jawline from ear to ear, lifting the muscles.

23. Repeat movement.

24. Scissor movement to forehead.

25. Using pads of the fingers tap gently around the eye area.

26. Repeat movement 13.

27. Repeat movement 1.

28. Slide the hands across to the temples and apply slight pressure to signify the end of the routine.

ACTIVITY

1. What adaptations could you make to the facial massage routine for a client with dry or sensitive skin?

2. How much time should you allow for the facial massage?

Face masks

Face masks complement the beneficial effects of the cleansing routine. They have deep cleansing qualities and may contain active ingredients to hydrate and soothe the skin.

Face masks are based upon different formulations which will vary according to the ingredients used and the action required. A sound knowledge of the action and effects of the basic ingredients will allow you to formulate preparations to suit the need of the individual. The timings for face masks within the 60-minute treatment schedule will vary depending on the type selected, however a face mask doesn't usually take more than 20 minutes.

The mask is generally applied at the end of the facial treatment. However, some facial routines may specify the application of the mask at a specific point, designed to achieve maximum benefit.

There are several types of mask used to suit all skin types:

- **Setting masks** – these masks dry on the skin. They include clay-based masks and peel-off masks (used on oily skin to remove excess oil and deep cleanse).
- **Non-setting masks** – these masks do not set but are cooling and soothing on the skin. They include biological and clay-based masks, to which oil is added.
- **Specialised masks** – these are masks that include paraffin wax, oil masks, gel masks, thermal masks and cream masks (used on specific conditions such as very dry skin).

Different face masks have many beneficial effects on the skin. They:

- soothe and calm
- soften
- improve desquamation
- moisturise
- deep cleanse
- have a slight bleaching effect
- remove excess oil
- stimulate circulation.

General contraindications to face masks are as follows:

- infections like herpes simplex or impetigo
- recent scar tissue

- cuts and abrasions

- highly sensitive or sensitised skin, for example through sunburn.

The mask should be applied onto skin that has been thoroughly cleansed and is free of all products. In some cases the mask may be applied over the massage medium when carrying out specialised treatments. However, the skin will normally be completely free of all traces of product. Earlier in this chapter skin analysis and inspection was discussed (see page 115). It is very important that you examine the skin thoroughly to enable you to make an informed decision about the most suitable formulation for the client.

The mask should be mixed with a spatula, not a brush. This will ensure an even distribution of ingredients. If a brush is used to mix, the neck of the brush becomes clogged with the formula. Masks can be applied with a brush or spatula depending on type. They should be applied evenly, especially clay-based masks mixed to a setting formula. If they are unevenly applied they can evaporate too quickly, giving a burning, itching sensation on the skin.

Soothing, refreshing eye pads made from witch hazel or water can be applied. However, client preference should be ascertained as some clients may feel claustrophobic and prefer to have their eyes open.

Setting masks
Clay-based masks

Clay masks are made from a variety of clay and powdered mineral ingredients. The basic ingredients are:

- **Calamine** – this is a pale pink powder. It is ideal for sensitive skin conditions. It soothes inflamed skin, calms high colour and has a very gentle effect. It is usually mixed with orange flower water or rose water.

- **Magnesium carbonate** – this is a bright white powder. It has slightly astringent properties and is particularly effective on skins with isolated blemishes. It is commonly used in conjunction with other powders because of its effects.

- **Kaolin** – this is a dull white powder, stronger in effect than magnesium carbonate. It has a drawing effect, which is deep cleansing. It increases blood circulation and removal of waste products.

- **Fuller's earth** – this is a greyish green powder. It is the strongest of all the powders and is usually mixed with witch hazel. Fuller's earth should only ever be used on oily or seborrhoeic conditions. It induces a fast vascular response and is very stimulating. It aids desquamation and has a deep cleansing action.

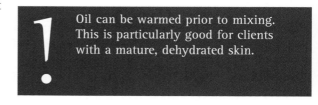

! Oil can be warmed prior to mixing. This is particularly good for clients with a mature, dehydrated skin.

A combination of these ingredients is mixed with an active liquid ingredient to form a paste. These liquids are as important as the powders and, therefore, should be prescribed with care. They include:

- **Witch hazel** – an astringent, which has a stimulating and drying effect. Used on oily skins.

- **Rose water** – a mild tonic effect. Used on dry skins.

- **Distilled water** – used on normal skin.

- **Orange flower water** – similar to rose water, but slightly stimulating.

Vegetable oils have a softening and moisturising effect. Especially good for mature skins and dehydrated conditions. A few drops can be added to the clay mask.

The face mask paste is mixed to a smooth, even consistency and applied to the face and neck using a sterilised brush.

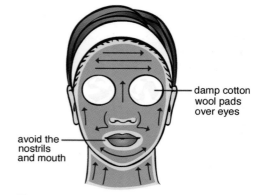

damp cotton wool pads over eyes

avoid the nostrils and mouth

Figure 7.6 *Applying a face mask*

Care should be taken to avoid the hairline, septum, mouth and eyes.

As the mask dries the moisture in the formulation evaporates and has a tightening effect on the skin. Impurities are brought to the surface of the skin and the clay powder absorbs excess oil and removes surface adhesions.

Once the mask has dried, it should be removed using warm water and sponges. Once all trace of the mask has been removed, the skin should be wiped over with dampened cotton wool.

Peel-off masks

Peel-off masks have become increasingly popular. They are not as strong as clay-based masks. Peel-off masks fall into two categories: those based upon waxes (paraffin wax), gums, latex and plastic resins, and gel-based ones.

They may be water-based or, for quicker drying, may contain alcohol. They are applied in their liquid state and left to dry on the skin.

This group of masks is easier to apply than clay masks and are gentler on the skin. The wax- and latex-based products form a seal on the skin, which induces heat and prevents moisture escaping from the skin enabling the moisturising product to be more readily absorbed. The effect on the skin is cleansing and, through the creation of heat, promotes an erythema (slight redness). They are suitable for all clients except those who are very sensitive or who have a couperose skin. Couperose skin refers to dilated capillaries found on the cheeks and around the nose. The walls of the capillaries lose their elasticity and remain permanently dilated, giving the skin a pronounced redness. Dilated capillaries appear on fine, sensitive, dry skin, or can be the result of years of exposure to extremes in temperature, i.e. cold winds and extreme heat. Spicy foods, alcohol and very hot drinks can also be contributing factors.

Gel-based masks are cooling and slightly astringent. Peel-off masks are designed to be lifted off the skin when dry, taking softened surface adhesions off the skin.

Non-setting masks
Biological masks

Non-setting masks are usually cooling and refreshing on the skin. They have different effects depending on the type of preparation used. Biological masks are those based on wholly natural ingredients such as herbs, vegetables, fruits, flowers and plant extracts. They are applied in a light film over the skin. This does not harden but becomes firm and drier depending on the binding agent, for example honey.

Biological ingredients can be sliced, chopped up and pulped and placed directly onto the skin or onto a gauze to aid removal. The ingredients may be mixed with honey, cream, egg white or yoghurt. This will lessen the astringent effect of some ingredients.

Most soft fruits have an acidic reaction on the skin and should be used with care. The enzymatic action of some fruits can soften and remove dead skin cells, but may also sensitise.

Herbs and vegetables can stimulate, balance and tone the skin. Plants can stimulate the circulation. Egg yolk whipped with honey has a moisturising effect. Whipped egg white or yoghurt has a drawing, tightening effect on the skin.

Specialised masks

These can be both setting and non-setting. They include:

- **Specialised cream masks** – these are usually part of a professional range that provides retailing opportunities for the therapist.
- **Paraffin wax** – an occlusive mask, particularly effective on mature skin types. Specialised products may be applied to the skin prior to application to enhance the effect.

- **Prescription masks** – usually gel based. These are a series of active products from which tailor-made masks can be created to suit the needs of the individual.
- **Thermal masks** – these masks either generate heat or require an external heat source.

Heat-generating masks are formed from a paste that is applied over a specialised cream or ampoule. The paste sets and generates heat as it hardens. The mask is lifted away in a solid form upon cooling.

Heat-reliant masks are preparations that include the use of warmed oil to mix and bind formulations. A gauze is placed over the application and an infrared lamp may be used to further increase the warmth.

ACTIVITY

1. List the uses and effects of a fuller's earth mask.
2. What is understood by thermal masks?
3. What is an occlusive mask?
4. What precautions should be taken when using biological masks?

ACTIVITY

1. Working with a colleague, design a face mask using biological ingredients.
2. List the formulation and the effect on the skin.

Aftercare

This chapter has discussed treatments designed to improve the condition of the facial skin. To ensure optimum effectiveness of the treatment, the client should be advised on how to treat the skin between visits for professional facials, thus maintaining the condition.

Remember if you are working in an assisting role you should ask the senior therapist if the finished effect needs any further treatment.

This advice should cover three aspects:

1. General care of skin at home.
2. Treatment of skin following professional treatment.
3. Other factors.

General care of skin

The client may have been carrying out a particular skincare regime for years. Their routine may require adapting or changing completely. It is quite common to discover that a client's skincare routine is actually the cause of the skin problem. The therapist should ensure that clients are aware that their skin type will not stay the same and that it may go through several changes.

It is very important that the therapist is knowledgeable about the product range available in the salon. You should read all available information, as this will increase your confidence when advising your clients. Most salons stock a professional range. This means that it is a range that can only be purchased through approved salons. It also means, as discussed earlier in this chapter, that there is a selling opportunity for the therapist (see page 117). The client will see a better result if the products used in the facial treatment are complemented by professionally prescribed products to use at home.

Treatment of skin

Aftercare advice should also relate to special treatment of the skin following salon treatment. Clients should be advised that any erythema caused by treatment will quickly disperse and is temporary. They should also be told what activities and products to avoid. This will depend on the type of treatment. However, it is wise to recommend that the client avoids using sunbeds, sunbathing, extremes of temperature or strong-scented products. Some facial treatments may carry on working for up to 24 hours and it is important for the client not to irritate the area, avoiding the application of make-up for several hours after treatment. Rough handling of the skin or using harsh, inappropriate products will only serve to undo the positive effects of the facial.

Other factors

The professional beauty therapy treatment will undoubtedly benefit and improve most skin conditions. It is important, though, that you consider other factors that may be the underlying cause of a skin problem or may influence the predicted outcome of the treatment.

Stress is thought to be one of the main causes of premature ageing. It can affect the client's sleeping pattern, lead to depression, weight loss or gain and sallow, dull-looking skin. Relaxation activities such as massage could be suggested to help improve the condition.

Smoking will also have an adverse effect on the skin. It can reduce the amount of oxygen reaching the skin, as the blood is polluted by the gases inhaled during smoking. This affects the oxygen reaching the cells and results in dryness and dilated capillaries. It will also cause the formation of premature lines around the lips. Of course, it has other very harmful effects on the rest of the body!

Diet also contributes to healthy skin. There has been a culture of change in dietary habits over the last 20 years. More food allergies, fad dieting and an increase in eating disorders have been seen. There has been a change in eating patterns and a greater reliance on snacks and processed foods. The effects of this change are evident in the increase in nutrition-related problems. A healthy body requires a balanced diet that contains a mixture of proteins, fats and carbohydrates. Fresh fruit and vegetables are a daily essential.

Exercise also affects the skin. If the client has a healthy, well-balanced diet and takes moderate regular exercise, they will look and feel better. They will have more energy and be less prone to tiredness and tension.

The therapist must understand the limitations of the professional salon treatment. It will help to improve the condition, but for how long depends on the client's willingness to bring about an alteration in lifestyle.

Ultraviolet light and the skin

The effects of the sun and sunbeds on the skin are well documented. Articles appear each year in journals and magazines just before the summer holidays or the ski season, offering wise and precautionary advice. It is important that, as a beauty therapist, you have an awareness and understanding of the long-term effects of exposure to sunlight.

Ultraviolet rays are damaging to the skin, although some types are more harmful than others. The amount of damage can be directly attributed to the length of time spent exposed to the rays. Damage can range from mild irritation to blistering, swelling and inflammation. Continued exposure to sunlight can cause permanent damage to the skin. The most severe and increasingly common danger is that of **melanoma** – skin cancer. Fair-skinned people are particularly prone to melanoma.

Facial treatments

The colour of skin, as discussed earlier in this chapter (see page 111), can be attributed to the amount of melanin present in the skin. The darker the skin, the higher the melanin content. Melanin protects the skin from the effects of sunlight. Therefore, darker skins are less prone to conditions such as melanoma and have more tolerance to ultraviolet exposure. It should be noted, however, that all skin types will suffer from the effects of overexposure: excessive dryness and premature formation of wrinkles.

The skin becomes drier following exposure to ultraviolet light and eventually the collagen fibres, which give the skin its elasticity, break up. This is exactly the same process that occurs during ageing. It is the prolonged exposure that speeds up this process, resulting in premature ageing. The effects of ultraviolet exposure cannot be reversed.

Psoriasis and acne are the only conditions that can be improved through controlled exposure to sunlight. This works by causing the surface of the skin to peel slightly, unblocking the sebaceous glands and increasing desquamation (removal of skin cells).

Sunscreens

The client should always be advised to use a sunscreen. Products will indicate a sun protection factor (SPF) number on the packaging. The SPF indicates the amount of protection provided by the product. Total sun block, for example, will range from SPF 60 to 95. Most make-up (foundations) have an SPF of 15 to 20. The choice of sunscreen will depend on the skin type, the activity (e.g. sunbathing, swimming, skiing) and the area of the world in which the client will be exposed to the sun.

The therapist must always advise the client on sunscreen products and use the opportunity to sell suitable products to the client. The following provides a guide on which level of SPF is needed for each skin type:

- very fair, freckled skin which burns easily – use SPF 30+
- fair to medium skin – use SPF 20+
- skin that tans easily – use SPF 15+
- children must be always be protected using SPF 50+.

The area of the world where the skin will be exposed to the sun is another important factor to take into account. The sun is strongest in very hot climates (i.e. the tropics and places like Australia). The Mediterranean is very popular for summer/beach holidays and the sun is also very strong there. Northern Europe and the UK are often regarded as safe areas for exposure to the sun. However, this is no longer the case due to changes in the ozone layer. The skin should always be protected from the sun, particularly around midday, and a minimum of SPF 15 should always be applied.

Fake tanning products

The known effects and dangers of the sun still fail to dissuade some clients. It may be prudent for the therapist to recommend fake tanning products. These used to be hard to apply, had a dreadful odour and invariably dried streaky. More recently, these products have become refined, effective and pleasantly scented! The professional application of these products has become a very popular service offered by the beauty therapist.

The skin should always be exfoliated and a light application of moisturiser applied. The skin should then be allowed to settle for a few minutes prior to applying the self-tanning product. Two or three light applications should be made to avoid streaking. The client should be advised to reapply after a few hours, depending upon the depth of colour required. When applying to areas of the skin prone to dryness such as knees and elbows, a small amount of moisturiser should be mixed with the self-tanning product.

It is important for the therapist to wash their hands thoroughly after application and the client should also be advised if they are going to use the product at home.

Most fake tans contain dihydroxyacetone. This adheres to the keratin cells and stains them an orangey-brown. As the skin desquamates the stained cells are shed, resulting in a gradual fading of the tan.

Chapter 8

LASH AND BROW TREATMENTS

LEVEL 2

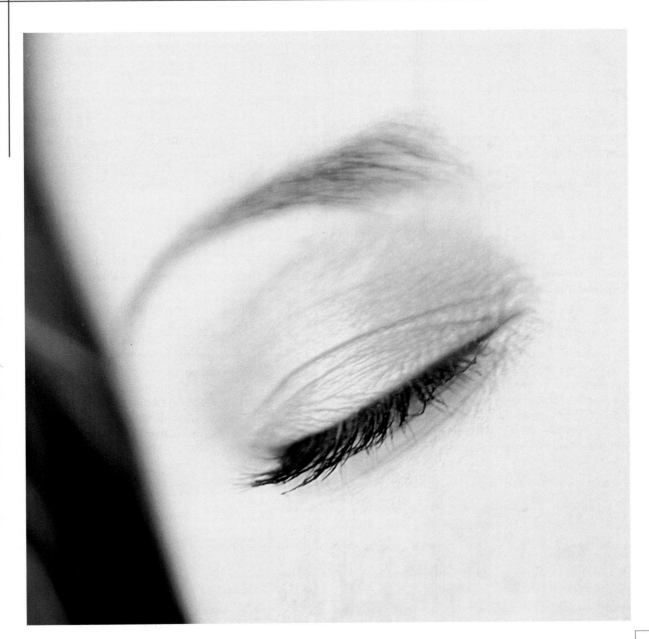

IN THIS CHAPTER YOU WILL LEARN ABOUT:

- Assessing the needs and requirements of the client
- Preparing the client and work area for lash and brow treatments
- Shaping the eyebrows
- Eyelash and eyebrow tinting
- Perming the eyelashes

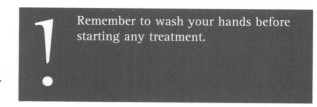

Introduction

The eyes are one of the most sensitive areas of the body. The texture of the surrounding skin is much finer and there is less subcutaneous fatty tissue offering support. Therefore the skin around the eyes can often look darker due to the fine texture and the skin being stretched over a bony prominence in the skull, thus creating a sunken area between the bone and eyeball. No matter how beautiful the facial features are, if the client has dark circles under the eyes, tired eyes, unkempt eyebrows or straight eyelashes, the beauty of the other facial features will be diminished. Treatments around the eye area are some of the most important of the salon services and they will have the most dramatic and immediate effect.

> **!** Remember to wash your hands before starting any treatment.

Assessing the client's needs

The assessment of the client's needs will depend upon the requested treatment. For many treatments around the eye area a **patch test** for sensitivity will be required. Popular salon treatments are tinting brows and lashes, and eyelash perming.

Patch-testing for lash tinting and perming

It is vital that a patch test is carried out at least 48 hours prior to any treatment in the eye area that involves the use of chemical preparations. This should be made clear to the client when they make their appointment. Your salon will have an established procedure for this, which will ensure that all staff who take bookings are aware of the policy and can advise the client accordingly. Clients may insist that it is unnecessary as they have had their hair tinted or chemically treated before with no ill effect. You must ensure that the client appreciates the sensitivity of the area and that it is common for different areas of the body to be more sensitive than others.

Procedure for patch-testing

1. Cleanse an area of skin either behind the ear or in the fold of the elbow.
2. Apply a very small amount of the chemical to be used to the area. This may be mixed tint or perm solution.
3. Leave for 5 minutes and then wipe over area (if applicable).
4. Advise the client to wash the area if an adverse (or positive) reaction occurs.

> It is important to note that strong products for wiping/cleansing the area are avoided as the client may be reacting to them rather than the applied treatment product.

Clients should be advised what to expect from a positive reaction: there may be redness and irritation in the area. The client should be told to inform the salon if a positive reaction occurs and to apply a cooling, soothing cream.

> **!** It is important to patch-test before **every** treatment as areas with a negative test result can become sensitised between treatments.

The date of the patch test and the outcome (positive or negative) should be recorded on the client's treatment plan or card (see page 74).

Eyebrow shaping

Eyebrow shaping is one of the easiest ways of giving definition to the eye area. It is only necessary to remove a few hairs to create a groomed appearance.

Preparation of work area for eyebrow shaping

The couch and trolley should be prepared prior to the client's arrival. There should be clean linen on the couch and the trolley should contain:

- a selection of cleansing and toning products
- a selection of bowls for cotton wool – dry and damp
- tissues
- spatulas
- an eyebrow brush or comb
- witch hazel
- surgical spirit – for wiping tweezers
- tweezers (manual and automatic)
- a hand mirror
- covered waste bin
- a steamer or facilities to prepare hot, damp cotton-wool pads
- treatment plan or record card.

All tools and equipment must be sterilised in the appropriate way and should not be brought to the trolley until they are required for use.

Preparation of client

The client should be in a semi-reclining position and the hair and clothing should be protected.

The area to be treated should be cleansed and toned. It is important to tone to ensure all cleansing product is removed from the area.

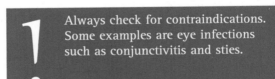

> **!** Always check for contraindications. Some examples are eye infections such as conjunctivitis and sties.

It is important to discuss the desired effect with the client before starting to remove the hairs. Consideration should be given to the natural brow shape and the shape of the client's face. You should also take into account whether the client has had their brows shaped before. If this is the first time it may be wise to shape them gradually over two treatments.

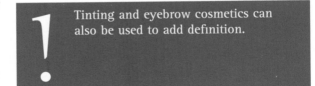

> **!** Tinting and eyebrow cosmetics can also be used to add definition.

Once the desired outcome has been agreed, the brow area should be brushed against the growth to separate the hairs and then brushed into their natural shape.

Shape of brows

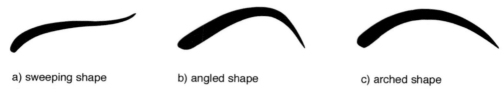

a) sweeping shape   b) angled shape   c) arched shape

Figure 8.1 *Corrective eyebrow shapes can be used to give definition to different facial contours*

Methods of eyebrow shaping

Eyebrows can be shaped using a variety of methods. They can be **waxed** using a small spatula and small strip for removal. Care should be taken when waxing such a sensitive area. The skin surrounding the eyes is very thin and delicate. This should be considered prior to using this method. This method would normally take 15 minutes to perform.

Tweezers are the most popular method. Manual and automatic tweezers are available. The automatic tweezer is designed for speed and for removing a lot of hairs.

Manual tweezers are used for final shaping and tidying the brows.

Fifteen minutes should be allowed for eyebrow shaping in the treatment schedule.

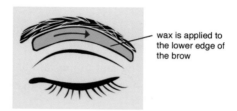

wax is applied to the lower edge of the brow

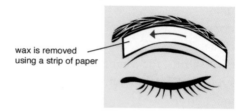

wax is removed using a strip of paper

Figure 8.2 *Waxing eyebrows*

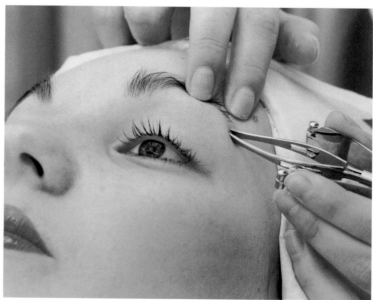

Figure 8.3 *Using automatic tweezers*

Procedure for shaping the brows

1. The brows should be warmed using either a steamer or hot damp cotton-wool pads.
2. The brows should be measured using the following guidelines.
3. Hold the skin taut and remove hairs only in the direction of growth.
4. Wipe over constantly with warm, damp pads.
5. Brush the brows regularly to ascertain developing shape.
6. Do not work on one brow only. Instead remove a few hairs from each brow to maintain balance.

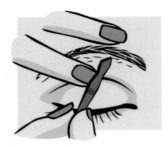

Figure 8.4 *Using manual tweezers*

> **!** Selection of the tweezer type should be left to the therapist. It is important that you feel confident with the selected tool.

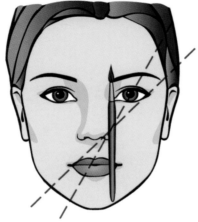

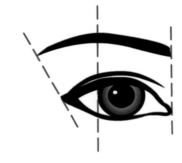

Figure 8.5 *Measuring guidelines for eyebrows*

7. Place removed hairs on a tissue. Do not leave on the skin.
8. When completed wipe over with a witch hazel pad to soothe the area.
9. Show the client the finished result.
10. Provide aftercare advice: avoid application of make-up until the erythema has gone and wipe over with soothing antiseptic cream.

> **!** Hairs should only be removed from underneath the brow line. Stray hairs at the temple area or above the brow should only be removed if they do not form part of the main brow growth.

Eyelash and eyebrow tinting

Tinting the eyelashes or brows can be one of the most natural and effective ways of enhancing and defining the eyes. It is particularly popular with clients for whom make-up is prohibited, for those who prefer a more natural look or who are going on holiday and do not want to wear make-up. It can also be effective if the client has changed their hair colour or if they have grey or fair hair and wish to add definition to the eye area. Eyelash tinting is complementary to eyelash perming and application of semi-permanent lashes.

You should allow 20 minutes for eyelash tinting in the treatment schedule and no more than 10 minutes for tinting the brow hairs. This will vary depending upon the client's natural colouring. Those clients who have a lot of red in their hair colour may require a longer processing time to achieve a satisfactory result.

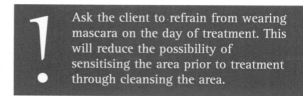

Ask the client to refrain from wearing mascara on the day of treatment. This will reduce the possibility of sensitising the area prior to treatment through cleansing the area.

Contraindications to lash and brow tinting

It is important to check for contraindications before tinting the eyelashes or brows. Contraindications include:

- positive reaction to the patch test
- cuts and abrasions in the area
- bruised (black eye) eye area
- conjunctivitis
- watery eyes
- sties
- inflammation or swelling
- known allergy to cosmetics.

Preparation of work station

The work station should be prepared prior to the client's arrival. The couch should have clean linen and the trolley should be prepared with:

- a selection of bowls – for damp and dry cotton wool
- tissues
- a selection of cleansing and toning products
- petroleum jelly
- a small glass or non-metallic dish
- a selection of eyelash tints
- preformed tinting shields
- 10 volume (3 per cent) hydrogen peroxide
- orange-wood sticks
- small brush
- spatulas
- eyebath and distilled water (for emergencies)
- a covered waste receptacle
- treatment plan or record card.

It is very important to ensure that the bottle of peroxide is kept tightly closed to maintain the strength of the peroxide.

All tools and equipment should be sterilised in the appropriate way.

Choosing the colour

Lash tint comes in a range of colours – black, brown, grey and blue. They can be mixed to provide a range of depth and tone of colour. As with all colour choice, the client may have a preference. However, certain considerations must be given to:

- colour of lashes
- age of client

- hair and skin colour
- client's usual make-up.

Applying black to a mature client with white hair would be harsh and would look artificial. However, black mixed with brown or grey would soften the colour. Young clients can take black or black mixed with blue to give depth to the lashes.

Particular care must be taken when choosing colour for the eyebrows. Do not be tempted to use the same colour as the lashes. Brown is the most commonly used colour.

Preparation of client

The client should be comfortably seated on the couch with their hair and clothing protected. The eyes should be cleansed and toned or a full cleanse carried out if the tinting is part of a facial.

Avoid cleansing the eyes with oily make-up remover as any oil or cream remaining on the lashes can prevent the tint from 'taking' properly.

Begin by confirming that the client has had a patch test (see page 142). Establish and record the outcome of the test before proceeding with the treatment. The desired effect should be discussed and you should inform the client of your recommendations. Always consider the different effects and depths of colour achieved by the various tints, depending upon the client's natural colouring. Pay careful regard to manufacturer's instructions as some may vary.

> If the client does experience any contra-actions to treatment, the tint should be removed immediately and the eyes rinsed using an eyebath and distilled water, followed by a cold-water compress to soothe the eye.

The client should be informed that, if at any time during the treatment, discomfort (a tingling or burning sensation) is felt, they should inform you immediately so that the tint can be removed.

Procedure for tinting the eyelashes

1. Place a dampened preformed tint shield under the lower lashes. It is advisable to coat the underside with petroleum jelly to help the shield to stay in place.

2. Using a clean, fine brush apply petroleum jelly to the upper eyelid and underneath the lower lashes.

3. The tint should now be mixed.

The formulation is usually 5–6 mm of tint to 2–3 drops of 10 volume peroxide (the tint comes out of a tube rather like toothpaste – you will need to squeeze 2–4 mm long). However, you should always refer to the manufacturer's instructions. Only a very small amount of tint is required. Do not waste products unnecessarily.

> The client may have fallen asleep during the process and could open the eyes if suddenly disturbed. It is therefore important to talk generally to the client, explaining each step in the procedure. It is also recommended that you inform the client not to open the eyes until instructed to.

4. Apply the tint to the bottom lashes on both eyes using a small sterilised dry brush. Ask the client to close their eyes and apply to the upper lashes.

5. Place warm, dampened (not wet!) cotton wool pads over the tint to create warmth. This will assist in the development of the tint and will also help to prevent the client opening their eyes during the processing time.

> Do not mix the tint until the client has been prepared. The tint will start working immediately and if it is not applied straight away the effect will be lessened. Always mix the tint formulation using an orange-wood stick. Never use the applicator brush to mix as the tint will clog at the top of the brush head, causing a messy application.

6. The tint should be removed following the manufacturer's recommended processing time. This is normally around 10 minutes.

7. The pad of cotton wool and the tint shield should be grasped and removed in a quick downward movement. This is carried out on both eyes. Ask the client to keep their eyes closed.

8. Dampened cotton-wool pads are then used to wipe the lashes. The area should be wiped until the cotton wool shows no evidence of any remaining tint.

9. The client should now be asked to open the eyes. Using a folded, dampened cotton-wool pad, gently wipe the base of the lashes. Continue until the pad wipes clean.

10. Wipe over the eye area with tonic to remove the petroleum jelly and show the client the finished result.

> **!** Care must be taken when applying the petroleum jelly. This will act as a barrier between the tint and the skin. However, it will also act as a barrier to the tint if it comes into contact with the hair, preventing the tint working on the lashes.

> **!** Make sure that you take the tint application as close to the roots as possible. Use a clean finger to gently lift the underside of the eyebrow to expose the roots of the lashes. This is particularly important in both the application and the removal process.

Procedure for tinting the brows

1. The brows should be brushed thoroughly to lift and separate them.

2. Petroleum jelly is applied to the surrounding area, taking care not to touch the hairs that are to be tinted.

3. The colour should be chosen carefully and mixed as for lashes.

4. The tint is applied to the hairs of the brows, not the skin, to avoid harsh lines, applying against the growth of the brows.

5. Apply to both brows and remove from the first brow immediately to assess the colour, which can 'take' very quickly. Then remove from the other brow immediately.

6. Discuss colour with the client using a hand mirror.

7. Reapply if colour is not dark enough.

8. It may take 3–4 applications to achieve the right depth of colour.

9. The area should then be wiped over with tonic pads to remove all traces of the petroleum jelly.

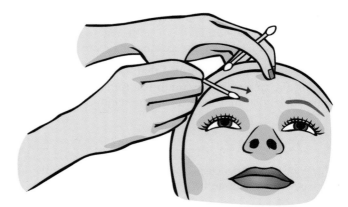

Figure 8.6 *Tinting the eyebrows*

> **!** Over-tinted eyebrows can look very unattractive. Use the technique described here to build the colour rather than trying to time 1 minute, which may be too long!

> **!** The brows must not be shaped beforehand and on the same day as tinting. The area will become sensitised following the shaping procedure and the application of tint could cause irritation. The client could have the brows shaped after the tint or could book a shape for the next salon visit.

Clients may choose to have a range of treatments on their eyebrows and lashes. The recommended timings for typical combinations are:

- Eyebrow shape and lash tint – 30 minutes.

- Eyebrow tint, eyebrow shape and lash tint – 35–40 minutes.

Eyelash perming

This technique has become a very popular salon treatment. It has revolutionised eyelash enhancement and is particularly effective for those with very straight lashes or those wanting a natural look while still defining the eyes. It is also popular

> ! Excess grease on the lashes from oily eye make-up remover will act as a barrier to the chemical, therefore preventing a successful treatment.

with clients who participate in sporting activities. Clients should always be informed of the limitations of the treatment and the expected duration of the perm. The effect normally lasts for 6–8 weeks.

The products use the same principles as those for the hair. The chemicals soften the internal structure of the hair, remoulding the shape, which is then fixed with the neutralising solution. These chemicals are strong and can damage the delicate eye area if incorrectly used. The chemical solutions for eyelash perming are in gel form, which is easier to apply and prevents seepage in the delicate eye area.

It is important to always refer to manufacturer's instructions.

Contraindications to eyelash perming

- Positive reaction to the patch test (using the perm solution).
- Inflammation of the eye.
- Excessively watery eyes.
- Sties.
- Conjunctivitis.
- Cuts and abrasions.
- Very dry skin.

> ! The lashes can be tinted prior to perming to enhance the finished effect of the treatment.

Procedure for eyelash perming

1. The lashes should be clean and free of any oil. An oil-free eye make-up remover should be used and wiped over the eye area with warm, dampened cotton-wool pads.
2. The lashes are combed and separated. Be careful to ensure the eyelashes are straight and not twisted or crossed.
3. A small pre-shaped dampened pad of cotton wool is placed under the lower lid.
4. The rods are 'sticky' and have been pretreated with glue. The rod should be bent slightly to a 'C' shape.

> ! The perm rollers (rods) are available in different sizes. Smaller rods for shorter lashes or a tighter finished curl.
> Medium is the most popular, with large used for longer lashes or a looser curl.

5. Place the glue from the kit onto the base of the lashes. This should cover at least twice the width of the rod and be of equal length. The rod should be secure at both ends and to the base of the eyelid.
6. Apply more glue to the top of the roller and, using an orange-wood stick, ease the lashes onto the rod.
7. The perm gel is then applied to the lashes and is covered with a damp cotton-wool pad. This will create warmth, which will aid the development time. A facial steamer may also be used at this point.
8. The treatment is left to process for 7–15 minutes. Using an orange-wood stick, check the curl by easing one or two lashes off the rod.
9. Using a dampened cotton-wool pad, gently remove the perm solution.
10. A fixing product (neutraliser) is then applied and left to develop. This stops the action of the perm solution. The area should be covered with a dampened cotton-wool pad and left for 7–15 minutes, depending on the time the perm solution was left for.
11. Apply the nourishing agent and leave for 5 minutes.

Lash and brow treatments

12. Gently wipe the upper part of the rod using a dampened cotton-wool bud, slowly rolling it downwards, freeing the lashes from the rod.

13. The lashes should then be thoroughly cleansed using warm, damp cotton-wool pads, and moisturiser applied.

Contra-actions to eyelash perming

Because of the very sensitive nature of the eyes the therapist must be aware of possible contra-actions and deal with them immediately:

- The alkaline solution can cause irritation to the eyes.
- Hydrogen peroxide used in the fixing (neutralising) process can cause irritation.

The lashes are then wiped over with damp cotton wool and a moisturising lotion is applied to the lashes.

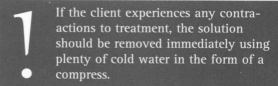

If the client experiences any contra-actions to treatment, the solution should be removed immediately using plenty of cold water in the form of a compress.

The lashes should be gently eased from the roller and the eyes rinsed using an eyebath and distilled water.

The lashes must be gently wiped to ensure all traces of chemicals are removed.

The client should be informed to apply a protective layer of petroleum jelly to the lashes if exposed to strong sunlight or humid conditions.

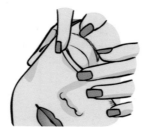
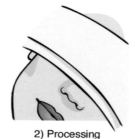

1) Securing the roller

2) Processing

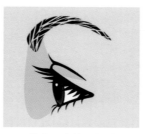

Before (side view)

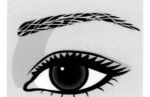

Before (front view)

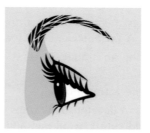

After (side view)

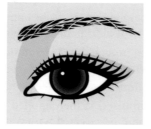

After (front view)

Figure 8.7 *Eyelash perming*

Chapter 9

DEPILATORY WAXING

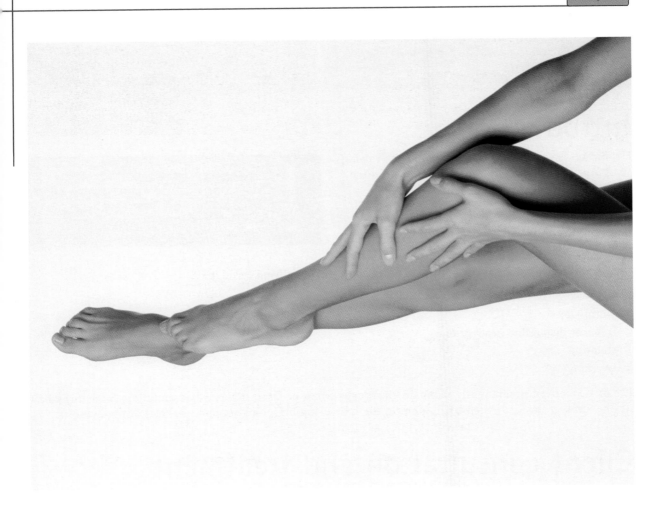

- Client consultation for safe hair removal
- Waxing products
- Preparing the work area for temporary hair removal
  - selecting products and materials for depilatory treatments
  - safety precautions
  - preparing the client for treatment
  - assessing clients and preparing a treatment plan
  - various methods of temporary hair removal
  - treatment methods for different areas of the body
  - erythema (cause and treatment)
  - aftercare advice
  - care and maintenance of equipment

Introduction

Depilation is the removal of superfluous hair using **temporary methods**. The hair is plucked from the follicle but the base of the follicle (the **papilla**) remains intact and can therefore provide nourishment for a new hair to grow. Temporary hair removal only lasts for two to six weeks, depending on the individual.

> ! It is essential that you have a clear understanding of the growth and structure of hair. Please refer to chapter 14, Related Anatomy and physiology, for full details.

Depilation uses a range of methods to pluck or pull the hairs from the skin:

- hot wax
- warm wax
- roller or disposable head system
- sugaring
- tweezing.

If hair is removed **permanently** using an electrical current or laser, this is called **epilation**. Sometimes hair on the arms or face is treated by **lightening the hair** using bleaching products instead of removing it.

Client consultation and treatment planning for waxing

A consultation should be carried out before every waxing treatment to establish:

- contraindications
- the client's expectations of the treatment
- the amount, type and area of hair growth.

When assessing the client for treatment, discuss the client's requirements and examine the area to be treated. Begin by checking for contraindications and examining the condition of the skin and hair.

Note the length, texture, colour and growth pattern of the hair. This will help you to decide on the method of treatment and the direction in which the wax is to be applied.

Some clients can be very sensitive to the products so it is important to check the record card to see if they have had hair removal previously and whether the skin reacted in any way. New clients should be questioned carefully to establish whether they have had any previous adverse reaction to treatment.

The treatment should be clearly explained to the client, giving some indication of how it might feel and how the skin may react and look for a short while afterwards. The normal skin reaction can come as a shock to some clients who expect smooth skin immediately.

Skin reaction from waxing
Normal reaction

The following may occur after waxing and are quite normal reactions:

- erythema in the area
- slight swelling
- tiny red spots around the hair follicles
- blood spots may appear during underarm or bikini-line waxing – this is due to the coarse nature of the hair and deep follicles, which have a rich blood supply.

Normal reactions will last anything from a few minutes to several hours, depending on the area treated and the skin type.

Abnormal skin reaction

The following signs may indicate an abnormal reaction to waxing:

- erythema or red spots on the skin that persist for more than a few hours (bikini line may last 24–48 hours)
- irritation, which may be an indication of an allergic reaction
- burning sensation accompanied by excessive erythema and possibly swelling
- bruising, which can occur when a poor technique is used – for example pulling the wax upwards, especially on the bikini line or on clients with loose crêpey skin
- pustules forming at the mouth of the follicles two or three days after waxing. This indicates poor hygiene.

Superfluous hair

Superfluous hair (unwanted hair), usually found under the arm, around the bikini line and legs, is regarded by some western societies as unattractive and unacceptable on the female. Many European women, on the other hand, do not regard this as a problem and do not remove hair from underarms or legs.

Smooth, flawless skin is much sought after, particularly during the summer when the body is more exposed or when clients are going on holiday. It is then that waxing becomes a very popular salon treatment. There are also clients who have waxing all the year round.

The amount and colour of superfluous hair will vary in individuals but is regarded as normal if it follows a normal growth pattern on the legs, underarm and bikini line, and can be seen as a family characteristic. The skin and hair characteristics of different races also influence the colour and amount of body hair: for example Asian characteristics are dark, fine hair on the body whereas people from the Far East have very little body hair. Hormones influence the amount of hair, with changes seen during puberty, pregnancy and menopause. Superfluous hair, however, may be unsightly because it is dark or grows thickly. This can cause embarrassment to the client and they may look to you for appropriate treatment.

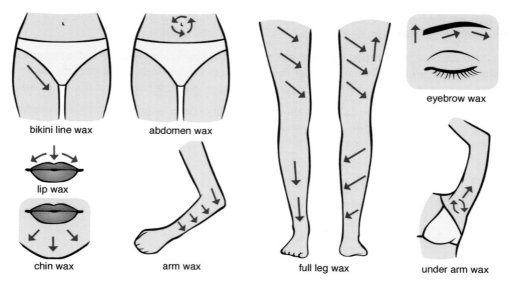

bikini line wax

abdomen wax

eyebrow wax

lip wax

chin wax

arm wax

full leg wax

under arm wax

Diagram to show the application of warm wax for different parts of the body (apply in direction of hair growth)

Figure 9.1 *Diagrams to show the wax application methods for different parts of the body*

Temporary methods of hair removal

For hair removal, the client may use a whole range of home treatments including:

- shaving using an electric or wet razor – this cuts the hair at the surface of the skin, leaving a blunt end which will grow through in 24–48 hours as rough stubble
- depilatory cream – this is made up of strong alkaline chemicals that dissolve the keratin in the hair and skin. The skin can become very sensitive after application. The hair is only removed to the surface of the skin so will reappear in 24–48 hours
- abrasive gloves or a pumice stone, which is rubbed over the skin in circular movements. This breaks off the hair at the surface of the skin. The skin may become sore with this method
- clipping or cutting may be used to cut hairs from moles (which should not be waxed or plucked) or to cut the hair close to the surface of the skin. A coarse stubble will be the result
- home waxing kits in the form of pre-waxed strips or roll-on wax are applied in the usual way to pull the hairs from the follicle. Home waxing can be very messy and the backs of the legs and underarms can be very difficult to reach.

Depilatory waxing products
Waxing

Hot wax has been popular for many years and there are still clients who prefer hot wax, particularly those with dark coarse hair. However, new products referred to as warm wax, which do not require heating to such a high temperature, are more popular and in many ways are more economical and hygienic.

Hot wax (hard wax)

Hot wax is mainly beeswax with resin added to make it more pliable. The wax may be a natural amber colour or have colour added to distinguish the product from those of other manufacturers. Sun-bleached beeswax is used by some manufacturers to increase the pliability of the wax. This product is usually opaque and coloured pale pink or lilac.

Beeswax liquefies when heated, which allows the wax to be applied to the area using a spatula or brush. The wax coats each hair and as it cools the wax contracts around the hair. The patch of wax is then pulled from the skin.

Warm wax (soft wax)

Warm wax is supplied in tins or plastic containers, which can be placed directly into a specially designed heater.

The product is mainly synthetic resins that are either water or oil soluble. Additives such as honey improve the sticky property of the wax. Warm wax may be a clear amber colour or opaque and coloured depending on the manufacturer. The properties of the waxes are similar to beeswax and work by coating the hair with the very sticky substance, which is removed using fabric (calico) or paper strips.

Ingredients such as azulene and camomile are added to help soothe the skin, or tea tree oil to help prevent infection. Warm wax is applied with a spatula or using a disposable roller system.

Sugaring techniques

The art of sugaring to remove hair from the body has been passed down by generations from very early times. The technique originates in the Middle East where it was the tradition to remove all the hair from the body of the bride before her wedding day. All the female members of the family would gather to prepare the sugar paste from a recipe that included sugar, water and lemon juice boiled together to a caramelised paste. The sugar was applied as a ritual to ensure that the bride's skin was perfectly smooth.

Sugar paste is now made commercially and can be obtained from wholesalers at a reasonable price. Traditional practitioners of sugaring may make their own paste using a special recipe, but this requires considerable experience because of the dangers involved in boiling sugar.

Advantages and disadvantages of temporary hair removal methods
Advantages

- Large areas can be treated.
- Instant results.
- Relatively low cost.
- Usually only slight discomfort to the client.

Disadvantages

- Some clients have problems with ingrown hairs.
- Needs to be repeated at regular intervals.
- There is a belief that hair growth increases due to the stimulation of the blood supply to the follicle.

Advantages and disadvantages of permanent hair removal (electro-epilation)

Electrical epilation using **short-wave diathermy** or **the Blend** (combining short-wave diathermy and galvanic currents) are the most commonly used methods for removing hair permanently. Each hair follicle is treated individually and the treatment is generally used for small areas of excessive hair growth (**hypertrichosis**). This treatment is suitable for facial hair, although some clients may request epilation to treat the bikini line or legs. However, this can be time-consuming and expensive.

Advantages

- Once an area has been successfully treated it will remain free from hair (unless new growth as a result of hormone changes occurs).
- Regrowth of hairs may occur after a follicle has been treated but these will be finer in texture and lighter in colour.

Disadvantages

- Skin reaction may occur.
- Some discomfort or even pain may be experienced by the client when working on sensitive areas such as the upper lip, or bikini line or around the nose.
- There is a high cost involved if large areas are to be treated.
- Treatment by poorly trained or incompetent therapists can lead to permanent skin damage, such as scarring.

Contraindications to waxing

Depilatory waxing must not be carried out if any of the following conditions are present in the area. Recommend to the client that the condition should be allowed to clear before waxing the area. If only a small area is affected (other than infectious conditions or allergies) waxing may be carried out by avoiding the problem area:

- cuts, open sores or abrasions
- sunburn
- recent scar tissue
- rashes or bites
- bruising
- known allergy to the products
- hypersensitivity
- thin, loose skin
- any infectious skin condition, e.g. herpes simplex (cold sores), conjunctivitis, sties (facial waxing)
- soreness, inflammation or swelling.

Where small lesions occur, waxing can be carried out if the lesion can be avoided or covered. Do not wax over:

- moles or warts
- unknown skin lesions.

It is advisable for the client to seek medical advice before having depilatory waxing if any of the following conditions are in the area to be waxed:

- legs: varicose veins
- underarm: mastitis or a mastectomy
- general: diabetes, severe psoriosis, eczema, oedema.

Preparation for waxing
Equipment and materials

The following things are needed:

- large secure trolley
- couch prepared with plastic sheeting and/or disposable bed paper (towels and sheets should not be used as the various wax products can be difficult to remove from bed linen)
- heater with sufficient wax for the treatment (roller heads prepared)
- surgical spirit/antiseptic
- cotton wool
- tissues
- talc
- tweezers placed in disinfectant
- soothing lotion
- fabric or paper strips for warm wax and strip sugaring treatment
- container for used wax strips
- disposable wooden spatulas for waxing and a metal spatula for strip sugaring
- after-wax lotion/cleanser.

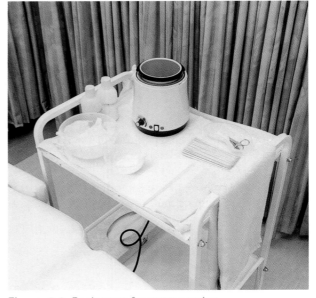

Figure 9.2 *Equipment for warm waxing*

Heating

It is essential that the wax is heated well in advance of the client arriving. If the salon uses a range of products for different hair types or areas of the body then these must all be ready for use. The client will be annoyed if they arrive for depilation treatment to find that have to wait for the wax to heat to the correct temperature or for it to cool to the working temperature because the heater has been left on.

Hot wax

Hot wax requires a thermostatically controlled stainless steel unit to which blocks or pellets of beeswax are added. The wax must be allowed to melt slowly to a working temperature of around 48°C, which will take approximately 40 minutes. Overheating, which can destroy the properties of the wax, must be

Depilatory waxing

avoided. Hot wax is usually a pale amber colour, but darkens as it is heated, especially if it is allowed to overheat.

All wax heaters must be thermostatically controlled. However, it is sometimes necessary to boost the temperature while working to keep the correct consistency of the wax. The consistency of the wax is an indication of the temperature. If the wax is thick like toffee it is not heated sufficiently and will be impossible to apply to the area evenly. If, on the other hand, the wax has a thin consistency, or is giving off fumes or smoke, it is an immediate indication of overheating and it cannot be used until cool. If overheated, the wax will be very runny and impossible to control on the spatula and can burn the client's skin. To ensure that there is no risk of cross infection, all waxing materials must be disposed of after each client. This includes spatulas, used wax, etc.

Warm wax

Warm wax (sometimes called strip wax or soft wax) will usually require heating to a temperature of 35–45°C. The wax may be heated in its own container in a specially designed thermostatically controlled unit.

Roller waxing systems using warm wax

Roller waxing systems use special thermostatically controlled heating systems and disposable cartridges of wax. Roller heads of varying sizes, for use on different areas, are fitted to apply the wax once it has been heated to the working temperature of around 40°C.

The heads can be cleaned using an oil-based after-wax cleaner or disposed of after use.

The disposable nature of the roller heads reduces the risk of infection and the equipment is easy to maintain. It is compact and, because of the sealed cartridges, very clean to use.

There are a number of systems available from different manufacturers.

Sugar paste

Heating sugar paste relies on achieving the right consistency and requires a special thermostatically controlled heater. Therapists who are experienced in sugaring can use a microwave for heating but it requires experience to ensure the paste does not overheat.

Whatever the product or method, it is important that you follow the manufacturer's instructions. Wax can overheat and there is a risk of burning the client. The heating must be controlled carefully. There are safety precautions for heating and testing the temperature (see below).

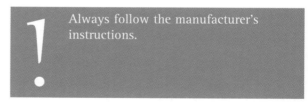

Always follow the manufacturer's instructions.

Hygiene, health and safety when waxing
Hygiene procedures when waxing

- The work area should be prepared with clean disposable paper and plastic sheeting.
- Spatulas and wax strips should be disposed of after use.
- Hot wax must be disposed of after each client to limit the risk of cross infection.
- The area of skin to be waxed must be cleansed with surgical spirit.

- Tweezers should be placed in disinfectant.
- Remember to wash your hands before and after treatment.

Safety precautions

- Wax that has been heated should not be moved around the salon.
- Wax heaters must be placed on a secure trolley.
- Heaters must have a thermostat to control the heating of the wax.
- Prevent leads from the heater trailing across the floor.
- You should test heated wax on your wrist before applying to the client. Remember to check the consistency of the wax. Overheated wax will be very runny and may emit strong fumes or give off smoke.
- The temperature of the wax must be checked throughout the treatment.
- Test the client's tolerance to the heat of the wax (particularly when using hot wax) by applying a small amount with a spatula to an area of the skin on which you will be working.

Posture and positioning for waxing

- The client needs to be comfortable and relaxed.
- For body waxing the client should be laid on the couch, either flat or semi-elevated. Pillows or rolled up towels can be used for support where necessary. The angle of the backrest of the couch or the pillow needs to be adjusted, e.g. for leg wax the client can be in a sitting position, for underarm waxing the client needs to lie flat with arms held above their head.
- The wax heater must be close to the therapist while working to avoid undue stretching, which can cause fatigue, and also to ensure the wax does not drip on the floor.
- There must be no trailing wires, or wires that are being stretched that could in any way make the wax heater unstable.
- The therapist should not have to overstretch or bend because of insufficient adjustment of the couch.
- Required positioning of the body may require the client to lie in unusual positions. Make sure the client is comfortable and at all times cover areas not being treated to maintain the client's modesty.

Preparing the client

Prepare the client by asking them to remove the necessary items of clothing. They should be allowed privacy and be provided with a gown or towels. Positioning the client for a bikini line wax is not very elegant so you must ensure that some means of cover is available to maintain the client's modesty throughout the treatment.

Protect the client's clothing using disposable bed paper or old clean towels (wax can spoil towels by getting into the fibres). Sugaring paste is easily removed by laundering the towels.

If you are applying wax to the face, protect the client's hair by placing disposable paper or a towel loosely over the hair.

Prepare the skin by wiping over the area to be treated with cotton wool soaked in surgical spirit. This acts as an antiseptic to cleanse the skin and remove oil and perspiration from the surface of the skin. This must be done thoroughly or the wax will not stick to the hairs. An antiseptic solution may be used, especially if the client is allergic to surgical spirit, but it will leave the skin damp. The skin must be allowed to dry before applying the talc. Surgical spirit evaporates immediately, making it a more efficient product to use.

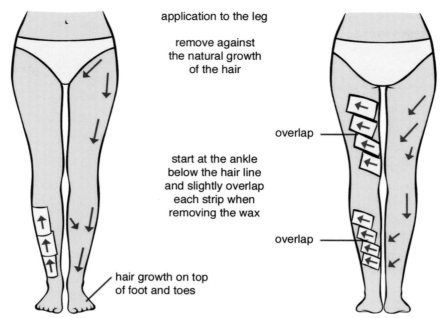

application to the leg

remove against the natural growth of the hair

start at the ankle below the hair line and slightly overlap each strip when removing the wax

overlap

overlap

hair growth on top of foot and toes

Figure 9.3 *Direction of hair growth on legs and strip/warm wax application*

Cleansing the skin should be done against the direction of hair growth to help to lift the hairs from the skin. At the same time, you can take note of the direction of the hair growth and plan how the wax needs to be applied. This is particularly important under the arm where the hair tends to grow in a swirl.

Talcum powder is applied to the area using a pad of cotton wool against the hair growth to ensure that the hairs are lifted from the skin.

Sensitivity test

Each individual has different levels of tolerance to heat, pain and sensitivity to products. It is therefore essential that a sensitivity test along with careful questioning of the client is carried out before starting treatment.

- Skin sensitivity to heat – ensuring the temperature of the wax is suitable for individual clients is essential at the start of each treatment.
- Allergic reactions to products used in waxing – it is essential to ask the client about previous wax treatments and whether they experienced a skin reaction and to observe the skin's reaction during the early stages of the treatment to ensure there is no adverse reaction.
- Removing the hair can be quite painful – clients will vary considerably as to their sensitivity to pain (pain threshold). Sensitivity can be increased when stressed, anxious or during menstruation.

> Different areas of the body will have different sensitivity. The skin around the bikini line area, for example, is very delicate and therefore will respond to temperature more quickly.

At the start of the treatment test a small amount of the wax on the client's skin in the area to be treated. Any reaction can be ascertained by:

- asking the client how it feels – any burning sensation or irritation must be noted
- looking for excessive erythema when wax is removed

- removing the small test area of wax and checking the client's pain tolerance by questioning them.

Any strong reaction must be noted on the client's record card and treatment suspended.

Procedure for waxing
Hot wax

1. Check the consistency of the wax before testing the temperature on your wrist. If it feels comfortable to you, apply to a small area on the client's skin and check the client's tolerance to the temperature.

2. The correct consistency of wax will enable you to control it on the spatula and apply it to the skin without dripping. Twisting the spatula will control the wax as you take it from the heater across to the client. It is essential that the heater is close by on the side of the couch nearest to your working hand. Do not reach across the client for the wax as it may drip wax on their clothing.

3. Apply the wax **against the direction of hair growth** in organised strips, following the growth pattern of the area. Ensure that the application of the wax is systematic. A disorganised approach will take longer and possibly leave hairs behind.

4. Hot wax needs to be applied thickly. This is done by building up one or two layers quickly, before the wax on the skin is allowed to cool. The aim is to achieve thick edges that can be picked up between the fingers, making it easy to pull off. If the application is too thin, the wax will cool rapidly and be too brittle to remove.

5. The wax can be gently pressed onto the skin as it cools to increase its attachment to the hairs.

6. To remove the wax, flick up the bottom edge of the strip, gripping the wax between the thumb and first finger, with the free hand supporting the skin. A long, quick movement is needed to remove the wax. It can be very uncomfortable for the client if it is done slowly. If the hand is lifted, pulling the skin upwards, this can cause bruising, particularly in the bikini line area.

7. Pressure should be applied to the area immediately after the wax has been removed. This helps to reduce the stinging effect.

8. As you gain confidence in applying the wax, you will be able to apply a few strips at a time, removing them in sequence. This will ensure that the treatment is carried out in a commercially acceptable time of 30 minutes for a half-leg wax, with an additional 15 minutes for other areas. Variations to timings depend on how coarse and dense the hair growth is.

9. Any small pieces of wax that remain on the skin can be lifted by using a piece of wax that has just been removed and pressing onto the area. If small pieces of wax are particularly stubborn, dip your finger into the hot wax pan and press it onto the wax remaining on the skin. This should lift it off.

10. If the wax has cooled and become difficult to remove, another layer of hot wax from the heater will soften it sufficiently to aid its removal.

11. Check that the area is free of hair. Odd hairs can be tweezed, but large areas will need a further application of wax. This must be done carefully because the skin will be more sensitive and warm from the previous application. Check with the client that the temperature of the wax is still comfortable before continuing.

12. Apply after-wax lotion either by using gentle effleurage massage or by soothing onto the area with the fingers, or with cotton wool for bikini and underarm areas.

Depilatory waxing

It is important to develop a technique that leaves the minimum of wax on the skin. This is achieved by:

- applying several layers of wax
- leaving thick edges to enable the wax to be lifted off in one go
- not allowing the wax to overheat and become brittle
- removing the wax when it is still slightly warm and pliable
- working in a methodical way over the area.

Warm wax

1. Check the consistency of the wax before testing it on yourself. Remember if the wax is allowed to overheat, it will become very runny and may give off fumes.

2. Test the wax on the inside of your wrist. If it feels comfortable you can apply a small amount on the client in the area to be treated.

3. Take sufficient wax onto the spatula, scrape one side of the spatula on the bar of the heater and hold flat as you move to the client to avoid drips.

4. Apply the wax with the edge of the spatula **following the hair growth** to give a **thin** layer.

5. The skin must be supported with the free hand to prevent overstretching the skin.

6. Take a fabric or paper strip and press it over the wax. Smooth over firmly with the hand to ensure the wax is sticking to the strip.

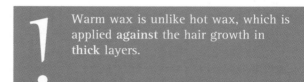

Warm wax is unlike hot wax, which is applied **against** the hair growth in **thick** layers.

7. Grip the bottom edge of the strip with the fingers and pull the strip away very quickly **against** the direction of the hair growth. Stretch and support the skin with the other hand. The strip must be removed parallel to the skin. If the strip is lifted up away from the surface of the skin, it will cause bruising and considerable discomfort to the client.

8. The same strip can be used again until it becomes thick with the wax and does not remove the hair. It can be disposed of by folding the wax sides together and placing in a suitable container away from the client. (The client does not want to see the removed hair lying around the work area.)

9. Aim to work methodically and cleanly.

Roller systems

1. Prepare the heater.

2. Remove the cap from a wax cartridge and attach the roller head. Screw down firmly but not too tightly, so the head can be removed easily.

3. Place the cartridge in the heater.

4. When sufficiently heated (check manufacturer's instructions) hold the cartridge upside down to allow the wax to flow to the roller head. The cartridge is now ready to use.

5. Hold the cartridge by its sides at about 45 degrees and roll **in the direction** of the hair growth.

6. Apply **one thin layer** of wax.

7. Return the cartridge to the heater to keep it at the working temperature.

8. Select a wax strip and place on the wax. Press firmly.

9. Pull the strip off **against the direction** of hair growth.

The routine and aftercare procedure is the same as for warm wax.

ACTIVITY

Compare the heating systems for each of the depilatory wax treatments. Give advantages and disadvantages of each.

If your salon does not use all the waxing methods, visit your local wholesaler and look at the equipment for waxing.

Procedure for sugaring

Hand sugaring

1. Test the temperature of the paste.
2. Take sufficient paste from the container with the fingers. It should be warm and pliable.
3. Spread the ball of paste on the skin using the middle three fingers in a strip about 6 inches long. When working on the legs or using less paste in smaller areas spread to an appropriate length.
4. The skin must be supported using the free hand (clean hand) by stretching the skin.
5. Remove the paste by flicking back along its length without lifting upwards. The process is repeated quickly on the next area until the paste loses its pliability, becomes full of hair and cools.

> ! The art of sugaring relies on the ability of the practitioner to adjust the paste to the correct consistency. This depends on several factors, such as the heat of the hands, the temperature in the room and the climate. Adding a few drops of water using a water spray can alter the consistency dramatically. Selecting a soft paste in winter or a hard paste in the summer can help to achieve the right consistency.

Strip sugaring

There are many similarities between warm waxing and strip sugaring techniques.

1. Apply the strip sugar very thinly using a flexible metal spatula in the direction of the hair growth.
2. Remove the strip sugar with fabric strips against the hair growth, supporting the skin below the strip to be removed.
3. Press the hand on the treated area immediately to help to reduce any stinging.

> ! This technique requires considerable practice. The paste will change from amber to a cream opaque colour as it is worked and cools. The used paste is placed in a palette ready for disposal simply by soaking in hot water. The sugar dissolves leaving the hair, which can be disposed of.

ACTIVITY

Look closely at the hairs you remove on the waxing strip and you will see some with a silver sheath. Others have no sheath, but a black blob on the end. Some hairs may appear straight across at the root as if they have been cut. They may have broken off.

The way the root looks can identify the stage in the life cycle of each hair. Turn to page 289 to read about the life cycle of hair.

Depilatory waxing

Treatment methods for different areas of the body

The majority of hair removal is from the legs and bikini line on the female client, and chest, back and arms on the male client, although the client may request removal of unwanted hair from other areas of the body. This will require a different approach to application and support for the skin. Figure 9.1 illustrates the application methods for different areas.

Bikini line

The skin in this area is very delicate and prone to bruising if too much pressure is applied. It is possible that there will be some bleeding from the follicles. This is because strong coarse hairs have deeper follicles. Make sure that any cuts or open wounds on your hands are covered by waterproof dressing and disposable gloves are worn to protect yourself from infection. Wipe the area to be treated with cotton wool and antiseptic. Dispose of the soiled cotton wool in a closed waste bin. Correct positioning of the client will assist in the easy removal of the hair.

Underarm

Positioning of the client to reveal the whole of the axilla is important. Take special note of the circular direction of hair growth. Follow normal preparation procedure.

Facial including eyebrows, lip and chin

When working on the face, the client's clothing and hair must be protected. The areas to be treated are small, so application must be very careful and neat.

Arms

The arm can be rested on the couch with the client sat on a stool. The hair may be quite long with a tendency to break off if a good technique is not used.

Abdomen

The area is soft, making stretching of the skin more difficult. The client should lie flat on the couch to stretch the area as much as possible.

Legs

Leg waxing can be a full leg or up to and including the knee, which is termed half leg. The toes and tops of the feet may also be included. A system of application must be used to avoid missing areas and to work cleanly and efficiently.

Completing treatment and aftercare

It is important to examine the area you have treated to ensure that all the hairs have been removed and that the treatment meets the client's expectations. If there are just odd hairs that have been missed, these can be removed with tweezers. Larger areas may need a second application, so do not apply any lotions to the skin until you are absolutely sure that the client is satisfied.

Reasons for poor hair removal

If the wax has not removed the hair successfully it could be that:

- the hair was too short for the wax to grip properly
- the area was not cleansed sufficiently to remove body lotion or natural oil on the skin
- warm wax was applied too thickly or allowed to build up on the paper strip
- the wax was applied incorrectly without following the natural hair growth.

Following treatment you should wipe over the area with after-wax lotion, depending on the product used:

- **Oil-soluble wax** will require an oil-based after-wax lotion to remove any traces left on the skin.
- **Water-soluble wax** or sugar paste can be removed by wiping over the leg with wet cotton wool and drying with disposable paper or tissue. Some practitioners recommend that sterile water is used (boiled water) to avoid any infection entering the open follicles.
- **Hot wax** tends to leave small particles of wax behind, so the area will require thorough cleansing with suitable after-wax lotion or surgical spirit, although this can be very harsh on the skin. A soothing cream is massaged onto the skin to cool and moisturise.

This is an ideal opportunity to explain to the client any skin reaction and to give her home care advice.

Contra-actions

It is essential that the therapist is vigilant throughout the treatment in case there are any adverse reactions to the treatment. A normal reaction will be slight erythema and small red spots at the mouth of the follicle in some areas such as the legs. It is possible that blood spots may occur in the bikini line or underarm areas. This is due to coarse terminal hair with deep-seated follicles being plucked from the skin, causing small blood vessels to rupture and bleed.

Adverse reactions (contra-actions)

- prolonged erythema
- burning sensation
- swelling
- irritation
- bruising
- pustules develop at mouth of the follicle a day or two after treatment (folliculitis).

Possible causes

1. Failing to recognise skin reaction following the sensitivity test.
2. Client sensitive to ingredients in the wax or preparation lotion.
3. Wax too hot can cause burns.
4. Wax left uncovered during storage allowing micro-organisms such as airborne spores to get into the wax, causing folliculitis. The wax is warmed providing ideal conditions for the growth of bacteria that cause infection.
5. Pulling the wax strip away from the skin during removal lifts the skin causing blood vessels to rupture (bruising). This is a particular problem in the bikini line area or on the legs where skin might be thin and loose (mature clients).
6. Bruising may occur if the skin is not supported and held firmly when removing the strip or hot wax.

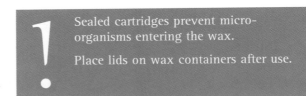

Sealed cartridges prevent micro-organisms entering the wax.

Place lids on wax containers after use.

How to identify histamine reaction to the skin

When the skin is injured, damaged or hypersensitive to a chemical, the mast cells release a substance called **histamine**. A histamine reaction causes the diameter of the blood vessels to increase (vasodilation) and the permeability of the blood vessel walls to increase also, producing a lowering of blood pressure. These effects, in turn, cause the familiar symptoms of an allergy:

- runny nose
- watery eyes
- pain
- swelling
- inflammation
- irritation
- blisters
- pustules.

When released in the lungs, histamine causes the airways to swell, a reaction designed to keep out the offending allergens. Unfortunately, the ultimate result of this response is the wheezing and difficulty in breathing seen in people with asthma or severe hay fever. Occasionally a deadly allergic complication can occur, which can kill, e.g. abnormal reaction to a wasp or bee sting.

A histamine reaction on the skin can be recognised by almost instant erythema, inflammation, localised swelling and irritation.

- **Erythema** is reddening caused by dilated blood capillaries in the dermis. Blood flow increases and speeds up the removal of the irritant and brings antibodies to the area to repair the problem.
- **Inflammation** is the body's natural reaction to infection or injury. The blood supply is increased, bringing extra white blood cells to fight the infection and promote healing Signs of inflammation are redness, swelling, area is painful to the touch and is hot.
- **Swelling** is caused by extra blood being brought to the area by the capillaries, allowing fluid to seep into the surrounding tissue. Blisters may form, or swelling and puffiness of the skin. Swelling acts as a cushion to protect the area from further injury.
- **Irritation** is caused by stimulation of the nerve endings. Severe itching can cause weals and areas of broken skin.

Aftercare advice

Explain the skin reaction to the client and that it will take several hours for the skin to return to normal. During the 24 hours after treatment they must avoid the following:

- wearing tight clothing over the treated area, especially the bikini line
- perfumed products such as deodorant
- make-up over the area treated on the face – tinted medicated lotion can be used if necessary
- sunbathing, sunbed treatment or hot bath – a warm shower is recommended, followed by a soothing after-wax lotion

! If any skin reaction lasts longer than 48 hours or progressively becomes worse, for example irritation or erythema, then the client should return to the salon for advice. The most likely explanation will be an allergic reaction to something in the product used. This can be treated with antiseptic soothing lotion and the condition noted on the client's record card.

Infection will appear as pustules at the mouth of the follicle (folliculitis), caused by bacteria entering the open follicle and indicating poor hygiene procedures by the therapist or incorrect home care by the client. This again can be treated by the use of antiseptic lotion. Serious cases may need to be referred to the doctor.

- swimming
- touching the area.

Clearing away after waxing

Waxing can be a very messy treatment because of the sticky products used. Ensure that the area and equipment are cleaned immediately.

Disposable collars are available for some heaters, preventing unsightly drips during treatment and making cleaning easier.

The wax heater must be thoroughly cleaned before returning to the store cupboard. Special cleaning products are supplied by the manufacturer, or use warm water for water-soluble wax, oil for oil-soluble wax and surgical spirit for hot wax. Sugar paste is water soluble and easily removed with hot water.

The roller system is particularly easy to clear away as heads are disposable or may be cleaned with after-wax cleaner.

Wax heaters should be covered by a lid when cool to ensure that the wax is not left exposed to the air. The warm conditions in the salon can encourage growth of micro-organisms and dust can settle on the surface of the wax. Ensure that there is sufficient wax in the heater before storing. This will save valuable time when you come to reheat the wax for the next client. Wax strips must be disposed of in the waste bin. The plastic bed cover and trolley should be wiped over.

ACTIVITY

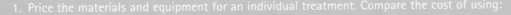

1. Price the materials and equipment for an individual treatment. Compare the cost of using:

   - roller system
   - warm waxing products
   - hot wax.

   Remember the time for treatment will be influenced by the amount of hair, the client's tolerance to the treatment and areas to be treated.

2. List the advantages and disadvantages of each method.

Chapter 10

MANICURE AND PEDICURE

LEVELS
1+2

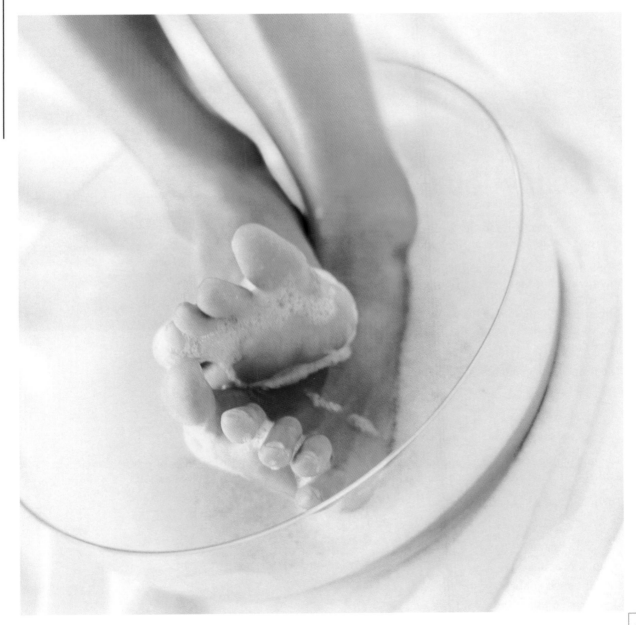

- Preparing the work area for manicure and pedicure treatment
  - tools and equipment
  - products and materials
  - hygiene procedures
  - preparation of the client
  - health and safety
  - codes of practice
- Assessing client needs by preparing a treatment plan
  - client consultation
  - types of treatments
  - contraindications
  - aftercare advice
  - client records
- Manicure and pedicure treatment methods
  - salon requirements – pricing – timing

Introduction

The word 'manicure' comes from the Latin *manus* (hand) and *curo* (care). It involves treatment to improve the appearance of the hands and nails.

Manicuring is a popular service offered in beauty therapy clinics, hairdressing salons and nail salons. The treatment can be offered as part of other salon services, e.g. hair styling, as part of a makeover in the beauty clinic or as preparation for nail extensions.

> **!** It is essential that you have a clear understanding of the growth and structure of the nails, the bones of the hands and feet, and the circulatory system of the hands and feet. Please refer to chapter 14, Related Anatomy and Physiology, for full details.

The purpose of manicure is to:

- recognise common nail disorders and disease
- provide a range of treatments to improve the hands and nails
- offer the client advice on nail care.

The manicurist has an ideal opportunity during the treatment to advise the client on other services available in the salon and to build a relationship with the client through conversation.

The manicure will include:

- filing and shaping the nails
- cuticle treatment
- hand massage
- nail polish application or buffing
- special conditioning treatments.

Client consultation and treatment planning for manicure

Client consultation is a very important part of the service offered to a client. It should be carried out prior to every treatment, whether the client comes for treatment regularly or for a one-off visit.

A client's health and circumstances can change between visits to the salon so it is important to go through the consultation process every time. It may be that you need to check progress against the treatment plan.

Details of client consultation and treatment planning can be found in chapter 5.

Assessing the client's hands and nails for manicure

First, clean the client's hands with cotton wool and surgical spirit. This will give you the opportunity to make a quick assessment of the overall condition.

Assessing the client for treatment involves:

- **Look** – looking at the hands
- **Touch** – touching the skin
- **Question** – questioning the client.

Look and touch

1. **The palms and backs of both hands.** Check for rough, dry patches of skin, any cuts or broken skin, sore areas where rings are worn and the colour of the skin, whether red and chapped or with pigmentation marks. The age of the client will affect the texture of the skin, and disease such as arthritis may be apparent.
2. **The cuticles.** The condition of the cuticle of the nails will immediately indicate whether the client cares for their hands and has regular manicures. Overgrown, torn and dry cuticles will require extra work during the manicure and home care advice to the client.
   Hangnail is a common condition where the cuticle becomes attached to the nail plate and it tears as the nail grows. Infection may then result. Biting the nails and cuticle also leads to thick and torn cuticle.
3. **The nails.** Inspect each nail for:

   - shape – there are many different shaped nails. A distorted shape may be the result of nail damage.
   - colour – slightly pink colour is an indication of healthy nails. Discoloured nails may be the result of smoking or may be caused by the client's work, as in the case of the hairdresser who works with products that colour the hair. (As hair and nails are of a similar composition, that is, made from the protein keratin, the nails will take on the colour in a similar way to the hair.
   - strength – nails will vary in thickness, flexibility and strength. This is normally a hereditary factor although illness, disease and certain drugs can severely affect the condition of the nails. Flaking and splits in the nail should be noted.

It is essential that you can recognise nail disorders and disease to establish contraindications. Refer to page 294 for details.

Question

Discussion with the client at this stage is a very important part of the consultation. If there are any conditions of the hands or nails that are contraindications and prevent you continuing with treatment, this must be handled in a very sensitive manner. An explanation of the condition and why it prevents you from continuing must be given to the client. This will usually be because there is infection present that could be passed on to other clients or therapists. It may be appropriate to explain to the client how the condition could spread and infect others in the home or workplace.

Manicure and pedicure

171

Gentle questioning will enable you to establish the lifestyle, habits and occupation of the client, all of which will have an effect on the condition of the client's hands and nails. You may be able to establish the cause of a condition by asking an open question:

- How do you look after your hands and nails at home?
- What kind of work do you do with your hands?

By talking to the client you will be able to identify their needs and expectations. You will be required to advise them on what the treatment entails, what the end result will be and whether you can meet their expectations. It is important that you discuss the cost of the manicure, especially if you have agreed to include a special treatment that will take extra time.

The questioning phase of the client assessment will allow you to build a rapport with the client and help them to relax, making the treatment more enjoyable.

All the details that you discover through looking, touching and questioning should be included in the treatment plan or record card.

ACTIVITY

1. Look closely at your hands. Write down what you see. Follow the look, touch, question routine. Now repeat the exercise on a colleague.

2. Observe as many different nail shapes as you can by looking at friends and family, and in magazines.

Contraindications to manicure

1. Infection in the area of the hands and nails recognised by the presence of **redness, swelling, pain** and **puss**.
2. Infectious nail disease.
3. Open cuts and abrasions.
4. Allergic reaction to manicure products, the symptoms being **itching, swelling, redness** or **raised blisters**.

ACTIVITY

A teenage girl appears at reception enquiring about treatment for nail biting. She reluctantly displays her hands to the manicurist, which shows severely bitten nails. She is a nervous and shy person. She explains that she is taking school exams at the moment but will finish school in two weeks' time.

1. Write a short paragraph on how you think this client is feeling as she discusses her hands and nails with the manicurist, how the manicurist should handle the client and what advice should be given.

2. Write out a treatment plan for this client to include both salon and home care.

ACTIVITY

Describe four adverse nail conditions, including clearly labelled diagrams of the nail and the nail bed.

Briefly describe for each condition:

1. Salon treatment.

2. Home care advice.

Preparing the work area for a manicure

As a manicurist you may be called upon to treat a client in a whole range of different situations: whilst the client is having other treatment in the beauty therapy salon or in a hairdressing salon, where it will be necessary to move to the client. This will require portable equipment, either a movable manicure station, which is a stool with a small table and drawers to hold products and implements, or a lightweight stool with products and implements carried in a basket.

Wherever you work, it is essential that:

- you ensure the manicure table and stool are at the right height
- seating for the client and manicurist is comfortable; you should not be in a slouching position as this can cause back problems over a period of time and will certainly cause fatigue
- there is good lighting – it may be necessary to have a magnifying lamp or an angle-poise lamp to hand
- there is adequate ventilation – when working with solvents it is essential that fresh air circulates freely (this applies particularly when using artificial nail systems).
- manicure implements are clean, sterilised and arranged in a neat and organised manner with everything to hand
- hot and cold water with liquid soap is available for washing your hands before and after treatment, for soaking the client's nails to soften the cuticle and to remove preparations from the nails during treatment
- there are plenty of clean towels available
- you have on hand disposable materials such as paper towels, tissues and cotton wool.

Client care and preparation

Before examining your client's hands ensure that you have washed your hands thoroughly using a medicated hand wash to minimise the risk of cross infection.

Ensure that your client is seated comfortably. Ask them to remove rings, bracelets or watches, which may hinder the manicure treatment, particularly the massage where hand cream could become lodged between the settings of the jewellery. The client's jewellery should be kept near the client, in a small bowl on the trolley.

The client's cuffs or sleeves need to be turned back and protected with tissue during massaging to avoid clothing coming into contact with manicure products, which may stain.

Before carrying out a manicure treatment the client must be consulted to establish **contraindications** to the treatment (see page 294).

Preparation and hygiene procedures

Preparation and hygiene procedures are an essential part of **all** salon treatments. Manicure implements are small items that can be cleaned and sterilised quite easily and some are disposable. The trolley, whether a specialised manicure trolley with drawers and compartments for storing tools and products or an equipment trolley, must be wiped over with disinfectant. Sterilised and clean tools need to be set out in an orderly way that allows the manicurist to have them close at hand while working. A manicure basket may be used by the mobile therapist.

Refer to chapter 1 for details on general health, safety and hygiene procedure.

Products, implements and equipment
Implements used in manicure

- **Nail scissors** – small curved blades for reducing the length of the nails.
- **Cuticle knife** – small, flat blade used to remove cuticle attached to the nail plate.

- **Cuticle nippers** – small scissor-like implement with a spring action to allow small movements, used to remove excessive, torn or damaged cuticle.
- **Buffer** – an implement that has a surface covered with chamois leather. It is applied to the surface of the nail plate to create a shine using brisk rubbing (friction).
- **Hoof stick** – orange-wood or plastic handle with a rubber end shaped like a hoof, used to gently push back the cuticle from the nail plate.
- **Nail brush** – used to remove all manicure products before the application of nail polish, may also be required to clean dirty nails.
- **Orange stick** – disposable wooden implement with one end slanted and the other pointed, which should be tipped with cotton wool before use. The orange stick has a number of uses: pushing back softened cuticle with the cotton wool-tipped end soaked in cuticle remover, to clean under the nails with pointed end tipped with cotton wool and to remove small amounts of preparations from their pots.
- **Spatula** – used to dispense products from pots (may be made from plastic material that can be washed easily or wood that can be disposed of after use).
- **Emery board** – has a dark side which is coarse and used when nails are to be shortened in length or for filing very strong nails. The light side is fine and used for shaping and smoothing the nails. The emery board should be flexible and 12–15 cm long to allow for good technique during filing of the nails.

> **!** Metal tools can be washed in hot soapy water and sterilised using an autoclave. They can be stored in an ultraviolet cabinet after sterilising. During the manicure small implements should be placed in disinfectant on the trolley.

> **!** The chamois leather cover can be wiped over after use with a damp cloth. The leather covers need changing regularly.

> **!** These items of small equipment can be washed in hot soapy water and placed in the ultraviolet cabinet for storage. The orange stick, spatula and hoof stick should be placed in disinfectant during the manicure.

> **!** Emery boards are made of fibrous board and therefore cannot be washed. They should be offered to the client for use at home or thrown away after use.

Products used in manicure

- **Polish remover** – a solvent that removes nail polish. **Amyl acetate** or **acetone** are the main ingredients in polish remover, with a small amount of oil added to help counteract the drying effect of the solvent on the nail plate.
- **Cuticle massage cream** – an emollient used to soften and nourish the cuticles. **Lanolin** or **mineral oils** are the main ingredients. Cuticle oil may be used in the same way.
- **Cuticle remover** – an alkaline substance that softens the keratin in the skin, allowing the cuticle to be lifted from the nail plate and excess to be removed using cuticle nippers. **Potassium hydroxide** is the main ingredient, which is caustic and very drying if not removed thoroughly after use. Cuticle remover also has a mild bleaching effect and can help to remove stains from the nails.
- **Buffing paste** – a mild abrasive substance which, when combined with the friction action of the buffer, gives the surface of the nail plate a shine. **Pumice, silica** or **stannic oxide** (jeweller's paste) is the main ingredient. Buffing may help increase the circulation to the nail bed and smooth ridges in the nail.
- **Hand cream/lotion** – an emollient that softens and nourishes the skin and assists in the application of massage. **Lanolin, glycerol** or **vegetable oils** are used to make an oil-in-water emulsion. Other ingredients include perfume, colour and some natural products such as aloe vera.

- **Nail polish: base coat, top coat and coloured varnish** – a plastic film that is applied to the nail plate. **Nitro cellulose** and a solvent such as **amyl acetate** are the main ingredients of all nail polish, with various pigments added to give colour, or guanine from fish scales to give a pearlised effect. Good quality nail polish lasts longer, has a good range of colours, has a good consistency for smooth application and dries quickly and evenly.

- **Base coat** – provides a smooth base for the application of coloured varnish, protects the nails from staining, which can be caused by colour pigment, minimises ridges or irregularities in the nail plate and prolongs the life of polish by helping to prevent chipping and peeling.

- **Top coat** – is used to give extra gloss to cream polish and to help the polish last longer by providing a hard surface, protecting the polish from chipping. Top coat is not required for crystalline polish as it can dull the finish.

- **Nail polish thinners** – a solvent used to thin down nail polish that has become thick. **Ethyl acetate** is the active ingredient and should be used very sparingly, otherwise the polish will not harden. Nail polish remover should not be used for thinning polish as the oil it contains will prevent the polish from drying.

- **Nail strengthener** – a product that hardens the keratin in the nail plate. **Formaldehyde** is the active ingredient in these products. Nail strengthener may also be an acrylic substance that provides a hard plastic coating to reinforce the nail.

- **Nail white pencil** – a pencil that is dipped in water before applying to the underside of the free edge. This whitens stained nails. **Titanium dioxide** is the main ingredient.

- **Quick-dry spray** – the cooling effect can speed up the drying process. A **solvent** aerosol spray that evaporates quickly is the basis of this product, although polish that is allowed to dry naturally is longer lasting.

- **Exfoliants** – a product containing abrasive ingredients that remove dead skin scale and help to smooth calluses and rough skin.

- **Masks** – can be adapted from facial products to draw impurities from the skin, soften and improve the texture of the skin.

- **Nail glue** – for minor repairs to the nail plate.

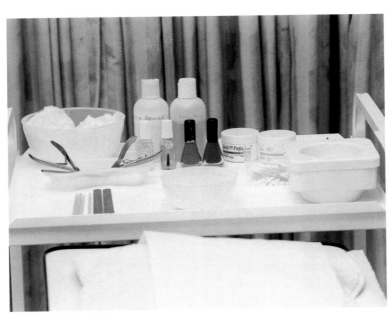

Figure 10.1 *Layout of the manicure trolley*

1. Familiarise yourself with the products used in your salon by reading the labels and manufacturer's instructions, checking the colour, consistency and smell.

2. Make a list of the products needed for a manicure.

3. Visit a department store or chemist shop and look at the range and cost of products and tools available to your clients.

General items of equipment and materials

As well as specialist items of equipment and products, you will need some more general equipment and materials that include:

- **Surgical spirit** – for cleansing the client's hands prior to examination and for disinfecting implements and surfaces.
- **Jar of sanitising fluid** – to hold manicure implements during treatment. This may be disinfectant or sterilising fluid.
- **Cotton wool** – for wiping over the hands when soaked in surgical spirit, for removing nail polish when soaked in polish remover and for tipping the orange stick before use.
- **Tissues** – for wrapping sterilised implements before use, for covering the towelling cushion during polish application to protect the towel.
- **Towels** – for drying client's hands during the manicure. A towel should be placed on your lap during the manicure for drying your hands.
- **Finger bowl** – filled with hot water and a few drops of medicated liquid soap for soaking the client's hands. (The water will have cooled sufficiently by the time the client needs to immerse their hand.)
- **Small receptacle** – for holding the client's jewellery safely while carrying out the manicure.
- **Waste bin** – for immediate disposal of waste materials. A small pedal bin is ideal.
- **Thermal mits** – used to keep hands warm during paraffin wax or mask treatments.

Disposable manicure pads are now available which, because they are disposable, prevent the spread of infection and ensure salon towels are not spoilt due to unsightly marks from nail polish.

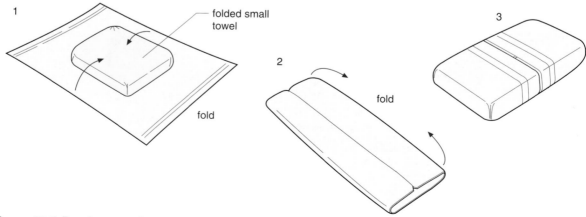

Figure 10.2 *Forming a manicure cushion with towels*

Hygiene procedures and care of small implements and manicure products

Small implements

Always buy good quality stainless steel manicure tools such as the cuticle knife and nippers, so that they can be sterilised without damaging them. Make sure blades are sharp, particularly the cuticle nippers, to avoid tearing the cuticle. Ensure that the hinge moves easily on the nippers to allow for the correct technique to be used.

All small tools must be sterilised after use, whether by autoclave or chemical sterilising fluid, as appropriate, (refer to chapter 1 for sterilising methods). The items should be dried and stored either in an ultraviolet cabinet or placed in a tool roll.

Products

Many manicure products contain solvents and must, therefore, be handled and stored carefully. The COSHH risk assessment for your salon will identify hazards when using these products. (For details of COSHH regulations refer to chapter 1).

It is important that tops are secure on bottles to avoid evaporation of polish remover and solvent in polish.

Particular attention is needed when caring for nail polish. Your clients will want to choose from a wide range of polish colours. Polish should be of excellent quality to ensure a long-lasting finish and good colours.

The necks of the bottles should be wiped after use to ensure that the top fits securely. When the solvent is allowed to evaporate from the polish, it becomes thick and impossible to apply to the nails. Polish will require thorough shaking before use to ensure a smooth well-mixed colour. Small beads are placed in some bottles to ensure thorough mixing. Slight separation may occur in cream polishes, leaving a white deposit or sometimes dark layers form at the top of the bottle.

Coloured polish needs to be stored upright, away from direct sunlight to avoid fading of colour pigments and thickening of the polish due to changes in temperature.

ACTIVITY

Tick the boxes as you prepare for your first manicure.

- Is the manicure area warm and tidy? ☐
- Do you have clean towels available? ☐

Implements
- cuticle nippers ☐
- cuticle knife ☐
- emery board ☐
- buffer ☐
- orange stick ☐
- hoof stick ☐
- spatula ☐

Materials and equipment
- manicure trolley/table ☐
- stool ☐
- water bowl ☐
- waste bin ☐
- cotton wool ☐
- tissues ☐
- manicure cushion ☐
- jar of sterilising fluid or disinfectant ☐
- bowl for client's jewellery ☐

Products
- polish remover ☐
- cuticle massage cream ☐
- nail scissors ☐
- buffing paste ☐
- hand cream ☐
- base coat ☐
- coloured polishes ☐
- top coat ☐
- nail strengthener ☐
- nail white pencil ☐
- quick-dry spray ☐
- French manicure products ☐
- mask ☐
- exfoliant ☐

Work method for manicure

Begin by cleansing the client's hands by wiping with surgical spirit, check for contraindications and discuss the treatment plan with the client.

Quick reference guide for manicure

The following is a quick reference guide to the work method for manicure. Each stage is explained in more detail later in this chapter.

1. Remove nail polish from the nails of both hands.
2. File the nails of the left hand (buffing can be done at this stage without buffing paste).
3. Apply cuticle massage cream.
4. Soak left hand in the bowl of warm soapy water.
5. Repeat steps 2, 3 and 4 on the right hand.
6. Dry left hand thoroughly.
7. Soak the right hand.
8. Treat the cuticles on the left hand by applying cuticle remover and pushing back the cuticle using a cotton wool-tipped orange stick and a hoof stick.
9. Remove excess cuticle using the cuticle knife and cuticle nippers.
10. Use the nail brush to rinse off cuticle remover and any loose cuticle. Dry thoroughly.
11. Repeat steps 6 and 8–10 on the right hand.
12. Massage both hands.
13. Remove grease from the nail plate on each hand using cotton and polish remover.
14. Apply nail polish. Base coat (once), coloured nail polish (twice) and top coat (once). If the client does not want nail polish, buff to a shine.
15. Allow polish to dry completely. Offer the client home care advice.

Procedure for removing nail polish

1. Apply nail polish remover to a pad of cotton wool. Hold between your first two fingers to avoid remover smudging polish on your own nails.
2. Press the pad firmly onto each nail and hold, allowing the solvent to dissolve the cellulose coating on the nail.
3. Slide off the nail in one movement, from the base of the nail to the free edge, to prevent the colour spreading over the finger.
4. It is sometimes necessary to repeat with fresh cotton wool or to apply remover to a cotton wool-tipped orange stick and remove colour from around the cuticle.
5. Ensure there are no traces of old polish as this will spoil the benefits of treatment and the final appearance of the nails.
6. Remember to place the top on the bottle of remover to prevent the solvent evaporating.

Shaping the nails

This is an important stage in the manicure. You must discuss the shaping of the nails with the client. They

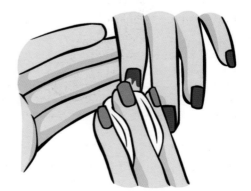

Figure 10.3 *Removing nail polish*

may have very strong views. There are a number of factors that must be taken into consideration at this stage:

- Natural shape and length of the nails – are they equal in length and shape?
- Condition and strength of the nails – are the nails brittle, dry, thin?
- Client's occupation – for example, a nurse cannot have long, pointed nails.
- Shape of the hands and fingers.
- **Oval** – the ideal shape as it provides strength to the free edge.
- **Square** – a square shape is popular, particularly for long nails and nail extensions.
- **Pointed** – pointed nails require shaping down the nail wall, which causes weakness to the free edge. Splits low down in the nail plate can result.

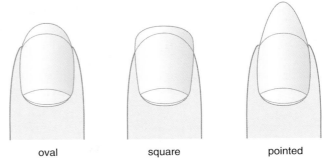

oval   square   pointed

Figure 10.4 *The effects of different nail shapes*

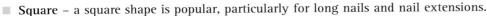
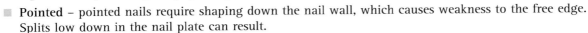

ACTIVITY

Look at nail shapes in fashion magazines to establish the latest fashion trends.

Shortening the nails

It may be necessary to shorten excessively long nails. This is best carried out using sharp, curved nail scissors, followed by filing. The nail should be supported while cutting the free edge. Very hard brittle nails may require soaking first. The nail should be cut straight across leaving it slightly longer than the finished shape to allow for filing.

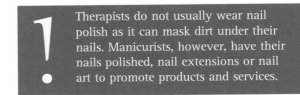

Therapists do not usually wear nail polish as it can mask dirt under their nails. Manicurists, however, have their nails polished, nail extensions or nail art to promote products and services.

Filing

Good quality emery boards should always be used. They should be flexible and 12–15 cm in length to allow long sweeping movements when filing. The emery board will have different degrees of coarseness on either side, indicated by the colour. The dark side is coarse and used for reducing the length of strong nails. The finer side is light in colour and used for shaping and smoothing the nails. The emery board should be held with the thumb on the side not being used and four fingers on the other side.

Nails must be filed in one direction, from the side to the centre of the nail tip, making an oval-shaped movement. Long, swift, rhythmical strokes should be used. Sawing movements backwards and forwards can damage the nail, particularly if soft and delicate. Filing into the corners of the nail by pulling back the nail wall will weaken the nails and reduce the support to the free edge. This can lead to splits and breaking of the nail.

Bevelling is used after shaping to remove any fragments left after filing and to smooth the edge of the nail. The fine side is used to file under the free edge at 45 degrees.

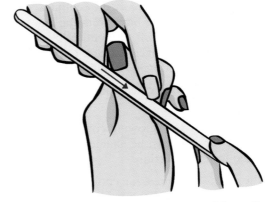

File in one direction to the centre of the nail

Figure 10.5 *Filing nails*

Cuticle treatment

The aim of treatment is to reduce dryness and overgrown, torn or thick cuticles, leaving the skin around the nail neat, soft and pliable.

Cuticle work is an important stage in the manicure. The treatment required will depend on the condition of the client's hands and nails. It may take several manicures to treat poor cuticles. This should be indicated in the treatment plan.

Cuticle massage cream is applied first. A small amount is dispensed from the pot using an orange stick and applied to each nail. The cream is massaged into the nail and surrounding skin. The emollient makes the cuticles pliable and the massage increases circulation to the tips of the fingers.

Soaking the fingers in hot soapy water will soften the skin and clean the nails.

Cuticle remover and using implements is the next stage of cuticle treatment. One of the major problems with untreated cuticles is that the skin adheres to the nail plate and becomes torn, causing hangnails. Cuticle remover and the use of special implements to remove cuticle from the nail plate and trim excess cuticle from around the nail is advised.

After soaking, the hands are dried and cuticle remover applied all around the cuticle and under the free edge. Cuticle remover is slightly caustic and breaks down the keratin in the skin, allowing the cuticle to be loosened. It may also remove stains from the nail plate.

A cotton wool-tipped **orange stick** is used to push back the cuticle. A rolling movement is used, starting halfway up the nail plate and rolling down to the base of the nail, gently pushing back the cuticle.

The **hoof stick**, with its flexible rubber hoof-shaped end, is designed to continue the lifting of cuticle from the nail plate. Use flat circular movements, working downwards to the base of the nail plate.

The **cuticle knife** should be held flat in the palm of the hand, not upright between the thumb and first finger, like a pencil. The flat position ensures that the length of the blade is used to gently 'scrape' any cuticle sticking to the nail plate, rather than using the point of the blade, which could damage the matrix.

The blade is stroked in one direction and must be moistened throughout by dipping into the manicure bowl. This prevents scratching the nail plate.

Cleansing under the free edge to remove dirt and dead skin is carried out using a cotton wool-tipped orange stick, taking care not to dig into the nail bed.

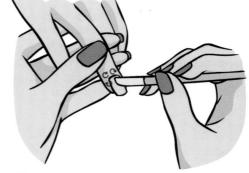

Circular movements pushing back the cuticle

Figure 10.6 *Pushing back cuticles*

The **cuticle nippers** are used to cut away excess cuticle that has been lifted from the nail plate during treatment or to cut off torn cuticle. Some clients require careful cuticle work at this stage, due to overgrown or damaged cuticles, often caused by the client biting the nails and surrounding skin or lack of care to hands and nails, resulting in dryness and damage.

Hangnail may be treated but special care must be taken not to pull at the skin, causing discomfort to the client.

Excessive forward-growing cuticle (**pterygium**) can be improved with very careful use of cuticle nippers. Cuticle nippers must be handled very carefully to avoid tearing the cuticle and causing bleeding, which could lead to infection.

The aim is to remove the cuticle in one piece so that there are no rough edges. This requires the correct holding of the nippers. They should be held in the palm of the hand with the spring between the handles moving smoothly. The nipper blades are then used in a 'nibbling' action in a curved movement around the base of the nail.

Pulling the cuticle as a result of poor technique or blunt blades will cause tearing and possibly bleeding. Trimming the cuticles too closely will weaken the protection they give to the nail and increase the risk of infection.

It is not always necessary to use the cuticle nippers. For example, clients who have regular manicures and a good home care routine may not accumulate a great deal of cuticle.

The **nail brush** is used next. Dipping the treated nails into the water in the manicure bowl, the brush is used from the cuticle to the free edge. This gets rid of the dead skin removed during this stage of the manicure and, most importantly, flushes away the cuticle remover, which is slightly caustic and, if left on the nails, would be very drying.

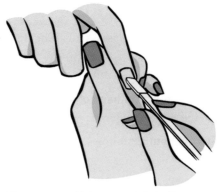

Figure 10.7 *Using a cuticle knife*

Inspect the nails and cuticles

When cuticle work is completed on both hands it is important to evaluate the treatment so far. Visual checks should include:

- Are the nails an even shape?
- Does the free edge of the nails need bevelling to remove any layers or snags left after filing?
- Do the nails require any repair?
- Are the cuticles pushed back exposing as much lanula as possible?

Any minor shaping or correcting rough or torn cuticle should be done at this stage.

You should gain the client's approval and refer to the treatment plan. Any future treatment to improve the nails and surrounding skin should be discussed and recorded in the treatment plan.

Hand massage

Hand massage can be the most enjoyable part of the manicure for the client. Allow sufficient time to ensure that the massage is not rushed and that the full benefits are experienced.

The benefits of hand massage are to:

- relax the client
- increase the blood and lymphatic flow to the hands and fingers
- improve mobility in the joints
- spread the hand cream or lotion
- nourish and smooth the surface of the skin by helping the skin to absorb the hand cream
- remove loose skin cells.

Massage of the hand uses:

- **Effleurage** – stroking movements using the palm of the hand or the tips of the fingers. These are flowing movements using very little pressure to spread the hand cream. Effleurage is applied in an upward movement, towards the heart and should start and end the routine.
- **Petrissage** – kneading movements, which are deeper and more stimulating. Petrissage increases lymphatic and blood flow and can aid the removal of loose skin cells.
- **Rotations** – circular movements applied to the joints to aid mobility.

Where possible the client should remove long-sleeved items of clothing or roll sleeves up to the elbow to prevent hand cream from soiling clothing. The client may wish to have massage to the lower arm and hand, in which case short sleeves are essential. Otherwise the massage is applied to the wrist and hand only.

Manicure and pedicure

Massage routine

The area to be massaged can be divided into:

- the forearm and elbow
- the wrist
- the palm and back of the hand
- the digits (fingers).

If your routine follows a set pattern it will make it easier for you to remember and ensure a thorough massage.

Hand massage

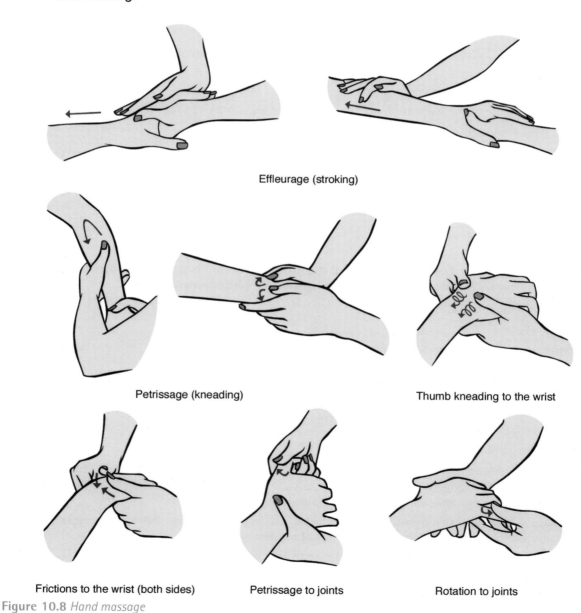

Effleurage (stroking)

Petrissage (kneading)

Thumb kneading to the wrist

Frictions to the wrist (both sides)

Petrissage to joints

Rotation to joints

Figure 10.8 *Hand massage*

Quick reference guide for hand massage

This is a quick reference guide to help you while you are practising. The full procedure follows.

1. Apply sufficient hand cream.
2. Effleurage from fingers to the elbow 3–4 times.
3. Petrissage (thumb-kneading) to the forearm (wrist to elbow) 3 times.
4. Thumb-knead the top of wrist (carpels).
5. Criss-cross thumb movements (friction) to the underside of wrist.
6. Rotate wrist 3 times in each direction.
7. Flex wrist 2–3 times.
8. Thumb-knead the back of the hand.
9. Thumb-knead the palm.
10. Thumb-knead the joints of the fingers.
11. Rotate fingers 3 times in each direction.
12. Finger 'snapping'.
13. Effleurage to finish.

The forearm

1. Take sufficient hand cream from the container using a spatula or pour lotion directly into your hands. Take care not to apply too much lotion as it becomes messy and your hands will not massage effectively if the skin is too slippery. It is also unnecessarily extravagant and wasteful.
2. Effleurage from the fingers to the elbow with a small amount of pressure to spread the cream evenly. Support the client's hand and mould your other hand around the upper surface of the arm as you move up to the elbow. Return, moving down the underside of the arm. It should not be necessary for you to alternate your hands, use whichever is most natural and comfortable for you. Repeat 3–4 times.
3. Petrissage (thumb-kneading) to the forearm using the thumb of one hand in circular movements, while supporting the client's arm with the other hand. Slide back down to the wrist and repeat.

The wrist

1. Thumb-knead the wrist using small circular movements, as if you were feeling for all the intricate little bones of the wrist.
2. Apply rapid thumb movements (friction) in a criss-cross action to the inside of the wrist. This stimulates the main artery (radial) leading to the hand.
3. Rotate the wrist by placing the client's elbow on the manicure cushion and, while supporting the forearm, grip the fingers and rotate in one direction and then the other. Repeat 6 times in each direction.
4. Flex the wrist by placing the client's elbow on the manicure cushion and, while supporting the forearm, interlock your fingers with the client's and push the hand back slowly and firmly. Repeat 2–3 times.

Palm and back of the hand

1. Thumb-knead the back of the hand from the knuckles to the wrist using both thumbs, in circular movements.
2. Thumb-knead the palm by turning the hand over and applying deep circular movements with both thumbs to the fleshy part of the palm.

The fingers

1. Thumb-knead the joints of the fingers and thumb.
2. Rotate fingers by supporting the hand and holding each finger individually, rotate first in one direction 3 times and then in the other.
3. Finger 'snapping' – use the first two fingers of your hand to twist and pull the finger from the knuckle to the fingertip, as if pulling blood through the vessels to the very tip of the finger.

To complete the massage

The final movement in the massage routine is to effleurage the hand and forearm 5–6 times, finishing with your hand slowly working to the tips of the client's fingers, placing them on the manicure cushion. The client's hand can be wrapped in a towel to keep it warm while repeating the massage routine on the other hand.

Effleurage can be used to link movements together or to warm up an area that has not been worked on for some time and may be getting cold.

Any excess massage cream/lotion left on the hands can be wiped off with a tissue. The client's hands should not be left oily or sticky.

Buffing

Buffing may be incorporated in the manicure at one of two stages in the routine:

1. After filing, without using buffing paste to increase the circulation to the nail, or with buffing paste to begin smoothing the surface of the nail plate. Nails with small ridges may benefit from buffing with paste as it is slightly abrasive. Deep ridges or damage to the nail plate will not be reduced by buffing.

2. After hand massage, as an alternative to nail polish:
   - for male clients
   - clients who want a natural shine to their nails
   - for those in occupations where polish would not be appropriate for hygiene reasons: nurses, those working with food.

Buffing method

1. A very small amount of buffing paste is taken from the container using an orange stick. Care should be taken not to use too much paste or to spread it onto the cuticle, as it is difficult to remove.

2. Place a small dot of paste on the centre of each nail plate of the hand being treated.

3. Spread the paste towards the free edge with the ball of the thumb before using the buffer.

4. Hold the buffer between the first two fingers, although this may depend on the style of the buffer. Holding the buffer correctly ensures that a light movement can be used, therefore avoiding thumping the nail.

5. Stroke the buffer fairly quickly **in one direction only**, from the cuticle to the free edge 15–20 times for

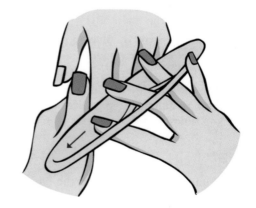

Buff in one direction only

Figure 10.9 *Nail buffing*

each nail or until you have created a shine. Ensure that buffing paste is not spread onto the surrounding skin.

Nail polish application

Choosing nail polish

You would normally discuss the colour and type of nail polish with the client during the consultation. The client may have definite views or rely on you to advise. The choice of colour should be recorded on the record card.

Points to be considered when choosing polish are:

- the age and colour of the skin – older hands that are uneven in colour and have red and blue tones do not suit orange and peach colours
- bright colours draw attention to the hands and require the nails to be an even length and shape
- dark nail polish will draw attention to the nails and make small nails look even smaller
- pearlised polish shows up any imperfections in the nail plate
- a special occasion may require matching of the polish to an outfit or other make-up colouring.

Nail polish application

The final stage of the manicure is the application of nail polish. Ensure that you have allowed sufficient time when planning the treatment for careful application. (See figure 10.11.)

1. Place a tissue over the manicure cushion to avoid spoiling the towels.
2. Ask the client to replace jewellery to avoid smudging the nail polish at the end of the treatment. Ensure that the nails are free from grease and manicure preparations by wiping over with nail polish remover on cotton wool. Make sure there are no cotton wool fibres left on the nails.
3. It may be appropriate to ask the client to pay for the treatment at this stage so there is no risk of damaging the finished application.
4. Apply a base coat first, followed by two coats of coloured polish and then a top coat. Pearlised crystalline and frosted polish do not require top coat, so a third coat of colour may be applied.
5. To avoid risk of smudging the polish during application it is a good idea for the right-handed manicurist to start with the little finger of the client's left hand and work towards the thumb, repeating on the right hand. (The left-handed manicurist should reverse the procedure.)
6. The way in which the client's finger is supported is important to prevent catching the nails during application.

The colours and style of application of polish will depend on fashion and to some extent the length and shape of the nails:

- the whole of the nail plate can be polished
- the lanula can be left unpolished
- the nail plate can be polished, leaving a gap at the sides, to give an illusion of length, which is particularly useful on broad thumb nails
- the nail plate can be polished natural pink, with free edge polished white (**French manicure**).

Allergic reaction to nail polish

Formaldehyde resin is thought to be the cause of allergy to nail polish. Itchiness and inflammation, followed by dry flaking skin, is likely to occur around the eyes or areas where the nails come into contact with the skin, such as the face and neck.

Removing excess polish

Polishing the nails is very skilled work and requires a great deal of practice. The most experienced manicurists sometimes make mistakes and too much polish on the brush can lead to flooding of the cuticle. This can be rectified by using a cotton wool-tipped orange stick dipped in polish remover to carefully work around the cuticle taking off any polish. This method should only be used when occasional mistakes are made during application. Aim to apply polish without catching the surrounding skin.

Drying

It is essential that the polish is completely dry before the client leaves the salon. If possible, each coat should be allowed to dry before the next one is applied. Thick and poor quality polishes or over-thinned polish may not dry in the time available, so should be avoided. The client may request repolishing if the polish smudges after a reasonable amount of time. Quick-drying aerosols can speed up drying time by the rapid evaporation of the spray on the nails. A fine film of oil is left behind, which reduces the tackiness of newly polished nails.

Repairing a smudge

It can be extremely annoying if the client or the manicurist catches the nails before the polish is dry. If the nail is badly smudged, then it is advisable to remove the polish from the nail and reapply, starting with base coat. Sometimes a minor smudge can be dealt with by applying polish remover to the nail. This must be done carefully by applying polish remover to the tip of your finger and smoothing over the smudged nail in one direction towards the free edge.

This may be repeated, taking care not to flood the nail with remover.

If successful, the nail should be left to dry and a further coat of coloured polish applied if necessary.

French manicure

The French manicure is designed to show off and enhance the natural appearance of healthy nails. A healthy nail has a pink nail bed, white lanula and free edge. (See figure 10.10.)

The manicure or pedicure follows the normal routine, with careful attention to cuticle work to expose the lanula and filing to provide a good shape to the free edge. The free edge is whitened by:

- using a white pencil under the free edge
- applying white tape to highlight the free edge
- applying white nail polish to the free edge. A stencil can be used to achieve a perfect line following the hyponychium (flesh line).

The whole of the nail plate is then polished with a pink translucent polish to complete the look.

Contra-actions to manicure

1. Allergic reactions can occur to many of the products used in manicure, e.g. lanolin in hand cream, colour pigment, perfume or the solvents used in nail polish. The reaction may occur on the hands or around the nails, but it is quite common for allergies to occur around the eyes, for example, or where the allergen has come into contact with the skin by touching, e.g. the face or neck.

A serious allergic reaction can be seen initially as:

- redness
- irritation
- swelling.

After a while the skin may become:

- dry and scaly
- blistered
- infected with weeping sores.

2. Infection around the nail where the cuticle has been over-trimmed or torn.
3. Staining of the nail plate due to overuse of strong-coloured polish or using strong-coloured polish without a base coat.

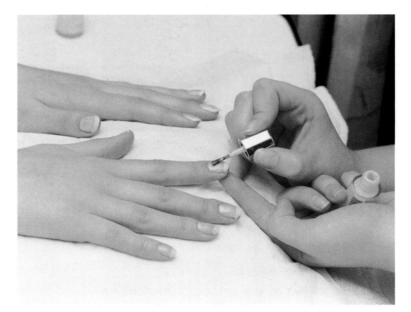

Figure 10.10 *French manicure*

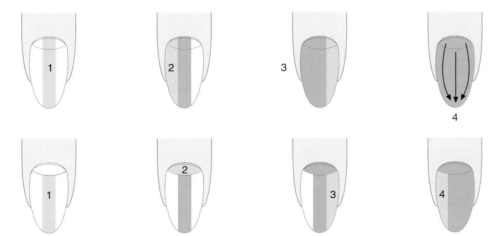

Figure 10.11 *Different polish applications*

Select a dark-coloured varnish and ask three friends or colleagues with different nail shapes and lengths to act as models. For example:

- short square-shaped nails
- long oval-shaped nails
- mis-shaped nails.

Begin by wiping over the nails with polish remover and apply a base coat. Do not choose old thick polishes just because you are practising. Apply two coats. Do not use an orange stick to remove polish from the cuticle.

Evaluate your polish application in each case using the following checklist and add a comment on the suitability of the dark colour for each of the models.

Polish application checklist	Yes	No
Was the polish a good consistency?	☐	☐
Did you start with the finger and work towards the thumb?	☐	☐
Did you use the minimum number of strokes to apply the polish?	☐	☐
Was the polish smooth on the nail?	☐	☐
Did the polish cover the nail plate evenly?	☐	☐
Was there any polish on the cuticle or surrounding skin?	☐	☐
Were any of the nails smudged?	☐	☐

Evaluation of the manicure

Always check the client's satisfaction in line with the treatment plan:

- Have you completed the treatment as agreed?
- Is the client pleased with the manicure? (always ask the client before they leave the salon)
- Do you have any recommendations for further treatment to maintain or improve the client's hands and nails?
- Was the treatment completed in a commercially acceptable time of 45 minutes?
- If extra treatment such as paraffin wax was included, was this completed in 15 minutes?

Aftercare advice

Offering the client aftercare advice is an important part of salon service.

You can use the opportunity to:

- advise on home care
- recommend further treatment
- retail cosmetics.

Advise the client to:

- wear protective gloves when doing gardening, housework and washing-up as detergents and chemicals will dry the skin and nails

- dry the hands thoroughly after washing and apply hand cream
- protect the hands in cold weather by wearing warm gloves
- use hand cream and cuticle cream just before going to bed
- not to use fingernails to open lids
- protect weak and brittle nails with nail strengthener
- always use an emery board for filing the nails, not a metal file as they create heat by friction and dry out the nail plate
- buff the nails as this will improve circulation to the nail bed and give the nails a natural shine
- ensure a good diet – calcium, iron and vitamin A are necessary for nail health.

Pedicure
Care of the feet

In general, people do not look after their feet. Women in particular will follow fashion trends in footwear at the expense of comfort and correctly fitting shoes. This can lead to long-term foot disorders such as bunions and calluses, as well as poor posture.

Choosing the correct shoes for everyday wear, particularly for work, is important. For example, the beauty therapist, who stands for long hours in a very warm environment, should choose shoes that support the foot. A good fit is necessary so that the toes are not cramped and the heels are not chafed, causing blisters and hard skin.

A low heel rather than a flat shoe gives support to the arch of the foot. Equally, very high heels are extremely tiring if worn for long periods of time. They tend to change the natural posture by throwing the weight forward.

The purpose of pedicure is to:

- improve the appearance of the feet and nails
- relax tired and aching feet
- reduce hard skin on the feet
- offer advice on care of the feet and referral as necessary to a chiropodist.

The pedicure will include:

- reducing the length of the nails
- cuticle treatment
- removal of hard skin
- foot massage
- nail polish application as required.

Much of the routine for manicure applies to pedicure.

The major differences are:

- the positioning of the client and therapist for treatment
- the treatment of hard skin and the implements and products used
- foot massage routine.

Contraindications to pedicure

- infectious conditions – clients may be unaware of conditions of the feet that require referral to a doctor or chiropodist (e.g. verrucae, athlete's foot)
- open wounds such as burst blisters, cuts or abrasions.

(See page 293 for details of nail disorders, which apply to feet as well as hands.)

Preparation and hygiene procedures for pedicure

All general hygiene procedures for salon treatments apply, as do the routine hygiene procedures for manicure relating to implements, equipment and the work area.

(Refer to pages 173 and 177 for details.)

Client preparation

Soaking the client's feet prior to thorough examination and treatment is essential. A quick visual check of both feet is required and you should question the client regarding any foot problems.

1. Prepare a foot bowl with warm water and antiseptic liquid soap.
2. Place both feet in the water for 3–5 minutes. This will help relax the client, as well as freshen the feet prior to treatment.
3. It is a good idea at this stage to dry the feet with disposable paper towels in case, after closer examination, infectious foot disease is present.

Clients are often unaware of conditions such as athlete's foot and you may not be able to see it without close examination between the toes. This can be carried out discreetly whilst drying the feet. The client can be advised and referred to a chiropodist or doctor. The treatment should be cancelled until the condition has cleared. The foot bowl will need to be disinfected, paper towels disposed of immediately and you must wash your hands very thoroughly.

Products, implements and equipment

Pedicure treatment will require the same products and implements as for manicure, with the following additions:

- foot bowl
- nail clippers or curved scissors
- cuticle trimmer
- callous file or corn rasp for removing hard skin
- exfoliating cream or hard-skin remover
- toe separators

(A buffer is not required.)

Procedure for pedicure

The basic manicure routine is followed throughout, except where extra treatment is required to deal with foot-specific conditions such as hard and dry skin and thickened nails. These are discussed later in this chapter.

Quick reference guide for pedicure

1. Soak both feet in warm soapy water.
2. Dry both feet with disposable paper and inspect the feet closely.
3. If there are no contraindications present continue with treatment.
4. Remove nail polish.
5. Replenish the water in the foot bath to ensure that it is warm.

6. Cut nails on the left foot with curved scissors or nail clippers as required.

7. File.

8. Apply cuticle massage cream.

9. Soak.

10. Repeat steps 6–9 on the other foot.

11. Dry the left foot thoroughly.

12. Soak the right foot (check with the client that the water is still warm).

13. Treat the cuticles on the left foot by applying cuticle remover and pushing back the cuticle using the cotton wool-tipped orange stick.

14. Remove excess cuticle with the cuticle knife and cuticle nippers.

15. Use a callous file or rasp, if required, to remove the build-up of hard skin, usually on the pads of the foot, heel and little toes.

16. Apply hard-skin remover to the sole of the foot, heels and tops of the toes, as required. Using the heel of the hand apply with vigorous rubbing to help exfoliate the hard skin.

17. Rinse off the cuticle remover, hard-skin remover and exfoliated skin in the foot bath using a wad of cotton wool.

18. Dry the left foot and wrap in a dry towel to keep warm.

19. Repeat stages 13–18 on the right foot.

20. Massage both feet (and lower leg as required).

21. Remove any remaining massage cream from the nail plate on each foot with polish remover on a pad of cotton wool.

22. Use toe separators or tissues twisted between the toes to separate the toes and prevent the polish smudging.

23. Apply polish. Base coat (once), coloured polish (twice) and top coat (once).

24. Allow polish to dry completely. This is absolutely essential before replacing tights/stockings and shoes.

25. Give home care advice to the client.

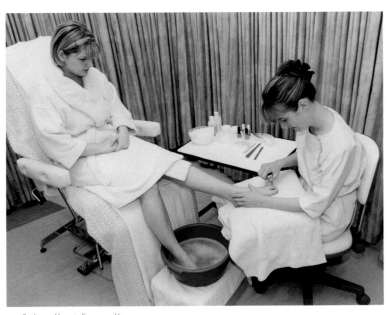

Figure 10.12 *Position of the client for pedicure*

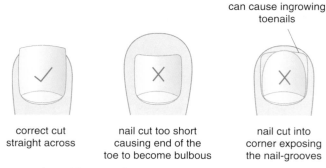

can cause ingrowing
toenails

correct cut
straight across

nail cut too short
causing end of the
toe to become bulbous

nail cut into
corner exposing
the nail-grooves

Figure 10.13 *Toenails cut correctly and incorrectly*

Cutting the toenails

Toenails should be cut straight across to avoid ingrowing nails. After soaking the feet to soften the nails, the nail clippers or sharp scissors can be used, followed by filing with the coarse side of an emery board.

Pressure from wearing shoes can cause the nails to thicken, particularly the big toenails. Thickened toenails are particularly common in older clients. It may be necessary to refer the client to a chiropodist for nails to be cut.

The nails protect the ends of the toes and should not be cut too short as this will cause discomfort and pressure on the ends of the toes. (See figure 10.13.)

Cuticle work

The cuticles on the toes are often quite thick and overgrown unless the client cares for their feet and has regular pedicures. The cuticles can be treated in the same way as in a manicure, but extra time will be needed for using the cuticle nippers or cuticle trimmer to cut excess cuticle from around the nails. The cuticle trimmer should only be used on hard raised cuticle. It is a small V-shaped implement. The V has a sharp cutting edge that trims excess cuticle as it is passed around the base of the nail.

Removing hard skin

Hard skin develops on the feet as a form of protection in those areas that receive the greatest pressure and rubbing. The balls of the feet and heels are commonly affected. You should remove or smooth only unsightly dry skin to improve the appearance of the feet. It is the job of the chiropodist to deal with excessive hard skin including calluses and corns.

A range of implements and products can be used for treating hard skin. The callus file and corn rasp are metal files used to lift dead hard skin from the foot using a quick filing movement (see figure 10.14). Hard-skin remover/exfoliants use chemicals or abrasive ingredients to remove hard skin.

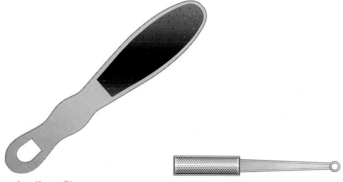

Figure 10.14 *Corn rasp and callous file*

Foot massage

Foot massage is very relaxing for the client. It is important that the client is positioned comfortably to avoid strain as pressure is applied during the massage. Refer to page 181 for the benefits of massage and massage movements.

It is usual to massage the feet and lower leg, but if the client is wearing trousers they may wish to have just the feet and ankles treated. Remember to protect clothing from the lotion by using tissues.

Remember to follow a sequence, as for hand massage, by dividing the area to be massaged into the:

- lower leg
- ankle
- top and sole of the foot
- toes.

See figure 10.15.

Quick reference guide for foot massage

1. Apply sufficient hand cream.
2. Effleurage from foot to the knee 6 times.
3. Petrissage (thumb-kneading) the front of the leg.
4. Petrissage the calf (palmar kneading).
5. Thumb-kneading round the ankle bone.
6. Thumb-kneading to the Achilles tendon.
7. Palmar kneading over the medial arch.
8. Thumb-kneading underneath the foot and toes.
9. Hacking to the sole of the foot.
10. Deep stroking of the foot.
11. Whipping of the toes.
12. Toe snatching.
13. Effleurage to the leg and foot 6 times.

Nail polish application

The procedure for applying polish is very similar to manicure, except the nails, apart from the big toenail, are often very small, making application more tedious.

Toes do not span naturally like fingers, so toe separators are required to keep them apart while the polish is drying. Toe separators made from foam can be obtained from beauty suppliers but, as they cannot be sterilised easily, it is more appropriate to use folded tissues that can be disposed of after treatment. Cotton wool may be used but the fibres may get onto the nails and spoil the finished polish application.

Aftercare advice

Offering advice to your clients after the pedicure will help them look after their feet between visits. It is also an opportunity to recommend retail products such as foot powders, sprays, foot baths and hard-skin remover.

Aftercare advice will differ for each client, depending on the condition of their feet. It may include the following:

- wash feet daily (more often if suffering from excessively sweaty feet and in hot weather)
- make sure feet are thoroughly dry after washing, especially between the toes

Manicure and pedicure

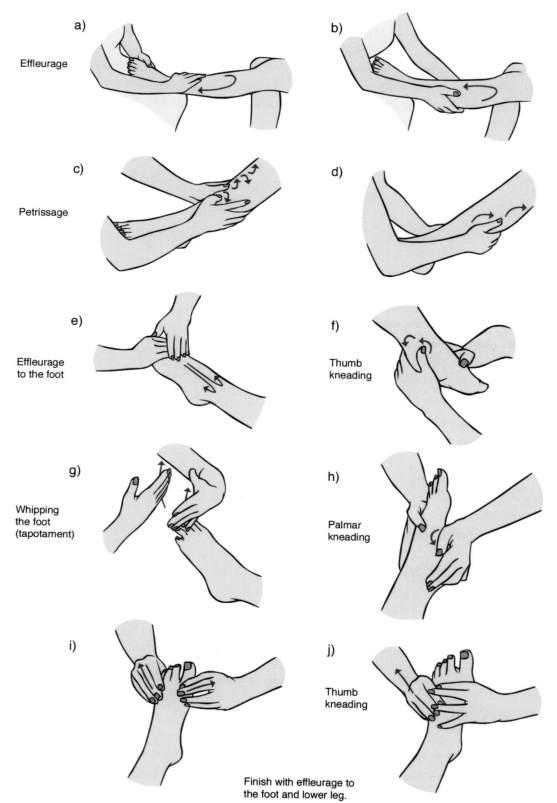

a)

Effleurage

b)

c)

Petrissage

d)

e)

Effleurage
to the foot

f)

Thumb
kneading

g)

Whipping
the foot
(tapotament)

h)

Palmar
kneading

i)

j)

Thumb
kneading

Finish with effleurage to
the foot and lower leg.

Figure 10.15 *Foot massage*

- change socks or tights daily
- allow the air to circulate around the feet by going barefoot whenever it is comfortable and safe to do so
- buy good quality shoes that fit properly (changing to shoes with different heels can help with tired feet)
- wearing very high heels over long periods of time should be avoided as they cause tired sore feet and poor posture
- avoid wearing synthetic shoes such as trainers over long periods of time as they cause the feet to sweat
- any infection or serious condition of the feet must be referred to a doctor or chiropodist (regular visits to a chiropodist may be necessary for some clients with ongoing foot problems).

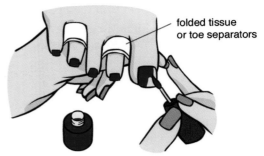

folded tissue or toe separators

Figure 10.16 *Applying polish to toes*

Evaluation of treatment

It is essential at the end of any treatment to evaluate the treatment against the treatment plan.

- Have you met the client's expectations? Are they satisfied with the pedicure? Have you done what you set out to do in your treatment plan? This could be special attention to the cuticle or hard-skin removal, for example.
- Was the pedicure carried out in a commercially acceptable time? A pedicure will take longer than a manicure because of the time needed to treat the cuticles and hard skin. A client who cares for their feet and has regular pedicures will require 30–35 minutes for treatment. If the feet require extra attention 45 minutes will be needed. The time you expect to take should be discussed with the client as part of the treatment plan.
- Was the pedicure of professional quality? You must aim to provide careful and accurate treatment in the best possible time to be commercially viable. Following your evaluation of the pedicure, was it the best you could do or are there things that require improvement and more practice?

ACTIVITY

Using the checklist on page 190 evaluate your pedicure treatment.

Evidence of your performance can be judged by:

- the client's comments – enter verbal or written comments in your diary or log
- colleagues in the workplace, who work with you and observe you – ask them to provide a written witness testimony
- your teacher or assessor who will mark your assessment book.

Special nail treatments
Manicure for a male client

It is necessary to adapt the routine of the manicure to meet the needs of male clients. Less time is required for varnish application and shaping the nails and more time may be spent on cuticle work and hand massage.

1. File nails to a shorter length and a gentle round or square shape.
2. Use unperfumed hand cream for the hand massage.

3. Use deeper movements in the massage and increase the time for massage.

4. Buff the nails with buffing paste to create a natural shine, rather than using polish. Some clients may wish to have a coat of clear polish.

Repolish

Regular manicure clients may on occasions request that their nails are polished without a full manicure. It may be that the client needs to change the nail colour between manicures to match an outfit or that they dislike the colour applied. Whatever the reason, a repolish must only be carried out on perfectly manicured nails to ensure that a professional finish can be achieved.

Repolish routine

1. Cleanse the client's hand with surgical spirit in the normal way.

2. Briefly check the shape of the nails and file if necessary.

3. All traces of polish must be removed on the left hand and fingers placed in the finger bowl to soak. This will remove all traces of polish remover and cleanse the nails.

4. Remove the polish from the other hand and place it in the manicure bowl, having removed the left hand.

5. Thoroughly dry the hand and check the cuticles. Remove any obvious bits of cuticle.

6. Apply hand cream and do a short massage routine to the hands.

7. Repeat on the other hand.

8. Wipe over the nails with polish remover soaked in cotton wool.

9. Apply nail polish in the usual way.

Nail repair

No method of nail repair will stand up to heavy daily work with the hands. As a temporary measure for a special occasion there are various methods of repairing fragile, split or flaking nails.

Causes of splits in the nail

A split may be in the free edge of the nail or below the free edge and may be due to:

■ nails being too long and catching on clothing or when doing jobs without wearing gloves
■ nails being filed to a point which are prone to splitting because there is less protection from the nail wall
■ chewing or over-trimming the cuticle so there is insufficient protection to the nail.

Causes of flaking/fragile nails

The nail is made up of layers of flat dead keratinised cells. Sometimes these layers separate at the free edge and peel back. This may be due to:

■ a hereditary condition – your client will tell you that they have never been able to grow their nails long without this happening
■ the diet
■ illness which can weaken the nails – damage may not be seen for several months
■ using strong chemicals or immersing the hands constantly in water, which will weaken the nails.

Nail strengthening

Products are available to help prevent nails from splitting. Nail-strengthening fluid applied to the free edge on a regular basis will harden the nails. These products contain formaldehyde and should be used with care following the manufacturer's instructions. Nail-strengthening polish is usually clear and can be used as a base coat. It provides extra coats of cellulose to the nail, forming a protective layer.

Nail repair products

Nail mending uses fibrous tissue and a fast-drying adhesive or nitrocellulose. Nail-repair glue or cement is also available.

Method of repair using mending tissue

The problem should be assessed during the client consultation and will be part of the treatment plan. Nail repair takes extra time and if you are planning improvement in the nails over a number of treatments this needs to be recorded. Nail repair is usually incorporated into the manicure during the application of the base coat. This method can be used as necessary between manicures but the nail must be free from polish or hand cream.

1. Wipe over the nail with polish remover.
2. Tear a small piece of fibrous tissue to the size of the split. (The tissue must be torn not cut to ensure that the edges are uneven. This allows the tissue to be blended onto the nail, disguising the repair.)
3. The nail-repair adhesive is applied to the nail plate, including under the free edge, and then to both sides of the tissue.
4. The tissue is placed over the split, allowing about a third to extend beyond the free edge. This is then tucked under the free edge using an orange stick that has been dipped in polish remover.
5. The tissue is smoothed onto the nail using the orange stick, which must remain moistened with polish remover. Smooth out any air bubbles, blending the tissue as close to the nail as possible. This can be achieved with a little polish remover applied to the pad of the thumb and carefully smoothed over the nail.
6. Turn the client's hand over and smooth the tissue under the free edge. Take care not to move the tissue and disturb the blending on the nail plate.
7. Apply a further layer of adhesive to the whole of the nail plate and allow to dry completely.
8. Coloured nail polish can be applied as required.

Broken, split and flaking nails can be remedied by the application of **nail extensions**. Many salons offer this service and you may wish to refer your client to a nail technician for specialist advice. (See also chapter 11, Nail extensions and nail art.)

1. free edge   2. below flesh line

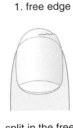 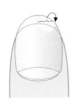   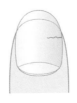

split in the free   nail mending tissue   nail mending tissue
edge   folded over the   placed over the split
                         free edge   on the nail plate

Figure 10.17 *Nail repair*

Heat treatments and skin conditioners for the hands, feet and nails

The therapist must make the most of opportunities for offering extra treatments to the client. This not only increases takings, but helps to keep the interest of the client as well as improving their appearance. A number of treatments can add to the enjoyment of a manicure and pedicure and also help to improve the condition of the client's hands, feet and nails.

Treatments used by the beauty therapist on other parts of the body, for example moisturising masks and exfoliating treatments, can be adapted for use on the hands and feet. The use of heat in conjunction with nourishing creams, oils or waxes can also be very beneficial. The heat required to increase the effectiveness and pleasure for the client can be supplied by:

- heating the material before application, as for paraffin wax or warm oil treatment
- applying hot towels that have been warmed either by soaking in hot water or by warming on a radiator or drying cabinet
- using electrical equipment such as an infrared lamp or thermastatically controlled electrically heated mittens.

Paraffin wax

Paraffin wax is solid and cloudy white in colour when cold. It is heated in a thermostatically controlled wax bath to a working temperature of around 49°C. Paraffin wax treatment is used to ease stiffness in the joints and to improve the texture, colour and condition of the skin. It heats the tissues by enclosing the area with warm wax.

This encourages:

- the skin to perspire
- erythema to develop
- increased activity in the sebaceous glands
- the pores to open, helping the nourishing cream, which has been applied to the hands and feet as part of the treatment, to be absorbed.

Some clients who suffer from rheumatism find this treatment helps to relieve pain and stiffness in the joints.

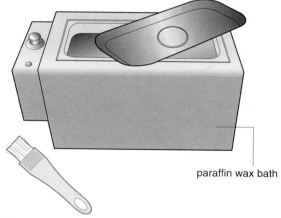

paraffin wax bath

Figure 10.18 *Wax bath*

Procedure for paraffin wax treatment

1. The wax must be heated in the wax bath at least 30 minutes before you need to use it. You will have to plan ahead to ensure the wax is properly melted and ready for use.
2. The manicure or pedicure is completed up to and including a brief hand/foot massage. A rich massage cream is applied and gently massaged into the area.
3. Test the temperature of the wax by first looking at its consistency. Then check the thermostat on the heater and apply wax to the inside of your wrist with a spatula.
4. Dispense the heated wax into a small bowl and quickly brush the wax onto the client's hands or feet (a small paintbrush is ideal).

5. Wrap the hand or foot in tin foil or a plastic bag and cover with a towel or use thermal mits or bootees.

6. This process is repeated on the other hand or foot.

7. The wax can be left on for up to 20 minutes, depending on how much time has been allowed for the manicure. Ten minutes is adequate. Make sure the client is seated comfortably and relaxed.

8. Remove the wax from the first hand or foot. The wax should peel off in one piece and be disposed of.

9. The hand or foot is now in an ideal condition for massage. A full massage of 10 minutes should be given to ensure that the client receives the full benefit of the treatment. Repeat on the other hand or foot.

10. Continue with the application of polish, taking extra care when wiping over the nails with polish remover to ensure that there are no traces of wax left on the nails which will prevent the polish adhering to the nail.

Safety precautions

1. Safety checks should be made on the electrical wax bath. The thermostat must be in good working order to ensure that the wax does not overheat.

2. Protect the client's clothing and the area around the wax bath during treatment. The process can be very messy.

3. Do not move the wax bath while it is hot.

4. Dispose of used wax immediately after use.

Oil treatment

The application of good quality warm vegetable oil to the hands and feet can be very beneficial in treating dry cuticles and nails. Almond oil is ideal, but because of the quantities required it can prove expensive for use in manicure and pedicure. Olive oil is most commonly used, although it tends to have a distinctive smell.

Procedure for oil treatment

1. Place sufficient oil to cover the fingers of one hand up to the first joint in a small bowl. Place this in a larger bowl of hot water on the manicure table.

2. When the cuticle work is completed on the left hand, the fingers are placed in the bowl of warm oil while the right hand is being treated.

3. The left hand is removed and placed on a tissue. It will be necessary to replenish the hot water to warm up the oil for the right hand.

4. The left hand can now be massaged using the oil. Pay particular attention to the cuticles and dry areas of skin. Massage would normally be confined to the hands and wrists.

5. As this is a remedial treatment, the client should be encouraged not to have polish applied. This allows the nails and cuticles to benefit from the oil soaking in. Any excess can be removed with tissues. If the client prefers, the hands can be wiped over with witch hazel on a pad of cotton wool. The oil treatment can also be used in an oil manicure as a substitute for soaking in soapy water.

Masks

The colour and condition of the hands can be improved by proprietary brand masks that hydrate the skin or remove unsightly sun spots by gentle bleaching. The masks are applied in the normal way, using a masking brush, and are removed after 10–15 minutes with warm water.

Exfoliating

Exfoliation is the removal of dead skin using mildly abrasive substances such as ground fruit kernels, oatmeal or salt. Exfoliation treatment for the hands removes dry dead skin scales, ingrained dirt and stains that tend to build up on hard-working hands.

Chemical exfoliants are more often used on the feet to treat the build-up of hard skin. An alkali breaks down the keratin in the skin, softening it. The product also contains grains that loosen the softened skin. The product must be rinsed off thoroughly to remove any traces of the alkali, which would irritate the skin. (Cuticle remover is a similar product that softens the cuticle to aid removal.)

Salt or oatmeal rub

Salt is mixed to a paste with water or oil and rubbed on the hands with the pads of the fingers, using gentle friction movements. Oatmeal mixed and applied in the same way has a similar effect, but is a little more gentle. The salt or oatmeal rub would come before hand massage in the manicure routine.

Chapter 11

NAIL EXTENSIONS AND NAIL ART

LEVELS
1+2

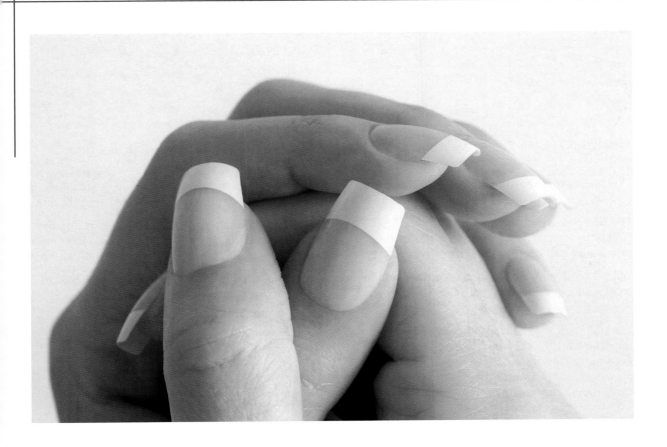

- Specialist products, chemicals, tools and equipment used in the application of nail extensions
- Health and safety
- Preparing the work area
- Assessing the needs of the client, client preferences and treatment planning
- Contraindications to the application of nail extensions
- Reasons for nail extensions
- Types of nail extensions
- Aftercare advice
- Removing artificial nails
- Contra-actions
- Nail art including preparation, techniques and design

Refer to chapter 14, Related Anatomy and Physiology, for the growth and structure of the nail, nail shapes and nail diseases and disorders.

The application of artificial nails has been around for many years. However, in more recent years the technology and products developed by manufacturers has brought a boom in demand for nail extensions.

The UK industry is growing in line with the USA, where nail care and extensions have been part of most American women's way of life for two or three decades. To support this expansion in demand, many more salons and nail bars have opened to provide up-to-date services in nail care, nail extensions and nail art.

When qualified in nail systems there are a number of career opportunities, from specialising as a nail technician, working in a nail salon or adding nail work as an extra dimension to treatments offered as a beauty therapist.

The nail industry is changing constantly so it is important for the therapist or nail technician to keep up to date through training courses and by always reading manufacturers' literature before carrying out any treatment.

 Before learning nail extension skills it is important that the therapist is competent in manicure.

Products, chemicals and equipment

There are quite specific products, tools and equipment used in nail extensions. In particular, the chemicals used can be toxic if not handled with great care.

- **Nail sterilisers** are alcohol-based sprays used to prevent bacteria and fungal growth occurring between the natural nail and the nail extension.
- **Primers** cleanse and dehydrate the nail plate. They draw moisture from the nail and remove surface oil and bacteria from the nail plate, and provide a surface for the acrylic to adhere to. Primers must be allowed to dry before continuing with the procedure.

 Nail primers are corrosive and must therefore be used sparingly.

Modern systems are being developed that do not require primer.

- **Acrylic powder and liquid** when mixed together create a chemical reaction that produces a substance that is durable and strong for creating an acrylic nail. The powder comes in a range of colours, e.g. pink and white, to create a French manicure.

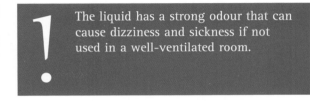

The liquid has a strong odour that can cause dizziness and sickness if not used in a well-ventilated room.

- **UV gel** is pre-mixed and when exposed to ultraviolet light (UV) it hardens.

- **Fibreglass/silk** mesh comes in strips that are cut to size. The strips may have adhesive backing to aid positioning on the nail.

- **Resin** is a liquid adhesive used with the fibreglass system to provide overlays on tips.

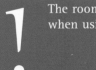

The room must be well ventilated when using nail extension products.

- **Resin activator** is a chemical that is sprayed onto the fibreglass and resin to speed up the setting/hardening process.

Tools and equipment

- **Cuticle tools** – the pusher or hoof stick is used to push and lift the cuticle from the natural nail plate. This is important to ensure that the nail extension fits as closely as possible to the natural nail. The cuticle knife removes any cuticle adhering to the nail plate that could affect the finished result of the nail system used.

- **Nail forms** – these are made of pliable metal, plastic or paper and enable a nail to be built up using a range of systems.

- **Brushes** – these are usually made of sable and are available in different sizes. They are an important tool for applying the products that form the nail. The brushes must be cared for by being cleaned immediately after use. A monomer liquid is best for cleaning brushes rather than soap and water, which dries out the sable hair.

- **Files and buffers** – there are various shapes and sizes based on a grading according to their 'grit' size. The coarser the surface, the lower the grit number, e.g. 60–100 are coarse files used for shaping; 100–180 are used on acrylic and UV gel; while 240 grit is fine grade and is used for blending and smoothing.

- **Tip cutters** – these are designed to give a clean cut when shortening tips.

- **Dappen dishes** – these are small glass or plastic screw-top containers that are used to hold small amounts of monomer liquid. The small neck of the dish reduces the surface area of the liquid exposed, limiting evaporation of the product.

Health and safety

Health and safety legislation and procedures for the beauty salon are covered in chapter 1, however nail extensions use a range of chemicals that require special health and safety procedures.

Control of Substances Hazardous to Health (COSHH) requires the employer to carry out risk assessment to ensure that therapists and clients are not put at risk by exposure to the chemicals used for nail extension systems. Overexposure to substances is a real hazard and every attempt must be made to limit exposure. The body can take in these substances in three ways:

- inhalation – breathing fine dust and vapours, causing dizziness, nausea
- ingesting – through the mouth into the digestive system, causing sickness
- absorption – through the skin or via open wounds in the skin, causing redness, irritation, rashes, blisters.

Preventing inhalation requires adequate ventilation through extraction units. Chemicals do not always have a strong odour but can be equally dangerous if handled incorrectly and inhaled. Some manufacturers recommend that the therapist wears a mask – this may be necessary if exposure is continuous in a nail salon. The fine dust from buffing and filling artificial nails can produce a substantial amount of fine dust. This can be kept to a minimum by changing the paper, tissues, etc.

> **!** If dust from buffing gets into the nail products or is left on the nail, the finished result will have a rough, gritty appearance.

Preventing ingestion requires the therapist and client to wash their hands thoroughly before eating food. Hot drinks should not be consumed at the nail station, as chemicals can be attracted to the hot drink, nor should food be stored or consumed anywhere near the chemicals.

Preventing absorption requires the therapist to use the correct techniques to regulate the amount of chemical used and avoid chemicals being allowed to stay on the client's skin for any length of time. Clients must be given good aftercare advice, especially if they attempt to glue back nails as they may be exposing themselves to chemical absorption.

The therapist must protect themselves by not allowing chemicals to get onto their skin, by covering open wounds on their hands and by washing the hands thoroughly should any chemical accidentally get onto them and after a nail treatment.

Care must be taken when dispensing chemicals to avoid spillages and absorption, ingestion or inhalation. Disposable gloves, a mask over the mouth and protective glasses should be worn for dispensing chemicals.

> **!** It is very important to read manufacturers' information carefully and always follow the recommended health and safety practice.

Preparation of the work area

The trolley should contain all the tools, products, materials and equipment required for the treatment. This saves time and avoids unnecessary disturbance to the client. The trolley should be covered with disposable, absorbent paper to soak up any spillages. A lamp is useful as the therapist has to carry out close and detailed work.

Both the client and the therapist must be sitting comfortably and at the correct height to avoid overstretching and bending, as the treatment can take up to one and a half hours.

Client consultation

The importance of professional appearance, personal hygiene and good communication skills is dealt with in chapter 5.

The specific requirements of consultation for nail extensions and nail art are to establish the client's needs, preferences and suitability for nail extensions and/or nail art. It is particularly important to carry out a consultation, to prepare a treatment plan and agree the finished look.

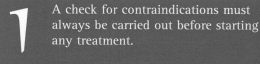

> **!** A check for contraindications must always be carried out before starting any treatment.

Contraindications

Not all clients are suitable for nail extensions because of their occupation. It is most important that the therapist checks for any signs of infection of the nail or finger, which may be bacterial, fungal or viral.

Bacterial

Paronychia (whitlow): This is an infection of the soft tissue around the nail. There is usually swelling, erythema, pus and tenderness in the area. A bacterial infection specific to nail extensions can occur between the natural nail and the overlay, giving a yellow-green colour. This will be discussed further in the section on contra-actions.

Fungal

Onychomycosis (ringworm): This is extremely infectious. The virus attacks the nail bed causing the nail plate to separate and become thick with yellow or white patches, starting at the free edge. It is also possible to see ringworm on the hands (tinea unguium) where round red patches occur on the skin.

Viral

Verrucae or warts: These are contagious viral infections. They are rough and hard lumps of horny tissue. They are found singularly or may appear in groups around the nail fold.

For other nail disease and disorders refer to chapter 14.

Other contraindications include:

- onycholysis: separation of the nail from the nail bed
- onychophagy: severely bitten nails
- allergic reactions to the chemicals and products used
- bruising of the nail or finger
- any cuts or torn cuticle around the nails.

The therapist will need to discuss the following with the client to enable them to give recommendations and prepare a treatment plan:

- reasons for wanting nail extensions applied
- occupation/lifestyle of the client to establish whether nail extensions are suitable
- suitability of each system
- nail shape and length required
- aftercare advice and maintenance.

Reasons for wanting nail extensions

- To enhance poor quality nails.
- For a special occasion.
- Out of curiosity.
- Fashion trends.
- For good personal grooming.
- Profession – model, celebrity.

Occupation/lifestyle of the client

There are certain professions/occupations, hobbies and activities where nail extensions would be unsuitable, for example:

- occupations: nurses, those working with food, cleaners, dentists, those handling money
- activities: most sports, caring for young children, housework
- hobbies: computers (word processing), playing cards, pottery, gardening.

Suitability of the system

The advantages and disadvantages will be discussed under each system.

Nail shape and length

Recently nail technicians have become more experimental by designing and creating the most dramatic look through new products, new technology and nail art. These designs are always great for fashion photography, competitions and styling, but most clients need a design that is natural and durable. The client's lifestyle and occupation will therefore influence the length and shape of the artificial nails applied.

There are a number of factors that the therapist must take into consideration when deciding the length and shape of the artificial nails.

Client's occupation

- Do they work with their hands all day?
- What type of equipment or tools do they work with?
- Are their hands in water for much of the day?

Hobbies

- Do they play sport, and if so, what type?
- Do they swim?

Lifestyle

- Is she a mother with children?
- Does she do a lot of housework?
- Does she have the time to maintain the extensions?

The Occasion

- Are the nails for a special occasion, i.e. a wedding?
- Are they for a holiday and will she be swimming?
- Are the nails to help her natural nails grow?
- Does the client intend to keep them on for a long period of time?

The natural shape and condition of the client's nails

- Some clients have natural nail shapes that are not suitable for nail extensions, or the condition of the nails is so poor the therapist has to advise the client to have regular manicures to improve the condition of the nails and cuticles before embarking on nail extensions.

By obtaining the above information a therapist can decide on:

- how best to meet the client's needs and preferences
- how long the nail extensions should be
- the best system to use
- maintenance requirements.

A client who works with their hands, be it at home or at work, may be advised to keep nails a more natural length and shape due to the stress and strain that may be applied to them. There will be less need to repair breaks and replace nails.

A client who is having the extensions applied for a special occasion, perhaps a wedding or a holiday, may prefer a more exotic design. Many clients request that nails are kept at the longest length possible. However, they must be advised that the nails may not be durable, are not as easy to maintain and are less practical.

A client who is having the extensions to help support their natural nail underneath, for example in the case of very brittle nails or if they are a nail biter, is best advised to keep the extension at the shortest length. This will give the natural nail beneath support and help the client to get used to the feeling of a longer nail.

A client who is having the extensions for a one-off occasion and does not intend to keep and maintain them can afford to have whatever length they desire. However, they should understand the restrictions very long nail extensions have in terms of everyday activities such as washing up. Long nails can easily be torn from the natural nail plate if they catch in clothing, causing damage to the natural nail and surrounding cuticle.

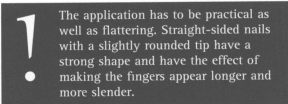
The application has to be practical as well as flattering. Straight-sided nails with a slightly rounded tip have a strong shape and have the effect of making the fingers appear longer and more slender.

The therapist must ensure that they follow manufacturer's guidelines to ensure the nails are secure and stable.

Types of nail extensions

Here we will focus on the application of nail extensions:

1. Tips.
2. Fibreglass (silk) system.
3. UV gel system.
4. Liquid and powder system (acrylic).
5. Sculptured nails.

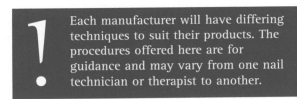
Each manufacturer will have differing techniques to suit their products. The procedures offered here are for guidance and may vary from one nail technician or therapist to another.

Nail preparation

This stage of the treatment is one of the most important and applies whichever system is being used. If this preparation is not followed meticulously the end result may not be of the standard your client will expect and the longevity of the nail extensions will be lessened.

For nail extensions to be successful the nail must be suitably prepared, i.e. cuticles softened, pushed back and trimmed.

A good nail technician will prepare the nail with great care and never forget or skip a process in exchange for speed.

Good nail preparation maximises adhesion of the artificial nail and most importantly reduces the risk of infection.

Nail preparation procedure

1. Prepare the work area by ensuring surfaces are wiped down with disinfectant and all tools are sterilised or disinfected as appropriate. Use disposable items wherever possible.

2. The therapist should begin by washing their hands thoroughly.

3. Ensure that the client has washed their hands and that they are clean and dry. The client's hands and nails must be wiped with isopropyl alcohol or a proprietary brand spray sanitiser. Surgical spirit should not be used for this purpose as it leaves an oily film on the nail plate that will prevent proper adhesion of the artificial nails. It is important to ensure that the hands are completely dry as water may be absorbed into the nail plate and it may lead to lifting of the nail extension at a later date.

4. A mini manicure should be carried out at this stage to ensure that the nails are fully prepared for the application of nail extensions.

- Remove any nail polish on the nails.
- Massage cuticle cream into the cuticles to soften.
- Push back the cuticle from the nail plate using either an orange-wood stick or hoof stick.
- A cuticle knife may be necessary to loosen any cuticle adhering to the nail plate. A clean nail plate is essential. If the cuticle is not removed fully the overlay product will not bond to the nail plate and lifting may occur.
- Remove excess cuticle if required.
- File the nails so that they are even in length and all of the edges are smooth. Doing this will also help the nail to fit the tip that is to be used.

The next step in preparing the natural nails is to remove the shine from the nail. Doing this gives optimum adhesion as the nail's surface is naturally smooth and shiny. Two shiny surfaces do not adhere or bond together effectively. It is necessary to slightly roughen the nail plate both to aid adhesion and to remove any trapped bacteria. This is done by using either a white block or a 240-grit file, lightly buffing from the base of the nail to the free edge, making sure the side wall area is buffed.

Dehydrating the nail plate is an important stage in the preparation. This is done to remove any traces of oil or moisture from the nail plate. Dehydrators that are used on the nail also act as sanitisers, removing oil and moisture as well as ensuring the nails are free from bacteria of fungal spores that could later cause problems. There are many dehydrators on the market and they must be applied following the manufacturer's instructions. Remember that the dehydration process is only effective for approximately 20–30 minutes and once this time has elapsed, the nail will naturally rehydrate and the process will have to be repeated.

The nails are now clean and prepared for the next stage of the treatment.

1 Nail tip application

There are many systems of nail extensions available today, and their application methods may vary. It is vital to follow the manufacturer's instructions to achieve the desired results.

Plastic nail tips originated from the traditional plastic false nail that covered the whole of the nail. Huge improvements in the manufacture of materials has brought a durable plastic tip that covers only a small part of the nail plate. The tips come in a range of different shapes and sizes, ensuring that those selected by the therapist meet the needs of the wide range of natural nail shapes of the clients. It is important to select the right tip to fit the client's nails to ensure a natural look and longevity of the nails.

Tip selection

There are certain characteristics that ensure a well-fitting and natural-looking nail tip. They should:

- be made from good quality plastic (look for ABS plastic)
- be flexible
- be a good natural opaque colour
- bond well with the adhesive
- be a good range of shapes and sizes
- be easy to blend to the natural nail.

These qualities are reflected in the cost of the tips. Cheap tips can be difficult to fit, look unnatural and are more prone to breaking.

When selecting the tips certain guidelines should be followed:

- Choose a tip that follows the same curve of the natural nail. Some clients may have a very flat nail, while others may have a curved nail. Look for the 'C' curve of the client's nails (see figure 11.1).

Matching the curve incorrectly could cause a number of problems, such as air bubbles between the tip and nail plate. This will show through the overlay and will look very unnatural. The risk of infection is increased as bacteria or fungus may grow in the spaces.

- Choosing a tip with the correct deep-stop point. This is the area of the tip that fits into the free edge of the natural nail. The correct contact area or well area is very important and must be large enough to fit snugly. The contact area on tips will vary. Some will cover a larger area of the natural nail than others. Some may have a 'V' cut into the well area to make blending easier. The weakest bond on a nail extension is between the natural nail and the tip, therefore it is vital that the tip covers only a small portion of the nail plate. If the nail is very short or bitten it may be necessary to use a tip with a smaller contact area. It is also important as a larger contact area used on the wrong shape nail will cause the tip to tilt upwards at an angle and this will look very unnatural.

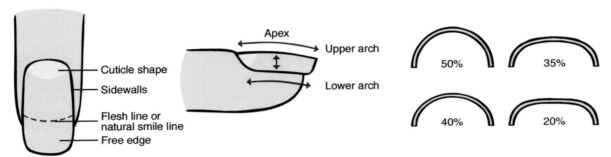

Figure 11.1 *The C curve of the nail*

- The side walls of the client's nails must be taken into account. If the tips do not fit perfectly into the natural nail grooves at the side walls the nail could lift and result in infection or the nail coming off.
- The nail tips come in 10 different sizes, 1 being the largest and 10 the smallest. When choosing the size of tip for each finger it is important that it covers the nail plate from side wall to side wall. If needed, a plastic tip can be filed to shape to fit the nail prior to application, so if necessary opt for the larger size to ensure the best fit. There should be no gap at the side walls when the skin is pulled back. Although it is not very noticeable when a new set is applied, as the natural nail grows the gap will become evident.

Tip application

1. Ensure that the correct tip is selected, by following the guidelines.
2. Carry out the nail preparation thoroughly.
3. Apply a small amount of adhesive directly onto the well of the tip. In doing this, rather than applying it to the natural nail, you are ensuring that the adhesive does not run onto the skin around the nail.
4. There should be no more than 30 per cent of the tip on the natural nail plate.

Nail extensions and nail art

5. Apply the tip to the nail at a 45 degree angle. Using a rocking movement apply it to the natural nail, making sure that you release any air bubbles and it forms a perfect bond. Hold the nail in position for about 10 seconds ensuring that your pressure is not too heavy. If you need to apply a lot of pressure you might find that the tip is too small.

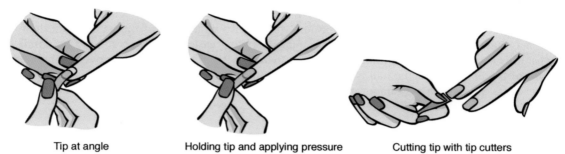

Tip at angle   Holding tip and applying pressure   Cutting tip with tip cutters

Figure 11.2 *Applying tips*

6. Ensure no excess adhesive is left under the free edge or around the side walls. It must be cleaned off before it dries.

7. Once all 10 tips have been applied, the length and shape must be decided upon. Consult the treatment plan and discuss once again. Always advise the client on the length that will suit their hands, occupation and lifestyle. Cutting the tip to size requires a sharp tip cutter.

8. The tips must now be filed to shape using a fine board of 240 grit or above. There are three different shapes that the client has to choose from, oval, rounded square or square, or squoval.

   Check the side walls and taper if necessary.

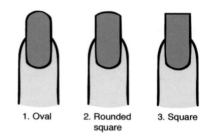

1. Oval   2. Rounded square   3. Square

Figure 11.3 *1. Oval 2. Rounded square 3. Square*

9. The next step is to blend the tip to the natural nail. Use a grit file of 240 to thin the entire tip. Blend in one direction and use long sweeps with the file to avoid friction to the nail bed. Begin at the free edge of the tip (zone 1), working down towards the seam (zone 2). When blending the seam line, make sure that the line disappears. Using very light pressure, file over the base of the tip near the seam, avoiding the natural nail. The contact area on the tip will become thinner and the nail will be translucent.

10. Use a white block to buff the area to ensure that there is no evidence of a visible seam line and the surface is smooth and free of scratches.

11. Check the tip application and remove any file dust from the free edge.

The next step is the overlay application. (Fibreglass – silk – system.)

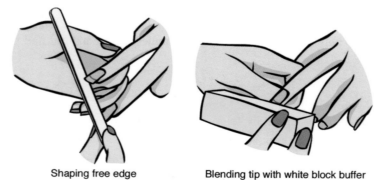

Shaping free edge   Blending tip with white block buffer

Figure 11.4 *Filing and buffing tips*

2 Fibreglass (silk) system

Fibreglass systems use a wrap and resin. Fibreglass mesh is used with a resin of ethyl cyanoacrylate or a liquid adhesive. Wraps and resins vary considerably so it is essential that the manufacturer's information and instructions are read carefully.

The fibreglass fabric is bought in strips, usually in a dispenser, to avoid dust or touching as oil will create a barrier to the resin. There are different weaves of fabric and some have a gentle adhesive backing to aid application.

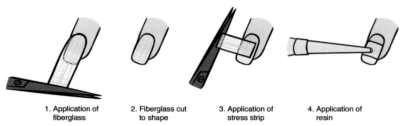

1. Application of fiberglass   2. Fiberglass cut to shape   3. Application of stress strip   4. Application of resin

Figure 11.5 *Applying fibreglass mesh*

Resins also vary in consistency and when they age they become yellow and brittle, which makes them unusable. Resins are hardened (cured) by an activator or accelerator which speeds up the time to set. The activator may be spray or brush-on.

Advantages

This system has always been known as the weakest of them all. However, there are many positive aspects of choosing this system over the others.

- It is a very gentle system for the natural nail as it requires very little buffing and there is no need for the use of primer.
- It can be soaked off very easily and in the minimal time (10–15 minutes).
- The overlay that is produced is not very thick and is flexible.
- This system is also useful for natural nail repairs as it is thin and will not look different to the other nails.

Disadvantages

- This system is recognised as being very fiddly and some therapists prefer not to use it unless requested by the client.
- The spray activator can cause allergic reactions such as breathing problems or skin reaction.
- The resin vapours can cause sore, watery eyes.

Application as an overlay on tips

1. Follow the nail preparation and tip application.
2. Using a pair of scissors cut the fibre or silk to the width of the nail. If adhesive fibreglass is being used remove the backing paper from the fibre, making sure not to touch the fibre as the oil from your hands will prevent the resin from soaking into the mesh.
3. Apply the fibre to the nail, making sure that it covers the entire nail and is not too close to the cuticle and covers right to the edge of the side walls. Use the paper to press it down onto the nail.

Trim the sides of the mesh so that it is slightly shorter than the nail tip. This allows the resin to seal the tip.

4. Apply a small strip of mesh onto the stress area of the nail. This is the join between the tip and the natural nail. This extra mesh will give the overlay added strength in this area.

5. Repeat this procedure to all fingers and thumbs.

6. Apply a small amount of resin down the centre of the nail. Using either a brush or a nozzle, work the resin into the mesh from side to side, ensuring all the fabric is sealed and becomes sheer. If a spray activator is being used, mist the activator over each nail.

7. Apply another layer of the resin to the nail ensure that the resin is spread evenly and that there are no traces on the skin surrounding the nail.

8. If a brush-on activator is being used, apply a small amount of resin to the nail as the activator will spread it. Spread the resin with the brush-on activator, making sure that you avoid the surrounding skin. Make sure that a brush cleaner is available to clean the brush between each application.

9. If spray is used, hold it at least 30 centimetres (12 inches) from the nails and spray once, making sure that all nails have been covered. Repeat for all nails.

10. Repeat steps 7 and 8 on all nails.

11. If more strength is required to the nails repeat steps 7 and 8 again.

12. The overlay should be smooth and require a minimal amount of buffing. To achieve a high shine use a soft file to buff, using a white block to remove any scratches and to refine the surface.

13. Remove all file dust with a brush and apply oil to the nail and cuticle.

14. Apply polish if requested and ensure that aftercare advice is given.

Maintenance

Fibreglass infills

Fibreglass nails should be maintained every 2–4 weeks depending on the rate of growth of the client's natural nails.

The system of infills is relatively easy and should take between 30 minutes and 1 hour unless there are problems such as lifting or lost nails. If the client is returning for an infill for the first time they may not need fabric applying in the growth area as the growth of the natural nail will be minimal.

Procedure

1. The same materials and equipment are required as for a new set of nails.
2. Ensure that all equipment is sanitised and available.
3. Sanitise both your own and your client's hands.
4. Use non-acetate polish remover to remove polish from the nails.
5. Using a cuticle tool, remove any new cuticle that has grown on the nail plate.
6. Replace any lost nails.
7. Using a 100-grit file, blend the edge of the overlay near the cuticle (zone 3) (see figure 11.7) until it is flush with the natural nail, taking care that the natural nail is not buffed during this process. It is at this stage that any area of lifting on the overlay is removed and buffed down.
8. Use a 240-grit file to buff away the surface shine from the whole nail and buff over the area with a white block to remove any scratches.
9. Apply a thin strip of fabric in the growth area (zone 3).
10. Apply a small amount of resin to the growth area of the nail (zone 3) and blend it to the rest of the nail.

11. Apply the activator as before.

12. Another thin layer of resin may be needed, followed by activator.

13. Use a white block followed by the three-way buffer. Buff the nails to achieve a high gloss.

14. Apply polish if required.

3 UV gel

The UV gel system uses a product that is pre-mixed and ready for use. The gel is acrylic and shares the same properties as the liquid and powder system. Gels have a thick consistency with a low odour when applying.

The system requires an activator to cure the gel. This may be ultraviolet light. The ultraviolet light must penetrate the gel completely so care must be taken not to apply it too thickly. A brush-on activator may be used where an ultraviolet light unit is not available.

This system is one of the easiest to use. It works very well for clients who have their hands in water a great deal because it cannot be soaked off. Removing the application can take some time: 30–45 minutes using buffing and files. Extreme care must be taken when removing the gel to avoid damage to the natural nail plate.

Advantages

- It is easy to apply.
- It cannot be soaked off.
- The nails can be slightly more flexible than with other systems.
- This system produces a permanent high gloss.
- When nails are applied well they look very natural.

Disadvantages

- Gels are not as strong and hard-wearing as liquids and powders.
- The nails are not easy to remove.
- Gels have a higher risk of allergic reaction.
- Some gels produce heat during the curing process.
- Very good ventilation is required.

 Low-odour products can be just as toxic as those that have a strong smell.

Application

1. Ensure the work area is well prepared and sterilisation and cleaning procedures have been completed.

2. Follow the nail preparation and the tip application procedure.

3. Ensure that all filing dust is removed by using a soft brush. If any dust gets into the gel it will cause a very bumpy overlay.

4. Take a small amount of gel and place at the tip of the nail using a clean brush. Apply a thin layer of the gel to the whole nail, leaving a small margin round the cuticle to ensure no gel touches the skin and cuticle. This is the base layer.

5. Turn on the ultraviolet lamp and ask the client to place their hand under it for the gel to cure for 2 minutes or however long is required by the manufacturer's instructions.

6. While the first hand is under the lamp, repeat steps 3 and 4 on the second hand.

7. Apply the second coat of gel to the first hand while the second hand is under the lamp. This second layer is the building layer. Place a large bead of gel in the centre of the nail. Spread the gel down the nail plate, leaving the bulk of it in the centre or stress area to give strength. Ensure that all sides of the free edge are sealed. As the second layer is thicker than the first it is important to make sure that no gel has come into contact with the surrounding skin. Cure for 2 minutes.

8. Repeat step 7 on the second hand.

9. Remove any residue from the nails with a nail wipe.

10. To get the perfect shape to the extension, the nail is buffed. Use a high-grit file.

11. Always check the shape of the nail by looking down the barrel of the nail to make sure it is even all over.

12. Use a white block to remove any scratches from the nail.

13. There are two ways of finishing the gel system. A three-way buffer can be used to produce a natural shine, or applying a very thin layer of finishing gel and curing for 2 minutes will produce a very high shine. Make sure that any residue is removed using a nail wipe if the nails are finished in this way.

14. Apply oil to the nail and cuticle area.

15. Apply polish if requested. Remember to remove traces of oil from the nail.

Maintenance

UV gel infills

UV gel nails should be maintained every 2–4 weeks depending on the rate of growth of the client's natural nails.

Gel infills should take about an hour to do, longer if some tips have been broken or your client has left it more than 2 weeks for their appointment.

Procedure

1. The same materials and equipment are required as for a new set of nails.

2. Ensure that all equipment is sanitised and available.

3. Sanitise both your own and your client's hands.

4. Using cuticle tools, remove any new cuticle that has grown on the nail plate.

5. If there are any nails missing these must be replaced.

6. Check the shape of each nail and length and carry out any corrections needed.

7. Gently buff the surface with a 240-grit file.

8. Using a 100-grit file, working in zone 3, blend the edge of the overlay until it is flush with the natural nail. Take care to ensure that the natural nail is not buffed during this process. It is at this stage that any area of lifting on the overlay is removed and buffed.

9. Remove all the shine from the surface and buff over the area with a white block to remove any scratches.

10. Remove file dust from the nails and use a nail dehydrator to cleanse the new growth.

11. Apply a small amount of the gel to the infill area and blend it onto the rest of the nail. If it is the second or third infill you may need to apply two layers for added strength. Cure for 2 minutes.

12. Remove the residue from the nails and buff as for the first application.

13. Use a white block to remove any surface scratches to the nail.

14. End with either a three-way buffer or a layer of gel as necessary. Remember that it must be cured for 2 minutes.

15. Apply oil and polish if required. Remember to remove traces of oil from the nail before applying polish.

Safety points when applying gel

- Always read and follow the manufacturer's instructions.
- Use extraction ventilation.
- Check the ultraviolet lamp regularly and change bulbs every 6–12 months, depending on use.
- Apply thin layers of gel.
- Always use strict hygiene procedures.

4 Acrylic or liquid and powder system

Acrylic is one of the most popular overlays, as it has strength, flexibility and it is extremely durable. However, it is one of the most difficult systems to master. Acrylic uses a mixture of both powder and liquid – a polymer powder in a range of colours and a monomer liquid. When the two are mixed together a solid is formed.

Practising product mixing is time very well spent for a beginner. The correct consistency for the liquid and powder must be achieved.

Each bead of product should be medium wet for ultimate performance (see figure 11.6). Beads that are too wet will undoubtedly lift, which will increase the risk of exposure to infection and will increase the work needed when infilling. Dry beads will be quite hard to apply and will be more prone to lifting and cracking.

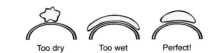

Figure 11.6 *It is essential the correct consistency is achieved*

The brush used to apply the product is very important because it will influence how much liquid can be held and this can alter the bead size. The brush should be good quality sable and tapered with no flared hairs to spoil the bead size.

Care of the brush is equally important. It should be cleaned with monomer after use and reshaped before storing. The brush should not be cleaned with soap and water as the detergent will dry out the sable hairs, making it difficult to use.

The key is to apply the product in a serious of zones to get a perfect uniformed shape. If too much product is applied per zone it will result in extra time buffing to thin out and refine. Excessive filing or buffing can cause great discomfort for the client and will also increase the risk of lifting by breaking down the structure of the overlay.

The Zones

- Zone 1: This is the free edge. The overlay must be thin on the edge so that the extension does not look artificial.
- Zone 2: This is the area over the smile line and just at the beginning of the nail bed. This is where the nail receives the most stress and so needs maximum strength.
- Zone 3: This is the area at the base of the nail, near the cuticle. This area should also be thin so that there is more flexibility in the nail and large ridges are avoided.

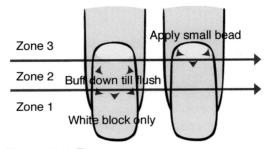

Figure 11.7 *The zones*

Advantages

- The nails are strong, flexible and hard-wearing.
- A permanent French manicure can be achieved.

- Maintenance is quick and easy.
- Irregular nail shapes can be corrected.
- When nails are applied well they look very natural.

Disadvantages

- The most difficult system to master.
- The nails take time to remove.
- Very good ventilation is required as odours can be a problem.

Application

1. Prepare the nails in the usual way.
2. Apply tips, shape and blend.
3. Follow the procedure for acrylic nail application as recommended by the manufacturer of the product to be used.
4. Apply a very small amount of primer at the base of the nails on one hand. The primer must be dry before applying the acrylic.
5. While the primer is drying ensure that the brush is prepared to begin the overlay. Fill a dappen dish with the monomer liquid. Clean the brush by submerging the bristles into the liquid to free it of air pockets and to prime it. Then wipe it on a paper towel.
6. Dip the brush back into the monomer and then press the sides of the brush against the dappen dish to release any excess liquid.
7. Start on the little finger of one hand. Pick up a bead of powder and place it onto zone 1. Wait for 5 seconds for the bead to set, then, holding the brush at an angle, press the bead with the tip of the brush using a combination of gentle patting and pressing motions to glide the product across zone 1. Check the shape by looking down the barrel of the nail to make sure the overlay is even.
8. Wipe the brush on a paper towel to remove any excess product.
9. Repeat stages 4, 5 and 6 for zone 2.
10. Then repeat stages 4, 5 and 6 for zone 3. Make sure that the bead is applied carefully to the cuticle area but leave a 1.5 mm gap. Gently press the overlay to thin the zone and create a good bond with the nail plate.
11. Apply the overlays to the other nails by following the same procedure. This application requires practice to ensure a smooth, even coverage is achieved.
12. By the time the overlays have been applied to both hands, the first hand will be ready for the next stage.
13. Wipe any excess product from your brush and clean it by dipping it into the dappen dish and brushing it on a paper towel.
14. Check that the acrylic has set by tapping the nail with the handle of the brush; if it is ready a clicking sound can be heard. If the acrylic has been applied carefully and not too thickly, finishing should not require excessive filing and buffing.
15. Using a 240-grit file, buff the surface of the overlay to help smooth out any bumps, ridges and unevenly distributed product. Check the overlay from all angles, not forgetting to look down the barrel, to ensure a perfect nail structure.
16. Use a white block to buff over the surface to refine and remove any surface scratches to the nail.
17. Use a three-way buffer, if required, to give a shine and seal the overlay.
18. Apply oil to the nail and cuticle to nourish the nail and surrounding skin.
19. Apply polish if desired.

Maintenance

Acrylic infills

The client should be recommended to return in 2 weeks. Acrylic infills should take about 1 hour to do, longer if some tips have been broken or if the client has left it more than 2 weeks for their appointment or if the natural nails have grown quickly.

Procedure

1. Ensure that all equipment is sanitised and available.

2. Sanitise both your own and your client's hands.

3. Using cuticle tools, remove any cuticle that has grown on the nail plate.

4. Look at the shape and length of the nails and adjust as necessary. Remember to check the treatment plan and discuss the length with the client. As the natural nail grows the nail extensions will get longer. This may not be what was agreed or recommended at the first treatment. If the client requests the nails to be left longer, remind them of the greater risk of breaking and lifting.

5. Use a 240-grit file to gently file down the side walls to straighten.

6. Continuing with the 240-grit file, blend the edge of the overlay until it is flush with the natural nail, making sure that care is taken and the natural nail is not buffed during this process. Remember the stress line has moved up the nail towards the free edge. Ensure that only the nail in zone 2 is buffed to avoid changing the shape of the rest of the nail. It is at this stage that any area of lifting on the overlay is removed and buffed down.

7. Remove all the shine from the surface and buff over the area with a white block to remove any scratches.

8. Ensure that filing dust is removed from the nails.

9. Apply a primer to the new growth area. Wait for this to dry before applying the overlay.

10. Apply a small bead of acrylic to zone 3 and press into shape, making sure that you blend it down to zones 1 and 2. Take care around the cuticle area and leave a gap of 1.5 mm.

11. Use a file to smooth the surface and buff around the cuticle area. Check the shape and look down the barrel to make sure that a perfect overlay is achieved.

12. Use a white block to smooth and remove any surface scratches.

13. Use a three-way buffer to seal and shine the nail.

14. Apply oil to the nail and cuticle area.

15. Apply polish if required.

5 Sculptured nails

Sculpting nails relies on a totally different technique than using a tip where the outline of the nail extension is easily created. Sculpting not only relies on a sound knowledge of the products and their application but also the correct placement of the sculpting form. Not all clients are suitable for sculptured nails, as follows:

- a flat natural nail shape makes it difficult to create a good shape
- bitten nails with the bulbous finger end are unsuitable because the sculpting form does not fit correctly
- thin or poor nail plates do not provide a sufficiently good foundation for sculpting
- ski-jump nails (nails that curve upwards at the tip) are not suitable as it is impossible to achieve a good shape
- clients who perform heavy work are not suited to sculptured nails.

Nail extensions and nail art

There are various types of sculpting forms made from:

- paper, with adhesive on the underside – disposable
- plastic – reusable
- metal – reusable.

Sculptured nails can be achieved using all systems. However, there are specific points to take into consideration relating to each system.

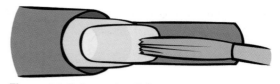

Figure 11.8 *A metal nail form*

Fibreglass

The curve and strength of the nail – a poor flat nail shape would be extremely difficult to sculpt.

Fibreglass cannot be extended very far beyond the natural nail because it is difficult to build a strong structure without a tip, so they would not last well.

UV gel

Gel can be successfully used with nail forms for sculpting although extra care must be given to placing the hands under the ultraviolet lamp to avoid dislodging the forms.

Liquid and powder (acrylic)

This is the most popular and effective of the systems for producing sculptured nails, as they are strong. The product is easy to use to build up shape and length. It is easy to correct chips or breaks in the nails and working on a form with acrylic allows more time to create a good shape than a tip because the form allows longer setting time.

Method of fitting the form

The important thing when choosing a form and fitting it to the client's nail is to produce a good 'C' curve. To do this the form must be bent to shape while placing it under the free edge.

> The C curve is not the same on every finger and the thumbs. It is important that the form fits snugly to avoid seepage of the product under the free edge of the natural nail.
>
> Only work on one finger at a time once the form is fitted.

Procedure

A basic procedure for sculpting nails.

1. Ensure the work area is well prepared and sterilisation and cleaning procedures have been completed.
2. Follow the nail preparation procedure.
3. Fit a sculpting form on one finger at a time.

> Follow specific manufacturer's instructions for application. When using a new product it is advisable to have training from the manufacturer in the correct use of their products.

4. Apply a bead of product to the centre of the free edge (zone 1). Press the bead with the brush into the centre and then to the side walls. Use the brush to create the lower arch.
5. Apply a second bead to zone 2. Smooth to meet zone 1.
6. Apply a final bead of product in zone 3 (cuticle area).
7. Repeat the process on each finger and the thumbs.
8. File and buff the surface of the nail to achieve a high shine.
9. Use a white block to smooth and remove any surface scratches.

10. Use a three-way buffer to seal and shine the nail.

11. Apply oil to the nail and cuticle area.

12. Apply polish if required.

Maintenance

The procedure for maintenance follows the system used. Refer to manufacturer's instructions.

ACTIVITY

Design an aftercare leaflet that gives the client clear information on the care of their hands and nails and the maintenance procedures required to keep the nail extensions looking immaculate.

Aftercare advice

The client must be informed at the outset of what is involved in maintaining the nail extensions. While some nails may be temporary, others remain on the nail as it grows and require infills to maintain a perfect shape.

Because of the pressure put on the tip of the nail they can come off or break. The longer the extension, the more likely this will happen. Replacing the nails will require a visit to the salon and a cost to replace the nail.

Make sure that the client is fully informed of the dos and don'ts and how to care for their nails at home. Stress to the client just how important it is that they follow a strict routine to maximise the life of the nail extensions.

An aftercare leaflet ensures that the client is clear about how to care for the nail extensions and will make them less likely to blame the therapist if the nails do not last or meet their expectations.

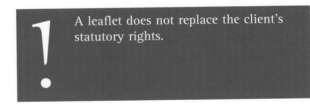

A leaflet does not replace the client's statutory rights.

The following points should be discussed with the client before they leave the salon.

- Contact the salon if any problems occur with the nails.
- If using polish remover ensure it is non-acetone.
- Always use a base coat before applying polish.
- Rebook for maintenance, infill treatments every 2–3 weeks.
- Apply oil or cuticle cream 2–3 times a day to the nail and cuticle.
- Use hand cream regularly to keep hands soft.
- Wear cotton-lined rubber gloves for daily housework jobs, especially if cleaning chemicals such as bleach and detergents are to be used.

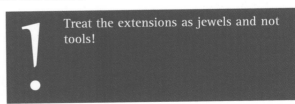

Treat the extensions as jewels and not tools!

- Take special care with fibreglass nails as they are not as strong and resistant to knocking.
- Take care not to catch the nails on clothing or grab at things as this can cause breakage and damage to the natural nails.

Removing nail extensions

Nail extension systems can only be removed using a solvent. Acetone is commonly used for this purpose although it should be used with care as it is extremely drying and can affect the natural nail plate and surrounding cuticle. The solvent breaks down the polymer chains in the chemicals. The easiest system to remove is fibreglass as the resin used has the weakest chains. The liquid and powder system is the next easiest to remove although it will take longer and requires some buffing. UV gel is substantially more difficult to remove. It has strong bonds and requires considerably more filing and buffing to remove the artificial nail.

Procedure

1. Place two glass or china bowls filled to about 3 cm with solvent. The bowls should be placed in hot water. The heat will accelerate the removal process.
2. Remove polish from the nails and cut back the length of the nails.
3. Submerge the nails into the solvent and cover with a towel to keep the heat in. It may be necessary to change the water to keep it hot. The process will take about 20 minutes.
4. Take one hand out of the bowl and gently remove the dissolved nails with an orange stick. Continue on the other hand.
5. The client will need to wash their hands to remove all traces of the solvent.
6. Check the cuticles and reshape the natural nails as necessary.
7. Reapply nail extensions or continue with hand massage and polish as required.

Another method of removal involves applying cotton wool soaked in solvent to each nail and then wrapping the hands in tinfoil to retain the heat. A plastic bag or heated mittens can be used to increase the heat and speed up removal.

Contra-actions specific to nail extensions

Clients sometimes complain that their natural nails appear thinner after extensions have been removed. This is mostly an illusion as they have become used to a thicker nail plate produced by the overlay.

If the correct procedures are followed, the therapist is skilled at the system used and careful consideration is given to the client's needs, the nail extensions should look natural and be long-lasting. However, poor practice when carrying out nail extensions can cause a number of problems.

Problem solving

Problem	Possible cause	Solution to the problem
Thinning of the natural nail	Constant buffing and filing, over-priming, nail plate not dehydrated before applying products, product has lifted and moisture is trapped between the layers	Use correct grit files, use a light touch when filing, apply primer very sparingly and allow to dry, always carry out meticulous preparation of the natural nails, do not soak the nails if giving a manicure before nail extensions
Splitting and flaking of the natural nail	Over-blending of tips, nail extension too long or too thick, client picks or bites the extension off, maintenance not carried out on time	Light touch when filing, advise client on appropriate length, make sure client is aware of maintenance needs and the correct removal of the extensions

(Continued)

Problem	Possible cause	Solution to the problem
Premature loss of the nail extension	Poor preparation of the nail plate, nail extensions too long, nails do not fit client's lifestyle, incorrect selection of system	Ensure good preparation, carry out a full consultation into client's lifestyle, occupation and expectations, consider the appearance and shape of the natural nail before selecting a system
Discoloration of the natural nail plate	Poor preparation of the nails, overuse of primer	Ensure thorough preparation of the natural nails before applying products, use nail primer sparingly and allow to dry
Obvious infills	Poor blending, too much product, client not attending maintenance appointments	Use correct infill technique, follow manufacturer's instructions, blend correctly, emphasise to clients the importance of keeping appointments to maintain their nails
Lifting from the natural nail	Nails too long, improper preparation of the nail leaving the nail moist or oily, maintenance appointments not kept, nail extension unbalanced, poor home care	A thorough consultation to establish how the client will manage the nail extensions in relation to their job and lifestyle, incorrect preparation of the natural nails, insufficient or too much product used
The finished nails pointing upwards or downwards	Incorrect placing of the tip or nail form	Check regularly throughout the application that the angles and curves are correct
The 'C' shape of the nail extension is irregular	Product applied unevenly or too much product applied, product too wet causing it to run	Practise to ensure high levels of skill, check throughout the application of the nails that the transverse arch and the 'C' shape are even.
Infection of the nail	Bacterial or fungal infection due to cracks or spaces in the extension, infection caused by the client picking, tearing or biting the nail extension leaving the cuticle and nail bed exposed to infection, lifting of the product at the free edge, side walls or cuticle allowing moisture to become trapped between the layers	Careful preparation, regular maintenance, advice to client on home care, skilful application to ensure there are no spaces between the natural nail plate and the extension

Nail art

The art of decorating the nails covers basic painting techniques, using one colour of nail polish, to embedding jewels into acrylic nails.

Polishing and buffing the nails to enhance the natural colour and shine are equally important techniques for the nail technician and therapist.

French manicure can be enhanced with delicate nail art application. See Figure 11.9.

Advanced techniques such as air brushing, 3D work and nail jewellery are beyond the scope of this book, but are an indication of the huge range of techniques available.

Nail art materials, tools and equipment

Good nail art relies on a creative ability as well as a good range of materials, tools and equipment. While a good wholesaler will have a range of material it is a good idea to visit trade shows and exhibitions to see the latest ideas, as new products and techniques are being developed all the time. Manufacturers will also provide a list of their products.

A wide variety of tools is available to the nail technician to help to create the different looks that may be requested by clients. For example, there are different types of brushes to help freehand drawing, striping brushes, small detail brushes and dotting tools.

The range of tools includes:

- brushes – good quality brushes are a sound investment as they last longer, do not lose hairs easily and can be moulded to achieve the finest point for fine work. A range of sizes and types are needed:
  - shading brush, which has broad square bristles for floating and shading colour
  - fan brush, which has the bristles fanned out to create swirling effects
  - fine detail brush, which has a fine tip used for precise detail
  - liner brush in different widths for creating thick or thin lines
  - glitter dust brush specifically to help avoid contaminating other products with the glitter. The brush should be sable and must be cleaned after use with nail polish remover.
- orange-wood stick – a standard piece of equipment for the manicurist and nail technician. It is versatile and used in nail art for picking up small items such as rhinestones
- marbling tool – also used as a dotting tool. A round metal end used to mix one colour into another. There is a different size metal part at each end of the tool to create dots of different sizes
- artist's palette – this is useful for mixing small amounts of nail paint.

The range of materials includes:

- nail paints – non-toxic, water-based, acrylic paints that can be diluted or mixed together to create a range of effects. These paints come in a range of colours and opalescent effects to give an iridescent shine to the nail. Nail paints can easily be cleaned off brushes because they are water based
- nail polishes or enamels – nitrocellulose in a solvent, such as acetate, which leaves a high gloss coloured finish to the nails
- base coat – nitrocellulose-based product that protects the nail from staining and provides a smooth base for the application of polish
- top coat – a thin, clear nitrocellulose nail polish used to provide a hard gloss protection for the polish, to seal nail art designs, and give the nails gloss.

Decorative materials include:

- rhinestones
- flat stones
- coloured powder
- transfers
- glitter dust
- glitter dust mixer
- foils.

Applying nail art

There are no set rules in applying nail art. The way to achieve the best results is to play around with ideas and have fun with the products.

By using a selection of techniques, gems and glitter, etc., the therapist can produce original designs or work from templates and pictures.

French manicure (see page 186) is the most basic type of nail art that a therapist will be asked to do for a client. This technique enhances the nail tip and the natural colour of the nail bed. The polish can be made to stand out even further by using different colours such as blue and white or red and yellow. The French manicure is a good base for nail art.

> Practice makes perfect and the simplest art can look just as effective as complicated designs.

A basic technique for freehand decoration

See Figure 11.11.

1. Polish all ten nails either with a coloured polish or a natural French manicure polish.
2. Select paint colours and a design.
3. Create a design by selecting from a range of freehand techniques: marbling tool to create dots of colour, a fan brush to create swirls, a liner brush for straight lines, a shading brush to mix colours on the nail.
4. Always keep the design simple for a striking effect. The surface available does not allow for complicated designs.
5. Allow the paint to dry thoroughly. The nail paint tends to look dull when dry so a top coat is needed.
6. Apply a top coat – one coat to fix the paint and give shine and a second coat to give added protection to the art work.

Opalescent paint effects

Procedure

1. A dark nail polish is used on each nail and a thin application of opalescent nail paint which complements the nail colour is applied.
2. The nail paint can be applied with a fan brush sweeping from side to side on the nail plate or a liner brush can be used following the same action.
3. The paint appears white during application but dries to give an iridescent effect.
4. Take care not to over-blend and lose the effect.
5. Allow the nail paint to dry and apply two layers of top coat.

Marbling

This is a simple technique using the marbling tool.

Procedure

1. Discuss the design and choice of colours with the client.
2. Apply the base coat and two coats of coloured nail polish, ensuring good coverage of the nail plate.

> The choice of colours will depend on the client's preference, perhaps to match an outfit, or the therapist's creative skill.

3. Place two different colours of nail paint on the artist's palette. Use only small amounts to avoid wastage.

4. Using the large end of the marbling tool place one drop of each colour on one corner of the nail.

5. Make sure the marbling tool is clean before swirling one colour into another to create a marbling effect. Do not overwork or the effect will look messy.

6. Allow the paint to dry and apply two coats of top coat.

Applying rhinestones and flat stones

Nail designs can be enhanced by the application of glitter, tiny stones and diamante (see Figure 11.9).

Procedure

1. Flat stones and rhinestones come in a vast range of colours, sizes and shapes.

2. The stones are applied to wet polish early in the application of a design or at the end of the design by using a dot of top coat, or during the application of top coat.

3. A selection of stones can be placed on the artist's palette and when needed they are picked up individually using an orange stick dampened at the pointed end with water.

4. Flat stones have a flat edge and sit well on the nail.

5. The design and the stones are further secured and protected with two coats of top coat.

Applying glitter

Applying glitter involves rolling the glitter on the nail with a sable brush that has been dipped in glitter dust mixer. See Figures 11.10 and 11.11.

Procedure

1. Discuss the design and choice of colours with the client.

2. Apply the base coat and two coats of coloured nail polish ensuring good coverage of the nail plate.

3. The glitter may be part of a design or complete the design.

4. Use the mixer product, allowing the glitter to stick to it and then apply by rolling the bead of glitter over the nail.

5. Circular movements are used to distribute the glitter rather than drag the product over the nails, which tends to separate the glitter particles.

6. Leaving some parts of the nail free from glitter allows the polish colour to shine through, giving a good effect.

7. Apply two coats of top coat.

Foils

Foiling produces a unique effect. There is no other technique that quite matches the effect achieved with foil.

The foil comes in rolls or sheets and is bonded onto a clear backing. The foil adhesive that is placed on the nail releases the foil from the backing, leaving the design made by the adhesive on the nail.

Procedure

1. Base coat and nail polish is applied to each nail. A clear nail can be achieved by using two coats of good quality base coat.

2. Ensure the polish is dry and apply foil adhesive sparingly in the area where the foil is to be placed. The adhesive is white, making it easy to see the design made, especially on dark polish.

3. Once the adhesive becomes clear it is ready for the foil to be applied.

4. Place the foil over the adhesive and rub the foil with a cotton bud to ensure it is firmly stuck to the adhesive.

5. Lift the backing away from the nails.

6. Apply two coats of top coat to seal and protect the design.

> ! Taking care of the tools and materials used in nail art ensures they will last for a long time.

Transfers

Applying designs to the nails using transfers is less time-consuming than freehand designs and does not require so much skill and creative ability. Transfers may be self-adhesive or released by moistening the back of the transfer with a wet cotton-wool bud. The transfer is applied to the polished nails and covered with two coats of top coat.

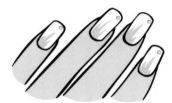

Figure 11.9 *A French manicure can be enhanced by using a rhinestone in the corner of each nail*

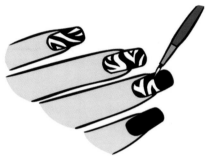

Figure 11.10 *Using the striping brush to paint animal stripes on a black nail can look effective. Glitter and design applied to a strong coloured polish can look very dramatic*

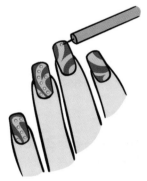

Figure 11.11 *The dotting tool can be used to create flowers and paw prints running across the nail*

The art of nail design

The range of nail designs is endless.

Figures 11.9 to 11.12 show just a few of the examples, but it is the creativity of the therapist or nail technician that comes to the fore when designing and applying nail art. By using the vast range of products, colour combinations and techniques available, the therapist can be as creative as their imagination and skill allow.

ACTIVITY

Use the blank nail diagrams in Figure 11.12 to create some of your own nail design ideas.

Don't forget when designing to take account of:

- the colours of nail paint and polishes you have available
- the material you have available
- the client's preferences
- the degree of skill you have. Do not attempt something too difficult and complicated. Simple designs often look the most effective.

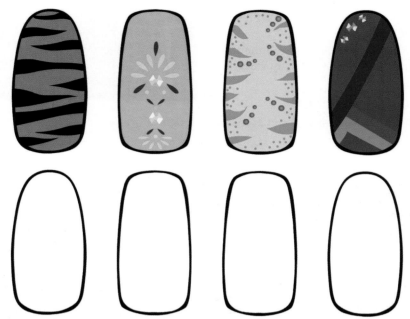

Figure 11.12 *Try out your own ideas*

Contra-actions

As with the use of all chemicals the client may be allergic to the products used. An allergic reaction would appear as swelling and irritation round the nails and on the hands, but also, as with any allergic reaction, the eyes may become red and watery or, in the worst cases, breathing difficulty may occur.

Because nail art is invariably applied to nail extensions, the health and safety measures for nail extensions must be taken into account (see page 203).

If the allergic reaction occurs when the client is having nail extensions or nail art applied the process should be stopped immediately and the products removed. If the reaction occurs some time later (the curing of nail extension chemicals continues for up to 48 hours after the nail application) the nails must be removed with acetone and it may be the solvents used in nail extensions that are causing the reaction. In severe cases medical advice is required before attempting removal.

Removing nail art

The polish and design are relatively easy to remove as the products are either water soluble or the polish is removed in the normal way.

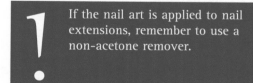

If the nail art is applied to nail extensions, remember to use a non-acetone remover.

EAR–PIERCING

LEVEL
2

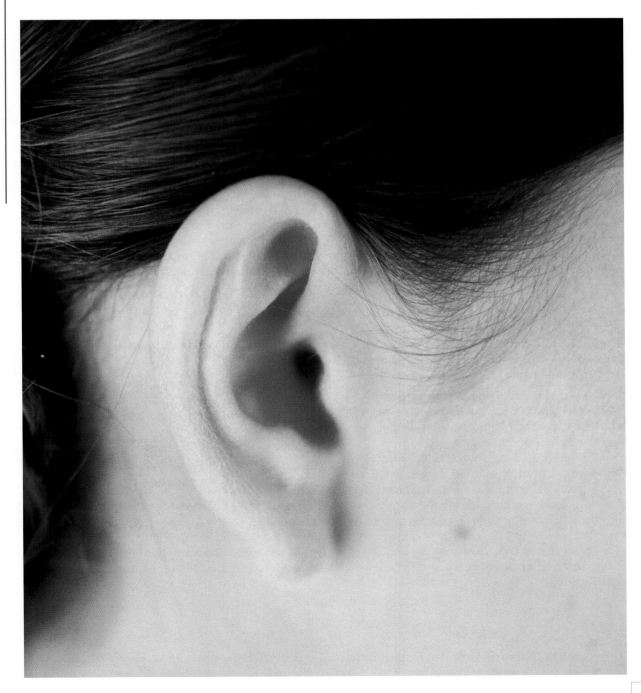

IN THIS CHAPTER YOU WILL LEARN ABOUT:

- Your responsibilities under relevant health and safety legislation
- How to work hygienically and safely
- Preparing the equipment and area for ear-piercing
- Client consultation
- Preparing the client for ear-piercing
- How to recognise and advise on contraindications
- Piercing the ear lobe
- Providing advice with regard to contra-actions and aftercare

Introduction

Ear-piercing is a quick, inexpensive and profitable treatment to perform, the standard service time being only 15 minutes with an average charge of £10–25. Although it appears as an optional unit to the NVQ qualification and can be performed by receptionists, jewellers and hairdressers as well as therapists, it should not be considered lightly. Ear-piercing is an **invasive treatment**, that is to say that the skin is broken, leaving the wound open to infection. Blood and serum loss may occur. There is a risk of cross infection by the AIDS and hepatitis B viruses. This has led to stringent control over the performance of this treatment, involving the salon registering with the local health authority, only disposable types of equipment being used and strict hygiene and waste disposal measures being implemented.

Legislation

Details of **Health and Safety at Work Act 1974** and the **Control of Substances Hazardous to Health Regulations 1992** and other relevant health and safety legislation can be found in chapter 1.

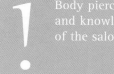

Body piercing requires specialist skills and knowledge and should not be part of the salon treatment.

Special attention should be paid to the **Local Government (Miscellaneous Provisions) Act 1982**, which stipulates that equipment for piercing the skin should be disposable or suitable for sterilisation by an appropriate method such as autoclave or chemical solution. Alternatively, the parts of the equipment that are in contact with the skin during treatment should be disposable. The Act also requires waste material from skin piercing be placed in yellow bin liners and marked as 'contaminated'. The contents have to be collected separately from other waste, then incinerated. Any needles and sharps should be placed in a yellow sharps box for special disposal. Your responsibilities under this and other Acts are to ensure that you know the content of the relevant legislation and carry out the recommendations stated within.

Hygiene and safety

It is essential to maintain high standards of hygiene and professionalism, as with all beauty therapy treatments. This is important to prevent cross infection and promote client confidence. Without such precautions insurance may become invalid. The following hygiene precautions must be carried out for ear-piercing:

1. Work surfaces should be wiped down with hot, soapy water or suitable sanitising solution, both before and after treatment.

2. The ear-piercing equipment should meet legal requirements by being disposable and sterile, ready for use.

3. Wash hands before and after treatment to prevent cross infection, even when disposable gloves are worn.

4. Open cuts or wounds should be covered with a sterile dressing.

5. It is recommended that disposable sterile latex or plastic gloves are worn.

6. The area to be treated is checked for contraindications.

7. Treatment is politely refused if there is infection or disease present. You should pay particular attention to ears that have been pierced previously, particularly multiple ear-piercings.

8. A non-toxic pen should be used to mark the ear lobe.

Preparing the equipment and area for ear-piercing

The ear-piercing system should be approved by the Environmental Health Authority under the Local Government (Miscellaneous Provisions) Act 1982. Stud earrings are more commonly used to pierce the ears due to the increased risk of infection from the ring or sleeper type, but modern gun equipment has eliminated this risk at the time of the treatment. However, the risk remains during the aftercare of the piercing.

The earrings are sealed in pre-sterilised packs, which should only be opened just before use. Where the system includes the use of a gun to pierce, plastic mounting devices are used so the earring remains untouched by hand. The sealed packs often have an expiry date or coloured seal that indicates when the pack should no longer be considered sterile.

There is a wide variety of earrings available: different shapes and those with small coloured stones in a variety of colours as well as the plain round gold type in large or small sizes.

Provide adequate ventilation and heating to ensure client comfort and minimise the risk of fainting. There should be plenty of light so you can see that you are performing the treatment safely and to the client's needs.

To perform an ear-piercing treatment you will need:

1. ear-piercing gun
2. earrings
3. non-toxic marker pen
4. medical wipes or swabs impregnated with alcohol to cleanse the ears
5. mirror
6. clean cotton wool
7. surgical spirit
8. lined waste bin
9. hair clips
10. disposable latex or plastic gloves
11. aftercare lotion and instruction leaflet

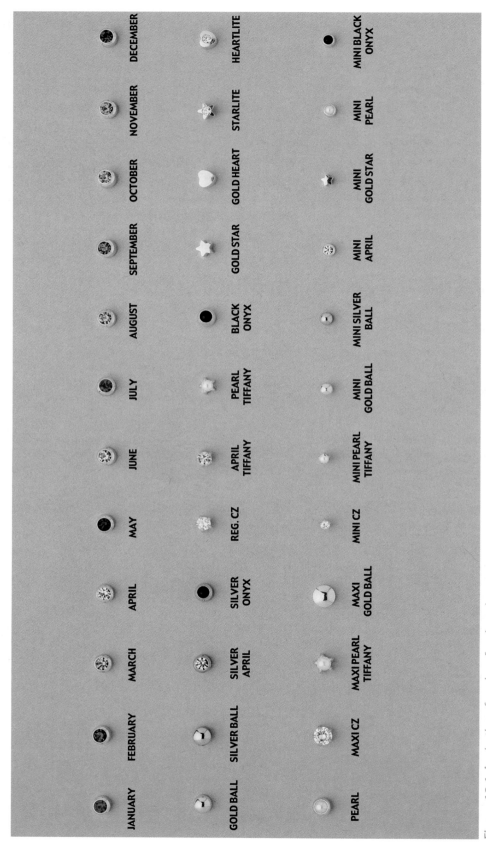

Figure 12.1 *A selection of earrings for pierced ears*

Client consultation

This process includes:

- consultation techniques
- agreeing the service and outcomes of the treatment
- maintaining the client's modesty and privacy
- recognising contraindications and the necessary action to take.

Consultation techniques

A consultation is important for ear-piercing to ensure the suitability of the client for piercing and to determine their needs. The client should be made aware of the procedure, cost, duration, healing time and aftercare before the treatment begins. The consultation must include the following:

1. The area to be treated must be checked for its suitability for piercing. Only the soft tissue of the ear lobe is suitable, as piercing the cartilage leads to a condition known as cauliflower ear, an overgrowth of cartilage. Infection of cartilage tissue is difficult to treat successfully. This chapter does not cover piercing of the nose and other areas of the body. Special insurance and equipment is required to perform these types of treatments.

2. The age of the client should be asked, as you are required by law to gain parental or guardian's consent in writing before piercing a child under 16. Some salons ask this of clients up to the age of 18 although there is no legal obligation to do so. Piercing the ears of a child of pre-school age is legal with parental or guardian consent, though some salons refuse to do this as part of their own salon policy.

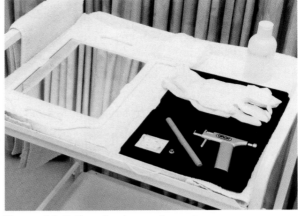

Figure 12.2 *Ear-piercing equipment*

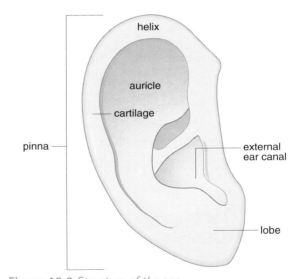

Figure 12.3 *Structure of the ear*

3. It is advisable to write the details of the treatment onto a record card and ask the client (parent or guardian if the client is under 16) to sign to say they have understood and agree to the treatment being performed. A leaflet explaining the treatment can be helpful, particularly as regards the degree of discomfort and the necessary aftercare procedures. Client records should be updated with accurate information on each visit so they can be referred to if necessary and kept confidential to maintain the client's privacy. Client privacy regarding records with reference to the Data Protection Act has already been discussed in chapter 1.

More can be found on consultation and communication techniques in chapter 5.

Information to be recorded includes:

- personal details – telephone number, etc.
- date of treatment
- client or parental signature
- details of the treatment – number of previous piercings, position of piercing (could be a diagram), procedure and aftercare advice given.

Contraindications

It is important that you can identify clients who are unsuitable for this treatment. For example, those requiring medical referral:

- diabetes, due to poor healing ability
- epilepsy, the stress and shock may induce a fit
- circulatory disorders, such as high or low blood pressure
- dysfunction of the nervous system, such as lack of sensation in the area.

Also those who have other conditions in the area that prevent treatment:

- scar tissue
- bruising
- swelling
- cuts and abrasions
- small ear lobe
- moles and warts
- inflammation
- ear infections
- skin diseases or disorders.

When a contraindication is apparent the therapist must use tact and diplomacy to inform the client that the service cannot be performed. If medical referral is required it should be made without naming the specific condition. The therapist should be able to recognise a possible problem but must not diagnose, as they are not qualified to do so. Some contraindications may prevent treatment at that time but it can be performed later when the condition has receded, such as inflammation. Clear and tactful communication is required to inform the client of the facts without causing them undue alarm or distress.

Preparing the client for ear-piercing

The client may be nervous so you must appear reassuring and confident in your approach.

1. The client should be seated at a height convenient to you. They must be comfortable and able to sit upright with the head level and facing forwards. The correct positioning of the client will ensure accurate piercing and minimise injury to you by poor posture, for example backache from bending.

2. Discuss the type and number of earrings required. No more than one pair of earrings should be fitted at one time because the risk of infection and the discomfort is increased. If only one ear is to be pierced, the remaining stud from the sterile pack should be discarded.

3. Secure the hair away from the ear with clips if necessary.

4. With the aid of a mirror, discuss the exact position of the finished result, ensuring this is in the fleshy part of the ear. If other

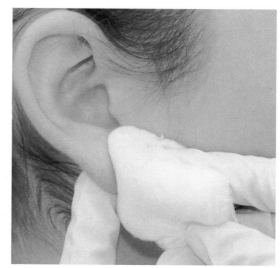

Figure 12.4 *Clean the back and front of each ear with a separate medical swab*

jewellery is present it should be removed at this stage.

5. Clean the ear back and front with a separate medical swab for each ear. Allow to dry.

6. Place a small dot on each ear lobe using the non-toxic marker pen to indicate the position of the earrings. Remember the dot should be placed in the fleshy part of the ear and not too close to the edge as this may cause tearing if caught accidentally. Ensure that the marks are level using the facial features as a guide.

7. Check the intended position with the client using the mirror. If incorrect remove the dot with a medical swab, allow to dry and try again. When both you and the client are happy, continue with the treatment.

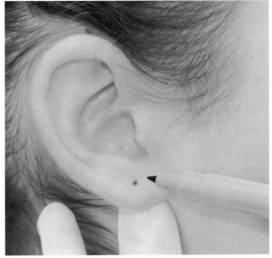

Figure 12.5 *Marking the position with a non-toxic marker pen*

Piercing the ear lobe

1. Load the gun with the earrings according to the manufacturer's instructions. Do not touch the earrings and ensure that all disposable guards are in place.

2. Hold the ear to be pierced with your free hand and with the gun in a horizontal position place the stem of the earring over the mark made on the ear lobe. Squeeze the trigger gently so the stem is closer to the ear. Check the position over the mark and if correct squeeze firmly to release the gun and pierce the ear. If the position is not correct, reposition and repeat.

3. Release the gun by gently pulling downwards while still holding the ear with the other hand.

4. Repeat on the other ear if required.

5. If the gun malfunctions the usual result is that the back of the earring is not secured to the stem. In this instance it is advisable to place the back into position by hand after wiping it with a

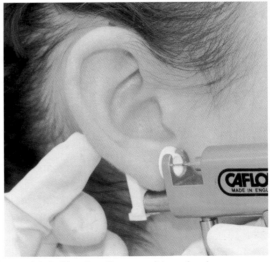

Figure 12.6 *Piercing the ear with a piercing gun*

clean medical swab. In the unlikely event that the ear is not pierced through, the earring should be removed, the area wiped with a medical swab, covered with a sterile dressing and the client asked to return when healed. This may take several weeks and they should be provided with aftercare lotion to bathe the area during the healing process. If any problems occur they should be advised to seek medical advice.

6. Show the finished result to the client in the mirror.

7. Instruct the client on aftercare.

8. Clean the gun with surgical spirit and store hygienically for the next use.

9. Remove all waste from the area including the gloves and place in a plastic bin liner in a covered bin.

Providing advice with regard to contra-actions and aftercare

1. Explain to the client that they will initially feel tingling and there may be some redness and slight swelling. If this persists, or any contra-actions such as irritation, soreness or weeping occur, the client must inform the salon so that advice can be given and notes made on the client's record card.

2. Advice on care of newly pierced ears is to be meticulous in keeping the area clean. Should any of the mentioned contra-actions occur, begin bathing with salt water or aftercare solution. If the problems continue the client should see a doctor.

3. The earrings should not be removed for 6 weeks to give the ears time to heal properly, preventing secondary infection. Premature removal will result in the hole closing up and/or infection.

4. The ears should be bathed twice a day with the aftercare solution or warm salt water. Undiluted antiseptic is not suitable for this as it is too strong and may cause irritation or chemical burns.

5. The hands should be washed before the ears are bathed and touching the ears or earrings between bathing should be avoided.

6. After bathing the earrings should be turned to avoid the ear healing onto the stud. To do this, hold the back of the earring with one hand whilst turning the stud with the other.

7. Avoid spraying the ears with hairspray or perfume and ensure that shampoo and soap do not accumulate around the earring.

8. After 6 weeks the earrings can be changed with others of a good quality metal. Care should be taken with cheap fashion earrings as they are made of metals that cause irritation and should only be worn for short periods of time.

9. If no earrings are worn then the holes are likely to heal over.

10. It is rare for a client to develop a condition called keloids, an overgrowth of scar tissue. If this does arise, the client should be advised not to have further piercing and to remove the earrings and seek medical advice if necessary.

11. If allergies occur at any time the earrings should be removed immediately and the client instructed to see a doctor if the condition is severe.

It is advisable to issue a leaflet on aftercare as well as verbally instructing the client.

ACTIVITY

Design an aftercare leaflet for use with clients who have had their ears pierced.

Chapter 13

SPA TREATMENTS

LEVEL
2

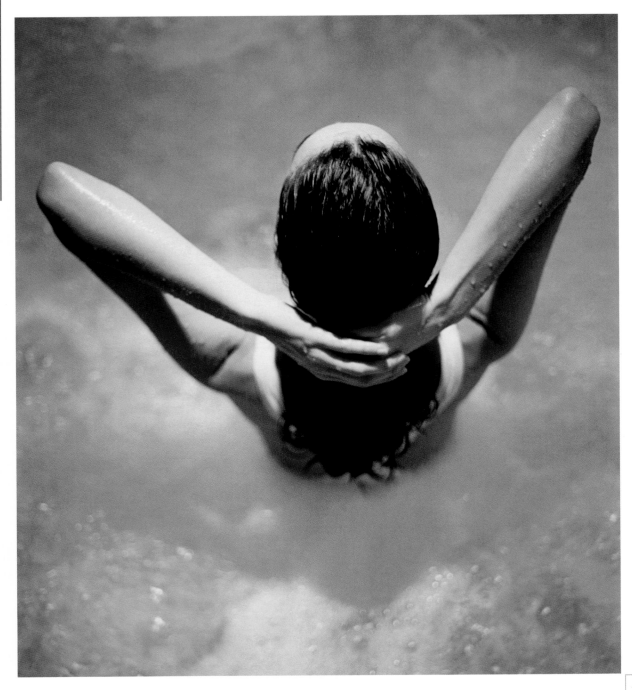

- Types of spa treatments available
- Effects of spa treatments on the skin and body
- Preparation and hygiene procedures for the client and the spa environment
- Maintenance procedures for the use of spa equipment
- Monitoring procedures for the use of spa treatment equipment
- Safe use of spa treatment equipment
- Possible contra-actions to spa treatments and the action to take if they occur
- Suitable aftercare advice
- Shutdown procedures to follow for spa treatments
- Legal responsibilities when using spa treatment equipment

Introduction

Spa treatments have become increasingly popular with clients. Originally available for the rich and famous at exclusive health farms, the increase in demand has led to their arrival in high street salons and day spas. As a therapist it is important to have knowledge of these treatments to increase your effectiveness and the chance of employment in every type of working environment.

Spa treatments, however, are not a new phenomenon. The benefits of such treatments were known in Roman times and even earlier, with the bathing rituals in Japan and northern European countries using heat and water for their therapeutic and relaxation effects.

Modern spa therapies include the traditional use of heat and water but with the addition of product application, wraps and flotation tanks for therapeutic effect.

Types of spa treatments

1. **Steam** – a moist heat treatment applied either in a specially designed room for use by several people or individuals can be treated in a steam bath or cabinet.
2. **Sauna** – a dry heat treatment applied using an insulated pine-panelled cabin or one made of logs for use by several people.
3. **Hydrotherapy** – the use of air and water jets to massage while heating the body. A **spa bath** is for use by individuals whereas several people can use a **spa pool** at once.
4. **Flotation** – the sensation of weightlessness created by this treatment induces a deep sense of relaxation and relieves aches and pains.
5. **Body wrapping** – allows the skin to absorb products for different effects, which is then enhanced by wrapping the body in specially designed bandages or thermal reflective sheeting.
6. **Relaxation rooms** – form an important part of the spa experience.

Effects of spa treatments

Many of the treatments listed above rely on the production of heat for their effect. It is essential to understand the effects of heat on the skin and body. Individual spa treatment effects will be discussed under each treatment.

We are aware of the relaxing and sedating effect of sitting in the warmth of the sun and need to understand what is happening inside the body.

Heat applied to the body, totally or in part, will result in a rise in body temperature. This triggers two processes to cool the body, **sweating** and **vasodilation** (dilation) of the blood vessels in the skin. Sweating, or diaphoresis, can result in 0.1–1.5 litres of water being exuded from the body. With the water, waste products are eliminated including sodium chloride (salt) and urea, therefore cleansing the skin and improving its tone and elasticity. In addition the kidneys are assisted in their function and it is thought that, combined with a calorie-controlled diet, weight loss can occur as a lot of this water is derived from the subcutaneous layer of the skin. Care should be taken, however, as dehydration can also result. A person already dehydrated, for example, someone under the influence of drugs or alcohol, should not have spa treatments.

Vasodilation promotes an increase in blood circulation, improved lymph flow and the exchange of nutrients and oxygen for waste products in the tissues. The skin and its structures and other tissues such as muscles are therefore nourished, promoting increased function. In the case of muscle tissue, the heat relaxes tense muscles and waste products, such as lactic acid produced after activity, are removed, promoting quick and efficient contraction and relief from aches and pains.

The increase in blood circulation is not localised to the skin and muscles. The general blood circulation is improved and results in an increase in heart and pulse rate and the lowering of blood pressure. These effects are similar to those produced when exercising and so there is also an increase in metabolic rate (the rate by which calories are burnt), adding to the potential for weight loss. However, unfit clients may feel exhausted after spa treatments due to this effect and so a period of rest after treatment is advised.

Other effects of heat are the soothing of sensory nerve endings promoting a feeling of thorough relaxation and comfort. With most spa treatments the skin is left hydrated, which allows for the effective application of electrical body treatments as the current passes easily through the hydrated epidermis. The relaxing of the tissues, especially muscles, makes them more receptive to treatments such as massage and passive exercise. For these reasons spa treatments are commonly used to preheat the tissues for another associated treatment as well as being a treatment in their own right.

In summary the effects of heat are:

1. Increases body temperature.
2. Induces perspiration.
3. Eliminates waste products.
4. Increases blood circulation with resulting erythema.
5. Lowers blood pressure.
6. Raises pulse rate.
7. Improves lymph flow.
8. Warms the tissues.
9. Relaxes muscles.
10. Relieves minor pain and stiffness.
11. Gives a feeling of relaxation and well-being.
12. Can be dehydrating.

Preparation procedures for the client

The preparation procedures for the client include:

- consultation
- client records
- hygiene and safety precautions.

Consultation

An effective consultation uses communication techniques to ascertain relevant information about the client regarding the use of spa treatments. The techniques used include questioning, listening and non-verbal communication such as body language. More can be found on consultation and communication techniques in chapter 5.

The consultation procedure should determine the indications and contraindications for treatment, and an explanation of the treatment procedure, the effects, any adaptations, duration and cost should be given. During this process the client must be made to feel at ease and reassured that their modesty and privacy will be maintained throughout the treatment. Time for the client to ask questions should be allowed in order that they may clarify or understand what you have said and allay any apprehensions before treatment commences. Allowing this time ensures their confidence and willingness to be treated.

Indications for the use of spa treatments

1. To ease stiffness after exercise.
2. For pleasure and relaxation.
3. To create a sense of well-being.
4. Part of a slimming programme to promote self-esteem.
5. Part of an anti-cellulite programme.
6. To cleanse the body.
7. To improve poor blood circulation – cold feet, swollen ankles, etc.
8. To prepare the tissues for other treatment (preheat).

Contraindications to the use of spa treatments

1. Cardiovascular conditions, e.g. angina, heart attack, etc.
2. High or low blood pressure.
3. Blood vessel conditions – varicose veins, thrombosis, phlebitis.
4. Skin diseases.
5. Respiratory disorders – colds, flu, bronchitis, asthma.
6. Pregnancy.
7. Fever.
8. Headaches or migraine sufferers.
9. Persons under the influence of drugs or alcohol.
10. Within 2–3 hours of a heavy meal or if no food has been eaten for several hours.
11. Diabetics.
12. Epileptics.
13. Recent scar tissue.
14. During the first two days of menstruation.
15. Severe exhaustion.
16. Severe bruising.
17. Hypersensitive skins.
18. Loss of skin sensation.
19. Sunburn.

Client records

To maintain a professional and safe spa environment it is important to update client records with accurate information after every visit. Accurate records ensure the safety of the individual without repeating information. This is particularly important if a different therapist is responsible for the client on another visit. A high level of service is therefore assured.

These records must be confidential; if logged in a paper-based system they must be stored under lock and key and if on a computer, they are subject to the Data Protection Act 1998. More on the Data Protection Act can be found in chapter 1.

Hygiene and safety procedures

1. Clients should be checked for contraindications and the appropriate action taken if present.
2. Clients should shower before using spa treatment equipment.
3. Remove make-up and hair lacquer to avoid entry into the eyes.
4. Clients should wear clean swimwear or disposable underwear as appropriate.
5. Do not leave client unattended in case of fainting.
6. Do not exceed temperature guidelines
7. Clients should be encouraged to rest after use.
8. Cool showers and/or plunge pools can be used to cool body temperature if desired.
9. Indicate source of heat in steam and sauna to avoid burns.
10. Duckboards, non-slip matting or towels should be used on floors.
11. Wipe up spilt water immediately.
12. Restrict duration according to treatment guidelines.
13. To reduce the risk of cross infection of foot-related diseases, such as athlete's foot and verrucae, disposable or washable shoes should be provided.
14. Jewellery should be removed as it will get hot during the treatment and may burn the client.

Preparation procedures for the spa environment

These include:

- hygiene and the principles of cross infection
- temperature and environment control including adequate ventilation
- preparation of equipment and area for use.

The moisture and warmth of the spa environment is an excellent breeding ground for micro-organisms. Airborne micro-organisms include viral infections such as those that produce colds and flu. They are spread in minute droplets of water in the airway of an infected person. Coughing and sneezing sends the virus into the humid air of the spa environment where another person can breathe them in. Food and drink can also be contaminated if the droplets fall onto exposed food. Waterborne infections can be spread by direct or indirect contact with infected surfaces or by being immersed in contaminated water. Bacterial, viral and fungal infections, such as athlete's foot, verrucae and cystitis, can be spread this way. It is imperative that strict hygiene procedures are maintained in order to minimise cross infection.

Hygiene and the principles of cross infection

A spa's floor and walls are usually tiled or lined with fibreglass or maybe marble. These surfaces are easy to clean with the appropriate disinfectant or hot water and detergent. Follow the manufacturer's/installer's instructions at all times to ensure adequate levels of hygiene. This is usually performed at the end of each working day or user session. This is very important as several people will use the facility at the same time.

Fibreglass is resistant to the growth of micro-organisms but should still be wiped with an appropriate disinfectant to prevent cross infection. A more detailed description of cross infection and the basic procedures to follow can be found in chapter 1.

The best way to avoid cross infection is to prevent anyone with an infectious condition from using the spa facilities. Strict application of contraindications by the therapist can greatly reduce the risks but this is not always possible with conditions that have yet to exhibit any symptoms. The application of good hygiene procedures performed at the correct interval of time can minimise the risks even further.

The following procedures are specific to the spa environment.

General hygiene procedures for the spa

1. Check the client for contraindications. Anyone with ear, skin, genital, foot or other bodily infection should refrain from using the spa.

2. All surfaces – floors, walls, benches, showers, etc. – should be washed down daily or more frequently if in constant use, with an appropriate disinfectant, in other words, one containing phenols, chlorinated xylenols or quaternary ammonium compounds and one that leaves no residue or smell. These should be used in a well-ventilated area following the manufacturer's instructions. Wearing personal protective equipment such as gloves, apron, mask and goggles will be necessary.

3. Clean, fresh laundry should be provided for each client, including a gown for personal use while visiting the spa. Laundry should be washed at the highest temperature possible with a suitable detergent.

4. A cut-out technique should be used where possible contamination of products or surfaces may occur. For example, clients should wear disposable shoes and towels to act as a barrier between clients and surfaces when cleaning the surface after each contact is impossible.

5. No food or drink should be consumed within the spa area but in specially designated areas only, such as the relaxation room. Water and fruit juice can be offered but should be provided by and under the control of the establishment. Such drinks should be kept in a refrigerator or sealed drinks dispenser and not left out in the spa environment. Any unused beverage should be disposed of at the end of the day.

6. Stagnant water is an ideal breeding ground for micro-organisms so pools of water must not be allowed to remain from condensation or spillage but should be mopped up immediately.

7. The possibility of external pollutants entering the spa on shoes and clothing can be avoided by providing changing facilities for both clients and staff. Therapists should not wear their work uniform outside of the spa environment.

8. Washing hands in hot soapy water before and after each client and after visiting the toilet is a simple yet effective way of reducing cross infection. Consider, also, washing hands after handling chemicals, even if gloves have been worn, and before handling beverages.

9. Strict records of cleaning regimes should be kept in order to maintain hygiene levels and easily satisfy a health and safety inspector. A simple way is to have a chart on the wall of each facility so that the person responsible signs in the appropriate space when the cleaning regime has been carried out. Some local authorities require strict procedures to be followed in public spas and swimming pools.

Cleaning procedure	Date	Time	Signature	Date	Time	Signature	Date	Time	Signature
Floors									
Showers									
Spa bath									
Sauna									

The following checklist will provide a routine to be followed:

1. Check for contraindications, i.e. skin diseases.
2. Clients must shower before use.
3. Clients must wear swimwear or disposable underwear during spa treatment.
4. Any cuts and/or abrasions should be covered with a waterproof dressing.
5. Place disposable absorbent paper on seats as well as towels.
6. Towels and paper should be changed after each client.
7. Towelling or paper should be placed on the floor of a steam bath or cabinet to absorb condensation deposited there.
8. The steam bath or cabinet should be wiped with a disinfectant solution after each client.
9. The sauna should be scrub-washed regularly with plain water only to avoid noxious fumes when the sauna is reheated.
10. The water in the sauna bucket should be changed after each client.
11. Hydrotherapy equipment intended for use by more than one person requires regular circulation of water to ensure the use of commercially installed filtration plants. The number of circulations before a hygienic level is achieved depends on the size of the spa pool. Be guided by the manufacturer's instructions.
12. Chemical treatment of the hydrotherapy equipment water with chlorine or bromine is essential. The aim is to produce a stable chemical condition that acts as a disinfectant but not so much as to be obnoxious to clients (causing eye problems, dry skin, unpleasant smell, etc.). The latest commercial installations incorporate automatic chemical treatment machinery, which can test regularity at short intervals. This should not replace manual testing (e.g. twice daily) and the appropriate records should be kept. These tests take the form of simple pH and chlorine level tests. It is important to maintain the correct level of pH to ensure effectiveness and no detrimental effects. A pH6 gives maximum disinfectant power but is unpleasant to bathe in; pH9 means that only a small percentage of chlorine or bromine is free to act as a disinfectant. An acceptable level is approximately pH7.4–7.6 to justify both criteria.
13. The pool itself should be drained occasionally and the acrylic surface wiped with a recommended cleaning agent (**not** detergent).
14. Spa baths are drained and cleaned for each individual user and therefore, generally, the water needs not to be treated.
15. Most baths are made of an acrylic material so the surface must be wiped after each use with a cleaner recommended by the manufacturer to avoid contamination of the recirculating water machinery.

Temperature control and adequate ventilation

A control panel away from the treatment area determines the temperature of a steam room. It cannot be adjusted to suit an individual and so a thermometer should be placed inside or the temperature displayed in order for the client to judge their tolerance level. In general men can tolerate a higher temperature than women and as the humidity is high the temperature is usually lower than that of a sauna.

The temperature and timing controls for a steam bath are usually found on the outside. These can be adjusted to suit an individual's tolerance level. Both controls are used to achieve the working temperature of 50–55°C.

Modern treatment saunas are panelled, usually made of pine, which is a material capable of absorbing the moisture from the air within, otherwise the air would become stale, smell unpleasant and be unhygienic.

The panels are packed with insulating material, which retains the heat within the sauna (saving electricity and preventing the alteration of the room's normal temperature). The air must be allowed to circulate around the sauna to permit an interchange of air within it. The heat is controlled by a thermostat, which should be placed outside the sauna to avoid interference by the clients. A thermometer indicates the temperature as near to the top of the sauna as possible. The correct temperature should be between 60–90°C at the top of the sauna. Generally, women prefer a temperature between 60–70°C and men 80–90°C. The heat produced is a dry heat so a water bucket and ladle are provided. Water is used to pour onto the stones to produce steam if the air becomes too dry. An essential oil such as eucalyptus may be used in the water to create a pleasant smell and give therapeutic effects.

Spa pool water temperature should not exceed 40°C as high water levels raise the body organ temperature to dangerous levels. At this temperature exposure should be limited to 15 minutes before cooling down. After this time further exposure can occur but for a shorter period. If prolonged exposure is desired, the water temperature should be reduced to normal body temperature (37°C).

Spa baths should be cooler than normal bathing temperature as the turbulence will raise the temperature beyond this level. The water should be comfortably warm on entering the bath.

Wet flotation tanks should also contain comfortably warm water so as to be pleasant and aid the relaxation experience, whereas in dry tanks the client lies on a waterbed or airbed wrapped in blankets and relies on the room temperature for comfort. Relaxation rooms should be of similar temperature, approximately 22°C.

Body wrap products often produce their own heat on application to the body, with the exception of paraffin wax, which must be melted before application. The temperature that is required for application varies a little with the amount being melted but should be approximately 49°C.

Ventilation

Spa treatments naturally produce a high level of humidity, which combined with the heat produces an ideal environment in which airborne and waterborne micro-organisms can multiply. By removing the warm, humid air and replacing it with fresh air the risks of cross infection can be greatly reduced.

It is thought that for this type of humid environment, approximately 17–20 cubic metres of fresh air are needed per hour for each person using the room. This is divided by the volume of the room to give the number of complete air changes needed per hour.

Example

In the relaxation room that measures 3 m high × 4 m wide × 10 m long there is the facility for 14 people to sit and relax. Seventeen cubic metres of air are needed per hour per person.

The calculations are:

Cubic metres of air: 17 × 14 = 238

Volume of the room: 3 × 4 × 10 = 120

238/120 = approx. 2

So the number of air changes needed per hour is 2.

Opening doors and windows can lead to draughts and work against the aims of the treatment. The best method of ventilation is air conditioning, an artificial form of ventilation. Modern units filter dust and other airborne particles, including micro-organisms, warm or cool air as desired and can moisten or dry air by the use of a control panel.

Preparation of equipment and area for use

Preparation of the spa environment involves general procedures and those specific for each type of equipment.

General procedures include ensuring an adequate supply of towels and other laundry and consumables such as tissue, couch roll, cotton wool, cleansers, etc. Each spa establishment will have its own routine to follow but each must be within legal requirements as described earlier to ensure hygiene levels. Regular stock controls should be in place to ensure availability and adequate laundry should be gauged by the number of clients booked for that day, with extra in case of emergency and late bookings.

Preparation procedures for the equipment involve the protection of surfaces with towels and paper in accordance with establishment guidelines and with most equipment the heating up procedures to efficient operational temperature.

Spa pools do not require preheating as the expense incurred to do this every day is great. Instead a thermostat, similar to that of an immersion heater in a domestic house maintains the pool's temperature. However, the water is not circulated overnight and so must start at the beginning of each working day. The water should be allowed to circulate the correct number of times as described by the manufacturer, depending on the size of the pool, to allow sufficient filtration to have occurred before the first client can enter it. This is a hygiene precaution that must be strictly adhered to.

Equipment	Warm-up period
Steam room	20–30 minutes
Steam bath/cabinet	10–15 minutes
Sauna	20–30 minutes
Paraffin wax (50 lb for a whole body application)	40–60 minutes

Body wrap preparation can involve preparing the couch with towels and thermal sheeting, placing bandages into special heaters or warming products in a water bath.

Relaxation rooms should be checked for warmth and comfort with magazines available, cushions and fresh beverages to aid the relaxation process. Lighting and appropriate music should also be considered.

Maintenance procedures for the use of spa equipment

These include:

- operational maintenance
- maintenance reports
- maintenance records
- chemical testing.

Operational maintenance

Efficient operational maintenance procedures ensure the smooth, safe and hygienic running of a spa and involve electrical and cleaning checks and maintenance of stock and water levels.

1. Electrical checks should be made by a qualified electrician as laid down in The Electricity at Work Regulations 1992, with frequent checks by the therapist for exposed wires and broken plugs. If faulty, the equipment should not be used. All electrical appliances should be switched off and disconnected from the mains when not in use. Due to the humid environment presented, a qualified person should install and maintain electrical equipment.

2. At the beginning of the day the correct function and the temperature of the equipment should be checked. The temperature can be checked simply with a thermometer being placed in situation. Any faults presented mean the discontinued use of the equipment.

3. Water levels are checked visually and these checks apply to steam and hydrotherapy equipment. A spa pool's water should be clear so that the bottom of the pool can be seen before the jets are running. Water must be maintained at the correct level so adequate filtration can take place. The water in pools should be drained and replaced according to the schedule laid down by the manufacturer.

4. Filter systems should be checked for operation but a professional fitter must perform maintenance.

5. Hygiene levels should be maintained throughout the day considering the frequency of use, levels of condensation and adequate supply of fresh towels, consumables and ventilation.

Modern professional hydrotherapy equipment that seats more than one person has suitable chemical testing equipment already fitted. However, this does not replace the twice daily manual checks using a testing kit recommended by the manufacturer. This is important in the case of testing equipment failure. Maintenance of the correct pH is important to provide adequate protection from cross infection. Always read and follow the instructions carefully. It is advisable to replace the chemicals in the testing kit once each year to ensure accurate readings. Test the water in your spa or hot tub with a reliable test kit on a schedule recommended by your spa or hot tub professional. Add the necessary chemicals according to the test results and the manufacturer's instructions. In the hot water environments of spas and hot tubs, disinfectants may rapidly break up and spread out, requiring more frequent water testing. Follow the manufacturer's instructions in this regard. The more people who use the facility, the more frequently you should test the water.

Remember:

1. Before using chemicals, read the labels and directions carefully. Follow label use instructions.

2. Keep all chemicals out of the reach of children.

Storage

1. Keep the original lids on all chemical containers and make sure the lids are closed tightly when not in use.

2. Do not stack different chemicals on top of one another.

3. Store spa or hot tub chemicals in a clean, cool, dry, well-ventilated area, preferably off the floor, to prevent contamination from other materials. Keep them away from other chemicals and equipment.

4. Keep liquid chemicals away from dry chemicals. Keep apart chemicals that are different forms of oxidising compounds. Physically separate all different forms of chemicals.

5. Do not store spa or hot tub chemicals where other flammable items may mix with them. For example, a mixture of these chemicals and fertilizer can cause a fire or explosion.

Maintenance reports

Following the discovery of a piece of faulty equipment, a clear label advising discontinued use should be attached and the fault reported to a senior member of staff. This should be entered into the equipment log and a professional contacted to instigate a repair if possible. The reporting of faulty equipment is a legal requirement and such reports should be made available for inspection if desired.

The unavailability of towels and consumables should also be reported to a senior member of staff so the provision can be made for their replacement. This can involve altering stock levels and reviewing the laundry procedures.

Maintenance records

You have a legal obligation to keep accurate records for the maintenance of spa treatment equipment. This includes water and chemical levels, frequency of testing and general maintenance and cleaning regimes. The local authority environmental health officer will inspect these records.

Chemical testing

Usage

1. Never mix two chemicals together. Use a clean scoop for each chemical, and avoid combining material from 'old' and 'new' containers.
2. Always add the chemicals directly to the spa or hot tub water, either in a suitable feeder, distributed across the surface of the water, or diluted and poured into the water. Follow label use instructions.
3. When preparing water solutions for feeder application, pour the chemical slowly into the appropriate amount of water, stirring constantly to provide mixing and dilution.
4. Always add chemicals to water. Never add water to chemicals.
5. Never add chemicals to the spa or hot tub water while people are using the facility.
6. Carefully clean up any spilled chemicals with large amounts of water, to dilute and wash away the chemicals. Disinfectants and pH adjustment chemicals can usually be sent to the sewer with large quantities of water, since they are intended for use at low levels.
7. Wash out empty disinfectant containers before disposal to eliminate danger of fire, explosion or poisoning.
8. Do not inhale dust or fumes from any chemicals. If necessary, use proper protective devices for breathing, handling and eye protection. Promptly wash off any residues that get on your skin.
9. Never reuse old chemical containers unless specified by the manufacturer.
10. If you have any questions regarding safe handling, storage or use of spa or hot tub chemicals, contact the manufacturer.

Monitoring procedures for the use of spa treatment equipment

This includes:

- monitoring of equipment and treatment area
- monitoring the client's well-being
- monitoring the client's modesty and privacy
- monitoring the presence of contra-actions and taking necessary action.

Monitoring of equipment and treatment area

Monitoring of the spa treatment equipment and the treatment area procedures has been discussed in some detail previously in this chapter. This includes checking:

- heat
- humidity
- water levels
- chemical concentration
- treatment times
- ventilation
- consumables
- ambience of the environment.

Treatment times are discussed as part of the safe use of spa treatment equipment later in this chapter.

Monitoring the client's well-being

The well-being of the client should be considered throughout the spa treatment to ensure their enjoyment and safety. This includes making enquiries as to the client's:

- comfort
- temperature
- needs
- presence of contra-actions.

When a client is enjoying the treatment they will be at ease and feel relaxed and comfortable. They may not realise, however, that they need to rest or drink water. Care should be taken with all clients, but especially those who presented a contraindication and have medical permission to have the treatment.

Monitoring the client's modesty and privacy

The client's modesty and privacy should be considered throughout the treatment to ensure their confidence, which in turn will guarantee their return custom. Consider:

- privacy of client records
- adequate changing facilities
- adequate and suitable gowns and covering
- security of personal belongings
- avoiding unnecessary exposure
- procedures for mixed gender usage.

Most clients will be a little shy about exposing their bodies and the therapist must use the verbal and non-verbal signs given by the client as a guide to the level of privacy they may need to feel comfortable. If the spa is being used by both men and women then the client should be informed. They should also be informed of the correct attire to bring with them when booking the appointment. Providing suitable changing facilities with individual cubicles for changing and the appropriate attire, i.e. a gown, will promote confidence. Avoid unnecessary exposure by careful towel handling when helping clients into and out of a piece of equipment.

Client privacy regarding records and security of personal belongings have already been discussed in chapters 1 and 5.

Monitoring the presence of contra-actions and taking necessary action

More on contra-actions and the necessary action to follow can be found later in this chapter.

Steam

Steam treatments can be administered in a steam room or Turkish baths and a steam bath or cabinet. Steam rooms are found in large health clubs and spas and steam baths are commonly found in beauty salons and smaller health clubs and spas. Steam rooms work on the same principle as the steam bath but on a much larger scale. Traditional steam rooms consist of a number of rooms with steam of different temperatures that clients can wander through according to their tolerance. Plunge pools are commonly found in steam rooms to help cool the client's body down. This creates a vigorous and stimulating effect but there is no additional benefit over allowing the body to return to normal temperature slowly whilst resting.

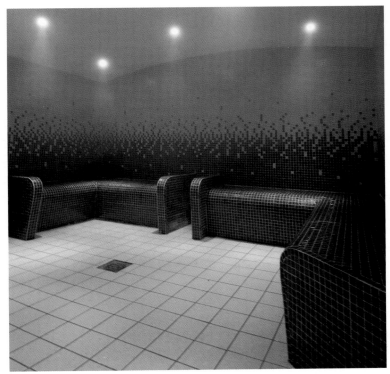

Figure 13.1 *Steam bath/cabinet*

Steam baths are usually made of fibreglass or metal. They have an adjustable seat inside that the client sits on so that their head is free when the steam unit door is closed. Underneath the seat is a container filled with distilled water. When the bath is switched on the water heats up and produces steam, which is trapped inside the bath. This provides a moist or humid heat.

Properties and individual effects of a steam treatment

1. High humidity (about 95 per cent).
2. Client breathes room air.
3. Heating costs are relatively low.
4. Body temperature rises but is less than in sauna.
5. Temperature changes occur relatively quickly.
6. Skin temperature is less than sauna.
7. Fibreglass is an easy material to keep hygienic.
8. Remember the client should be supervised at all times.

Procedure for steam bath application

1. Fill the reservoir of the steam bath to within 1 cm (½ inch) of the top or at least 5 cm (2 inches) deep.
2. Place towels and tissue on the seat and floor of the steam bath so that the client's legs are protected from the steam but do not block the flow of steam. Clients should be advised to place their feet on the covered teak floor treads and not to the rear of the steam bath to avoid burning.
3. Place a towel and tissue on the floor outside the steam bath.
4. Set the thermostat to the required position, approximately 8–9 on dial (see manufacturer's instructions).

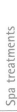

5. Place a towel over the opening for the head and switch on by setting the timer control to 15 minutes. Leave to warm up. This should be done before the client is ready. While waiting, perform step 6.

6. Clients should be checked for contraindications.

7. Clients should shower first.

8. Clients should wear protective head covering (a towel or bath cap) to protect their hairstyle.

9. Clients should remove all jewellery as it will become hot and may burn.

10. When the bell sounds the steam unit is ready for use. The steam bath will immediately begin to cool so it is important to get the client in the bath quickly.

11. Remove the gown or towel and help the client into the steam bath.

12. The towel used to cover the opening for the head is now placed around the client's neck for comfort.

13. Set the timer for the required number of minutes, maximum 25, less if it is the client's first treatment.

14. The timing should only be a guide. If any discomfort is felt, then the client may end the treatment. Remember that clients have different levels of heat tolerance.

15. After treatment duration, the client is helped from the steam bath. A clean towel should be available for the client to dry themselves.

16. The client should be encouraged to shower after a steam bath, before continuing other treatment, for hygiene reasons.

17. If no further treatment is required the client should be encouraged to rest for 15 minutes before getting dressed. Water or herbal drinks should be offered at this time.

18. Steam baths should not be taken more than once every other day.

The sauna cabin

The sauna originates from Finland and is based on the 'log cabin', which uses solid wood, usually pine, to form a free-standing unit that can be erected on any suitable flat floor. Modern treatment saunas are panelled versions, usually made of pine with insulating material, which retains the heat within the sauna. Air must be allowed to circulate around the sauna to permit an interchange of air within it. Heat is provided by electrically powered stoves, which heat special stones placed in a recessed tray above the stove. Small stoves for small saunas can be plugged into the normal electricity supply but larger ones need a special power cable and must be installed professionally. Seated on the stoves are special stones that emit the heat, rising on convection currents. Water is poured onto the stones to produce steam if the air becomes too dry. An essential oil such as eucalyptus may be used in the water to create a pleasant smell and give therapeutic effects.

No special plumbing is needed for a sauna, although running hot and cold water are useful in order to provide showering facilities and to hose down the sauna at regular intervals.

Properties and individual effects of sauna treatment

1. Low humidity (moisture).

2. Client breathes hot, dry air.

3. Heating cost requires use by several clients at one time for it to be cost-effective.

4. Considerable rise in body temperature, varying with the individual.

5. Temperature changes occur very slowly.

6. Skin temperature becomes very high.

7. Wood is difficult to clean so special hygiene precautions are necessary.

Remember the clients must be supervised at all times.

Procedure for sauna cabin application

1. Switch the sauna on. Small cabins take 20–30 minutes to heat up, larger ones, up to an hour.
2. Prepare the water bucket, adding essential oil if desired.
3. Prepare towels and tissues on benches (to be replaced after each treatment).
4. Clients should remove all make-up, jewellery and hair spray and wrap hair in a towel or cap.
5. Clients should shower before taking a sauna for hygiene reasons. If the client has difficulty in perspiring, being still wet from the shower will help.
6. The client may retain the towel or wear swimsuit/bikini bottoms in the sauna.
7. Encourage the client to sit on the lower benches away from the stove, then to progress to higher benches when warmed.
8. Encourage the client to breathe through the mouth rather than the nose, as it is more comfortable.
9. Clients may ladle a little water onto the stones to raise the humidity – make them aware of the increase in temperature this will create.
10. Advise the client they may periodically leave the sauna to shower or rest before returning.
11. Clients should have a cool shower after a maximum treatment time of 30 minutes.
12. The client should rest at room temperature for about 30 minutes, depending on the body temperature reached in the sauna, to allow the heart rate to return to normal.
13. The client should be offered water to drink during rest period.

Hydrotherapy – spa pools ('jacuzzis'), spa baths and hot tubs

Spa pool

Spa pools vary in size, accommodating from 4 up to 20 people, however it is common to find spa pools that seat up to 8 people. Spa pools look like miniature swimming pools with a submerged seat all round the inside edge. Air is compressed and forced into the water causing bubbles, and water in the form of jets increases the turbulence. These jets have a similar effect on the body tissue to massage.

The area around the spa pool should be non-slip as clients will be wet when they leave the pool. The area must also be kept warm to prevent clients from feeling cold. Around the edge of the spa pool is an overflow that allows water to be channelled away as the client steps into the pool instead of spilling out onto the floor. A good filtration system also helps to keep the water clean and hygienic. As more than one client at a time uses the pool, the addition of chemicals and strict water checks must be done to ensure hygiene.

Spa baths

These work on the same principle as a spa pool except that the bath will seat only one client at a time. This allows privacy for the client if they feel uncomfortable using shared facilities.

As the spa bath is used by one client at a time, the water is drained and the bath cleaned for each individual, therefore eliminating the need for chemical additives and filtration equipment to circulate the water at all times. This makes the running of a spa bath less expensive than other hydrotherapy equipment.

Hot tubs

A hot tub is traditionally a vertical, wooden structure allowing 4–8 people to stand upright in close contact. Being made of wood, it is impossible to keep hygienic and the close proximity of the bathers encourages cross infection. Modern hot tubs are made of acrylic or fibreglass and the name is now interchangeable with spa pool.

Spa treatments

249

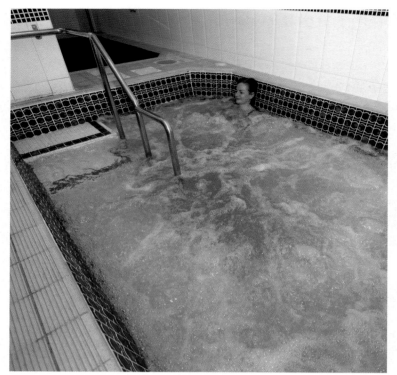

Figure 13.2 *Spa pool*

Power-jet massage

The massage effect achieved when water is applied under pressure to form a jet, or series of jets, can be as invigorating as some aspects of a manual massage, with the associated effects of warmth, steam and aromatherapy products. If spa treatment is not suitable, a similar experience can be achieved with a power-jet massage shower or impulse shower. The treatment can be provided within the confines of a shower cubicle, with the client regulating the jets for a range of effects on the body. These types of showers are fitted in top-quality hotels and are becoming common in the home.

Properties and individual effects of spa treatment

1. High humidity.
2. Client breathes air that is hot and humid.
3. Presence of air and water jets provides a massaging effect not obtained with steam or sauna.
4. Considerable rise in body temperature.
5. Skin temperature is also very high.
6. Client can regulate the jets of water.
7. Hygienic measures should be strictly adhered to with careful cleaning of the shower cubicle.

Remember clients should be supervised at all times.

Procedure for spa pool and hot tub application

1. Prepare the area as previously described ensuring the water has circulated the correct number of times according to its size.
2. Prepare the client.
3. Ask the client to hold onto the handrails of the pool, stand and step down into bottom of the pool.

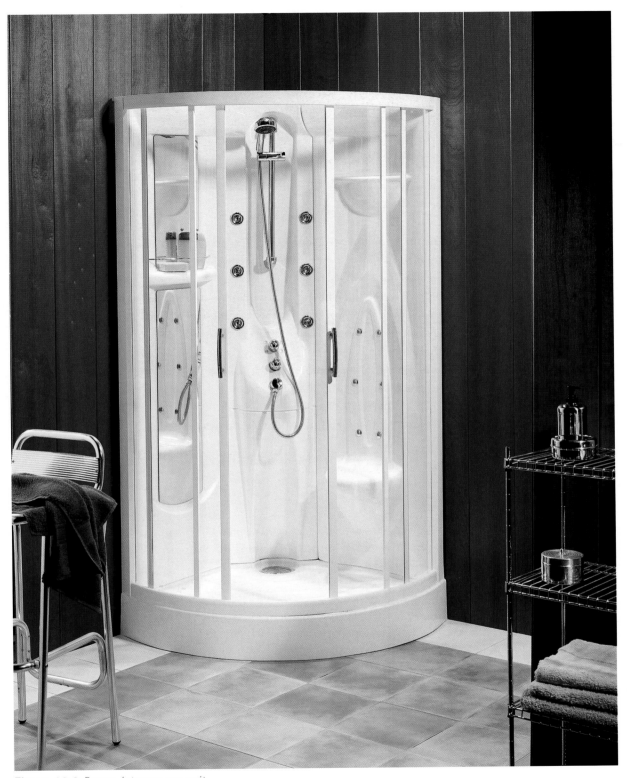

Figure 13.3 *Power-jet massage unit*

4. Ask the client to sit down on the seat.

5. Do not leave the client unattended.

6. After 15 minutes at a temperature of 40°, or longer if lower, the client must be helped out of the pool.

7. Provide a towel for the client to dry themselves and encourage rest for 30 minutes.

8. If further treatment is required, this can be performed during the rest period.

9. Provide water for the client to drink.

10. If no further treatment is required, after rest, the client should shower before getting dressed.

Procedure for spa bath application

1. Prepare the bath with warm water, enough to cover the highest water jet by 2.5 cm (1 inch).

2. Prepare the area with paper and towels.

3. Prepare the client.

4. Seat the client on the end of the bath and ask them to swing their legs onto the bath seat.

5. Ask the client to hold onto both sides of the bath, stand and step down into the bottom of the bath.

6. Ask the client to sit down on the bath seat.

7. Once the client is comfortable, turn the air jet control to minimum and start.

8. When the client is comfortable with the air, turn the water jet control to minimum and start the water jets.

9. Increase the turbulence using the air and water jet controls to suit the client's tolerance.

10. Do not leave the client unattended.

11. After the treatment time, a maximum of 30 minutes, switch off the air and water jets.

12. Ask the client to reverse the process of getting into the bath.

13. Provide the client with a towel to dry themselves and encourage them to rest for 30 minutes.

14. If further treatment is required, this can be performed during the rest period.

15. Provide water for the client to drink.

16. If no further treatment is required, after rest, the client should shower before getting dressed.

Flotation treatments

Compared with the invigorating and sometimes exhausting hydrotherapy, flotation treatments are psychologically relaxing and soothing. They rely on weightlessness for their effect and clients are treated individually in a secluded environment with the senses cut off from external disturbances and stimulated only by relaxing stimuli.

A wet flotation tank or pool has only a few inches of warm water in which the client reclines to allow the water to support the body weight. In most instances, this water is rich in salt and other minerals for absorption to provide rejuvenating and revitalising effects. When completely enclosed inside it is dark but for small lights that appear like stars in a sky. Relaxing music or sounds such as waves crashing on the shore are played and sometimes aromatherapy oil is added to aid the relaxation effect.

Dry flotation baths rely on a waterbed or airbed to produce the weightlessness with warmth being provided by thermal sheeting and/or blankets. Body packs or masks containing beneficial substances are applied before the treatment begins to give detoxifying, deep-cleansing and revitalising effects.

Properties and individual effects of flotation treatments

1. Extreme relaxation is induced.

2. Stress relief.

3. Mineral absorption.

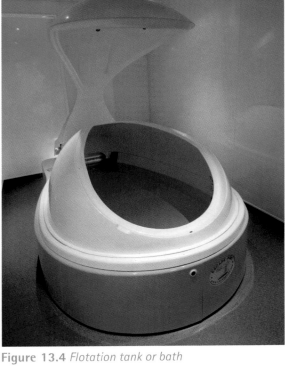

Figure 13.4 *Flotation tank or bath*

4. Improved blood and lymph circulation.

5. Improved skin tone and texture.

6. Detoxifying.

7. Alleviates fluid retention.

8. Relief of muscle aches and pains.

9. Deep cleansing.

Body wrapping

Body wrapping is a way of using natural body heat to aid absorption of products applied to the skin. Additional heat can be applied in the form of lamps and blankets after the body has been wrapped in bandages, clear plastic, stockings or thermal sheeting. The effects are varied depending on the products used. Some generate heat when applied to the skin, for example those containing extracts from plants, essential oils and including seaweed for their mineral and vitamin content. The products are available in many forms but gels, mud, salt rubs, creams and packs are popular. All claim to have similar effects, listed below, and are aimed at reducing cellulite and stretch marks and improving poor skin tone and texture. Some restore moisture levels and may have antibacterial or anti-allergen effects. Claims from others to lower cholesterol levels and stimulate the thyroid gland to produce weight loss have no medical confirmation.

Properties and individual effects of body wrapping

1. Mineral absorption.

2. Improved blood and lymph circulation.

3. Improved skin tone and texture.

4. Detoxifying.

5. Alleviates fluid retention.

6. Relief of muscle aches and pains.

7. Deep cleansing.

The treatment begins with cleansing and exfoliating, perhaps in the form of dry brushing, to maximise product absorption when the active product is applied. After being wrapped, the client can be exposed to additional heat in the form of radiant heat lamps or the application of an electric blanket. After a period of time, usually between 30 and 60 minutes, the product is washed off, sometimes with a power-jet massage-type shower attachment. Moisturising the skin then follows or the treatment can be concluded with another treatment, such as manual massage.

Relaxation rooms

The purpose of a well-thought-out relaxation room is to provide a place where the client can rest, returning the body temperature slowly to normal and maximising treatment effect. Careful consideration should be made to the temperature and facilities available. Water and/or fruit juice should be offered as refreshment as well as providing hydration. The ambience of the room, with soft music and lighting, comfortable seating and non-offensive décor can add to the client's spa experience.

 It is advisable that written instructions as to the use of spa treatment equipment are displayed in the relevant treatment area.

Possible contra-actions to spa treatment and the necessary action

The following contra-actions may occur after a heat and bath treatment:

- fainting/giddiness/light-headedness
- nose bleed
- excess erythema
- nausea
- sweating
- breathing difficulties
- allergic reactions
- dehydration.

It is the therapist's responsibility to prevent these contra-actions from occurring. This is achieved by carefully considering the treatment timings and temperatures for each client's individual needs and monitoring the client closely.

Fainting, giddiness and **light-headedness** are caused by a condition called **blood shunting**. This is where large volumes of blood are directed by the constriction of blood vessels and the dilation of others. In this case the blood is directed to the skin to reduce body temperature, leaving other areas with less blood. The area with less blood can be the head, due to its position and the blood having to work against gravity to reach it. Less blood means less oxygen is reaching the brain and it is this that causes the fainting, giddiness, etc. Blood shunting is a natural condition, which occurs every day in all people, but clients with heart disease, low blood pressure, who are overweight or who have eaten a heavy meal are prone to fainting due to the body being unable to cope with the heat and these other circumstances. So they are contraindicated for treatment.

Nose bleeds and **breathing difficulties** are often experienced in the sauna and steam room where the client breathes in the 'atmospheric conditions'. Recommend instead the use of spa pools, baths and steam baths where the client breathes 'normal' air.

Sweating and **erythema** are thought of as expected with the use of such therapies but if in excess or prolonged, discontinue use.

Dehydration is an unseen but likely contra-action so clients who may already be dehydrated, for example after consumption of alcohol or use of drugs, should be discouraged to have the treatments. The clients should always be provided with water for consumption.

Nausea may be experienced if a heavy meal has been taken before the spa treatment as blood is directed away from the digestive system to the skin, and the reverse applies where the client has not eaten for 4–6 hours – faintness and nausea may result. Discontinue treatment and allow the client to rest.

Allergic reactions to products should be soothed with cool water after discontinuing use. If severe or prolonged, seek medical advice.

Suitable aftercare advice

Aftercare advice should always be given and the client should be aware of further treatment recommendations.

The clients should be advised to:

- rest after treatment
- cool the body using showers or plunge pool
- drink plenty of water or fruit juice to hydrate the body.

Inform clients:

- that erythema should disappear 1–2 hours after treatment
- to soothe any allergy with cool water
- that if there is prolonged vomiting, nose bleed and breathing difficulties or if allergic reaction is severe, they should seek medical advice
- they should eat a light meal after treatment.

Shutdown procedures to follow for spa treatments

This section covers:

- hygiene procedures
- removal of condensation/water
- circulation of air
- disposal of waste
- liaison with colleagues.

Hygiene procedures

At the end of the day it is important that all equipment is cleansed according to the manufacturer's instructions using the appropriate disinfectant, and dirty laundry is removed and washed according to instructions. Water and chemical levels should be checked as well as cleaning of general surfaces such as walls and floors.

Removal of condensation/water

Water, if left to remain and stagnate, is a breeding ground for micro-organisms and can lead to the growth of unsightly mould so should be mopped up from floors, walls and equipment at the end of every day.

Circulation of air

Fresh air should be allowed to circulate to provide good ventilation after the spa area has ceased trading. Steam rooms and baths should have doors left ajar to allow the air to enter and prevent musty smells and the spread of airborne diseases.

Disposal of waste

Correct disposal of waste is a legal obligation of the therapist and includes making special provision for the disposal of contaminated waste in a yellow bin liner for incineration. Non-contaminated waste should be placed into black bin liners and placed in an agreed place for collection, away from the spa treatment area.

Liaison with colleagues

All of these procedures should be performed together as a team and require liaison with the other members of staff to avoid duplication and to ensure that all the necessary tasks are carried out.

Legal responsibilities

The legal responsibilities of the therapist include:

- record keeping
- disposal of waste
- cleaning regimes.

The relevant legal obligations have been noted throughout the text of this chapter and the relevant safety legislation has been discussed in chapter 1.

The following are additional associations and legislation that pertain particularly to spa treatments.

Swimming Pool and Allied Trades Association (SPATA)

SPATA is the trade association for the swimming pool and spa industry in the UK. Its 250 or so members comprise pool builders, retailers, designers, service engineers and trade suppliers in the UK and overseas. It covers both domestic and commercial installations.

Safety in swimming pools – Health and Safety Executive (HSE) and local council by-laws

Legislation on health and safety for swimming pools and spa pools was published in 1999 by the HSE. It provides best practice procedures and standards for the operation of pools and spas, including identifying risks that may lead to drowning, chemical safety and general poolside safety. Many local councils provide a code of practice for public pool operators.

Professional codes of practice for beauty salons and health spas

The various beauty therapy organisations and health and fitness club operators provide an industry code of practice along with membership and insurance cover.

Chapter 14

RELATED ANATOMY AND PHYSIOLOGY

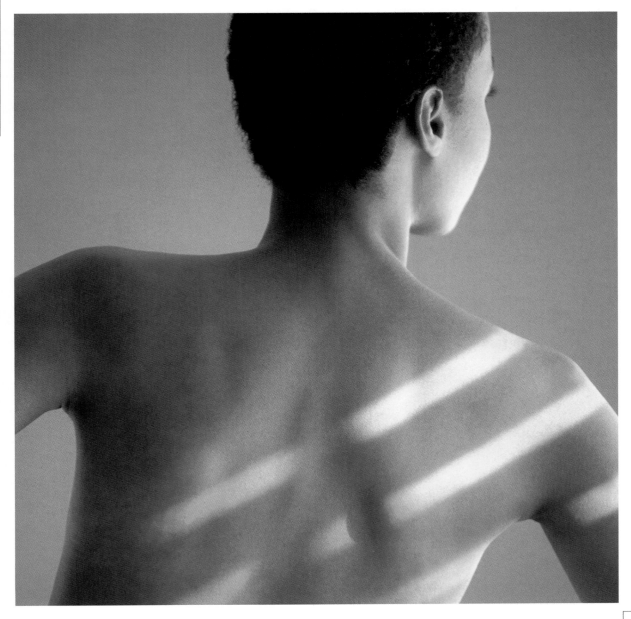

- The skeleton
- The muscles of the face, neck, shoulders, lower arms and legs and hands and feet
- Skin structure and functions
- Skin conditions
- Hair structure and growth
- The structure and growth of nails
- Nail conditions
- The composition and functions of blood
- Blood circulation to the head, neck, arms and legs
- The composition and functions of lymph
- The nervous system

Introduction

In this chapter we will explore the anatomy and physiology relating to the areas of the human body that the beauty therapist treats. This is important in order to provide professional treatments, understand the effects and possible contra-actions of these treatments and provide suitable home care advice, including product use.

Anatomy is the study of the parts of the body, or structure, involving the names and position, whereas **physiology** is the study of how those structures work, in other words their functions.

The information contained within this chapter is suitable for both NVQ levels 1 and 2 and the following table shows the relevant units cross-referenced with the areas listed.

		LEVEL 1		LEVEL 2						
		BT2 Assist with facial treatments	BT3 Assist with nail treatments on the hands	BT4 Improve and maintain facial condition	BT6 Provide make-up treatments	BT7 Remove hair using waxing techniques	BT8 Provide manicure treatment	BT9 Provide pedicure treatment	BT10 Provide nail art service	BT11 Extend and maintain nails
B O N E S	Head, neck, shoulder			•	•					
	Forearm and hand						•			
	Lower leg and foot							•		
M U S C L E S	Face, neck, shoulder			•						
	Forearm and hand						•			
	Lower leg and foot							•		

(Continued)

		LEVEL 1		LEVEL 2						
		BT2 Assist with facial treatments	BT3 Assist with nail treatments on the hands	BT4 Improve and maintain facial condition	BT6 Provide make-up treatments	BT7 Remove hair using waxing techniques	BT8 Provide manicure treatment	BT9 Provide pedicure treatment	BT10 Provide nail art service	BT11 Extend and maintain nails
S K I N	Structure and function	•		•	•	•	•	•	•	•
	Non-medical conditions	•		•	•	•				
	Diseases	•		•	•	•				
	Disorders	•		•	•	•				
B L O O D	Composition and function			•						
	Circulation to head and neck			•						
	Circulation to arm and hand						•			
	Circulation to leg and foot							•		
L Y M P H	Composition and function			•						
H A I R	Structure					•				
	Types					•				
	Growth					•				
N A I L S	Structure		•				•	•	•	•
	Growth						•	•	•	•
	Non-medical conditions						•	•	•	•
	Diseases						•	•	•	•
	Disorders						•	•	•	•

The skeleton

This section includes:

- functions of the skeleton
- the skull
- the neck and shoulder girdle

- the forearm and hand
- the lower leg and foot.

The skeleton is made up of two types of tissue: **cartilage** and **bone**. Cartilage is less rigid than bone and is slightly flexible. It is found on the articulating (moving) surfaces of bones, e.g. at movable joints, in the ribcage, nose, ears, larynx and windpipe. Bone is a rigid structure composed of water, living tissue, mainly collagen and inorganic salts, chiefly calcium phosphate. Bones are living structures with a blood and nerve supply and are influenced by changes in diet, hormone levels and stresses they are exposed to, such as an injury or overuse.

Where two bones come together a joint is formed. There are three main types of joint:

- **fixed joints** – also known as immovable and fibrous joints. As the name suggests, no movement occurs. e.g. the sutures of the skull
- **cartilaginous joints** – slightly movable and distinguished by the presence of a pad of cartilage between the bones, e.g. the bones of the vertebral column
- **synovial joints** – freely movable to allow a wide range of movements, e.g. the knee, elbow, hip.

Functions of the skeleton

1. **Shape and support** – there is a similarity between the shape of the skeleton and that of the external body, which can also be seen on other animals. The axial skeleton, that is the skull, vertebral column and ribs, supports the limbs of the appendicular skeleton. Together the skeleton and muscles hold the body upright and give us our posture.
2. **Protection** – the cranium and vertebral column protect the brain and spinal cord respectively, the ribcage protects the heart and lungs, and the pelvis protects the reproductive organs in the female.
3. **Production of blood cells** – the blood brings the required nutrients and oxygen necessary for red blood cell formation, which occurs in the bone marrow of long bones, e.g. femur.
4. **Calcium storage** – the blood supply of the bones provides nutrients that are stored and removed depending on the demands of the body, e.g. calcium, phosphorus and fat.
5. **Muscle and tendon attachment** – there are bony protrusions and rough surfaces of bones that allow for adhesion of muscles and tendons.
6. **Movement and locomotion** – by using joints and with the contraction of muscles the body is able to move, e.g. walking.

The skull

The bones of the skull are divided into two groups: the **cranium** and the **face**. Most of the bones of the skull form fixed joints called **sutures**. The only free-moving joint is that between the mandible – the lower jaw – and the temporal bones, which allow the lower jaw to move up and down, when chewing.

The cranium

Eight bones form the cranium, a box-like structure that protects the brain.

Name of the Bone	Position of the Bone
Frontal	One bone forming the front of the cranium including the forehead and upper eye sockets.
Parietal	Two bones forming the top and sides of the cranium.

The cranium bones

(Continued)

Name of the Bone	Position of the Bone
Occipital	One bone forming the back and floor of the cranium.
Temporal	Two bones forming the sides of the cranium, above and around the ears.
Sphenoid	One bone forming the floor and the sides of the cranium at the temple region and the back of the eye sockets.
Ethmoid	One bone forming the front floor of the cranium, the roof of the nasal cavities and the inner sides of the eye sockets.

The cranium bones

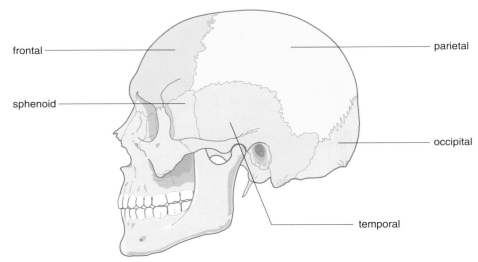

Figure 14.1 *The lateral view of the skull showing the bones of the cranium*

The face

There are 14 bones forming the facial structure and features.

Name of the Bone	Position of the Bone
Zygomatic	Two bones forming the cheekbones and the floor and side wall of the eye sockets.
Maxilla(e)	Two bones forming the upper jaw, the front part of the roof of the mouth, the sides of the nose and the floor of the eye sockets. The upper teeth are embedded in the maxillae.
Nasal	Two bones forming the bridge of the nose.
Mandible	One bone forming the lower jaw in which the lower teeth are embedded.
Lacrimal	Two bones forming the inner walls of the eye sockets.
Palatine	Two bones forming the back part of the roof of the mouth and sides of the nasal cavities (not shown in illustration).
Vomer	One bone forming the central division of the nasal cavities.
Turbinate	Two bones forming the side wall of the nasal cavities.

The face bones

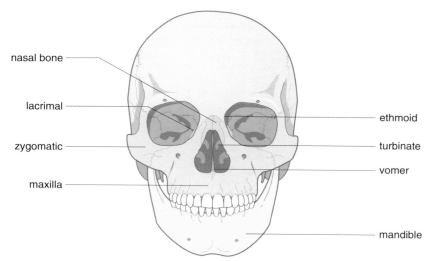

Figure 14.2 *The anterior view of the skull showing the bones of the face*

The neck and shoulder girdle

The neck

The neck forms part of the vertebral column, which is a series of irregular-shaped bones stacked on top of each other to form a column. Each vertebra is separated from the one above and below it by a disc of cartilage, which prevents the bones rubbing against each other and acts as a cushion or shock absorber for stress administered from the upper body to the lower or vice versa. The bones are named after the area in which they are situated, hence the neck bones are called the **cervical vertebrae** and there are seven of them in total. The upper two vertebrae nearest the skull are specialised and have a different structure to the others. The top vertebra is attached to the underneath of the occipital bone of the skull and has a hole through which passes a peg-like structure of the second vertebra. This arrangement forms a type of synovial joint called a **pivot joint** that allows rotation of the head. Figure 14.3 shows the relationship of the cervical vertebrae with the skull and shoulder.

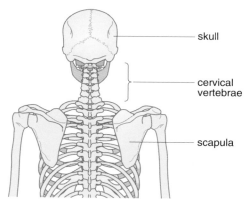

Figure 14.3 *The relationship between the cervical vertebrae and the skull and shoulder*

The shoulder girdle

The shoulder girdle is made up of the **clavicle, scapula** and **humerus** bones. The clavicle or collarbone is situated at the front of the body and forms a joint with the **sternum** or breastbone. The scapula is situated at the back of the body and forms a ball-and-socket joint with the humerus, the upper bone of the arm.

Name of the Bone	Position of the Bone
Clavicle	Two long bones, a left and a right, found at the front of the body from the shoulder to the sternum.
Scapula	Two flat bones, a left and a right, found in the upper back of the body at the shoulder.

The shoulder girdle bones

(Continued)

Name of the Bone	Position of the Bone
Humerus	Two long bones, a left and a right, forming the upper arm with joints at the shoulder at one end and the elbow at the other.
Sternum	One flat bone found centrally at the front of the body in the chest forming joints with the clavicle at the top and the ribs along its length.

The shoulder girdle bones

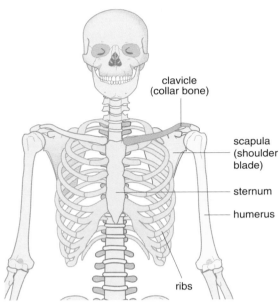

Figure 14.4 *The shoulder girdle bones*

The forearm and hand

The humerus extends from the shoulder to form the upper arm. The lower end forms a hinge joint, with the elbow, with the bones of the forearm. These bones are called the **ulna** and **radius** and they articulate with each other to form a pivot joint that allows the palm to turn forwards and backwards. At the lower end of the radius and ulna is the wrist or **carpals**, eight irregular-shaped bones arranged in two rows of four. The **scaphoid, lunate** and **triquetral** form condyloid joints with the bones of the hand, the **metacarpals**. The bones glide or slide over each other to allow a variety of movements. The metacarpals articulate with the small bones of the digits known as the **phalanges**. The joints between the phalanges are hinge joints.

Name of the Bone	Position of the Bone
Ulna	Runs down the little finger side of the forearm.
Radius	Runs down the thumb side of the forearm.
Scaphoid	Top row of the carpals on the thumb side.
Lunate	Top row, next to the scaphoid.
Triquetral	Top row, next to the lunate.
Pisiform	Top row of the carpals overlapping the triquetral on the little finger side.
Trapezium	Bottom row of the carpals on the thumb side.
Trapezoid	Bottom row, next to the trapezium.

The forearm and hand bones

(Continued)

Related anatomy and physiology

Name of the Bone	Position of the Bone
Capitate	Bottom row, next to the trapezoid.
Hamate	Bottom row, next to the capitate.
Metacarpals	Five long bones of the hand, one relating to each of the digits.
Phalanges	Fourteen bones of one hand, arranged with three bones to each finger and two to the thumb.

The forearm and hand bones

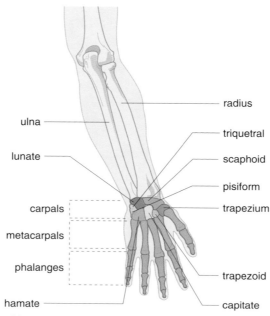

Figure 14.5 *The forearm and hand bones*

The lower leg and foot

The **femur** extends down from the hip to the knee where it articulates with the **tibia** to form a hinge joint. 'Floating' over the knee is the kneecap or **patella**, which is embedded in the tendon of the front thigh muscles, the quadriceps. The tibia forms the main bone of the lower leg and running parallel to it towards the outside of the body is the **fibula**. The tibia and fibula form a hinge joint with the **talus** of the ankle. The seven bones making up the ankle are collectively known as the **tarsals**. These support and distribute the body weight throughout the foot by a series of arches and articulate with each other to form gliding joints that allow movements at the ankle. The **calcaneus** forms the heel and attaches the strong muscles of the calf to the foot and enables walking, etc. Gliding joints are formed between the tarsals and the metatarsals, and condyloid joints are formed between the metatarsals and the phalanges of the toes. The joints between the phalanges are hinge joints.

Name of the Bone	Position of the Bone
Tibia	Found to the inside of the lower leg, from knee to ankle. Its function is to support the body weight.
Fibula	Found to the outside of the lower leg, from knee to ankle. Its function is to provide muscle attachment.
Patella	Found at the knee joint, commonly called the kneecap.

The lower leg and foot bones

(Continued)

Name of the Bone	Position of the Bone
Calcaneus	Forms the heel at the back of the ankle.
Talus	Found at the front of the ankle, articulates with the tibia and fibula.
Navicular	Forms part of the top of the foot and lies distal to the talus.
Cuboid	Lies to the outside of the foot.
Outer cuneiform	Lies between the cuboid and the middle cuneiform.
Middle cuneiform	Lies between the outer and inner cuneiform.
Inner cuneiform	Lies next to the middle cuneiform to the inside of the foot.
Metatarsals	Five long bones making up the length of the foot.
Phalanges	Fourteen bones of the toes of one foot. Two in the big toe and three in the others. Often found fused together in the little toe.

The lower leg and foot bones

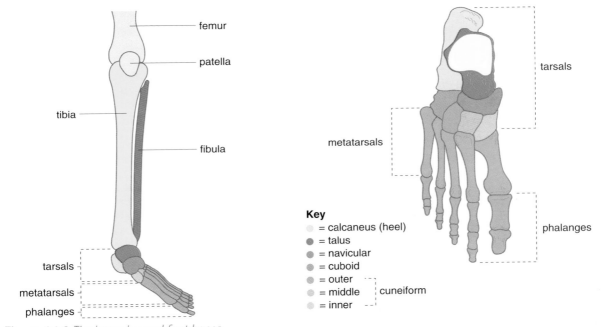

Figure 14.6 *The lower leg and foot bones*

Muscles

This section includes:

- the muscles of the face
- the muscles of the neck and chest
- the muscles of the neck and shoulder
- the muscles of the upper arm
- the muscles of the forearm and hand
- the muscles of the thigh
- the muscles of the lower leg and foot.

Introduction

Muscle is a special type of tissue that is able to contract. When it does so it usually becomes shorter, fatter and harder to the touch. There are three types of muscle tissue:

- **Voluntary muscle** brings about movement and locomotion. It is also called skeletal muscle as it is attached to and moves bones about the joints, or **striped** or **striated** muscle due to its appearance under a microscope. Voluntary muscle is under conscious control and the muscles discussed later are all of this type.
- **Involuntary muscle**, also called **smooth** muscle, is under subconscious control and is found in organs and systems of the body such as the blood circulatory system.
- **Cardiac muscle** is found only in the heart.

Voluntary muscle contraction is brought about by a series of events. First, the central nervous system, the brain and spinal cord, send a message in the form of an electrical impulse along a **motor nerve** to the muscle. When it reaches the muscle the nerve divides so that a nerve fibre serves each muscle fibre. This area is called the **motor point**. The message is passed from the nerve to the muscle fibres and the muscle contracts.

The ends of the muscles attached to bones across a joint bring about movement at that joint. In the face the muscles can be connected to bone at one end and skin or another muscle at the other. This allows the skin to move and create facial expressions.

To reverse a particular movement another muscle must contract. For example, the biceps muscle bends the elbow and the triceps straightens the elbow. These are known as antagonistic pairs and virtually all movements of the body are brought about in this way. The correct terminology used to describe muscle movements can be found in the glossary.

The muscles of the face

Name of the Muscle	Position of the Muscle	Action of the Muscle
Occipitalis	Found at the back of the head, attached to the occipital bone and the skin of the scalp.	To move the scalp.
Frontalis	At the forehead across its width, attached to the skin of the eyebrows and the skin of the scalp.	Wrinkles the skin of the forehead and raises the eyebrows creating a surprised expression.
Temporalis	Surrounds the ear and lies over the temporal bone, passing under the zygomatic arch to attach to the lower jaw.	Raises the jaw when chewing.
Corrugator	Between the eyebrows, attached to the frontalis muscle and the frontal bone.	Brings the eyebrows together creating frowning.
Procerus	Between the eyebrows, attached to the nasal bones and the frontalis muscle.	Draws the eyebrows inwards creating a puzzled expression.
Nasalis	At the sides of the nose attached to the maxillae bones and the nostrils.	Dilates and compresses the nostrils.
Orbicularis oculi	Surrounds the opening of the eye socket attached to the bones at its outer edge and the skin of the eyelids at the inner.	To close the eyes as in sleeping, winking, squinting and blinking.

The face muscles

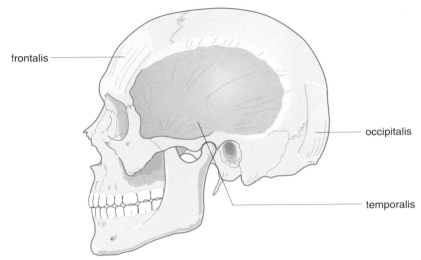

frontalis

occipitalis

temporalis

Figure 14.7 *Lateral view of muscles to the face 1*

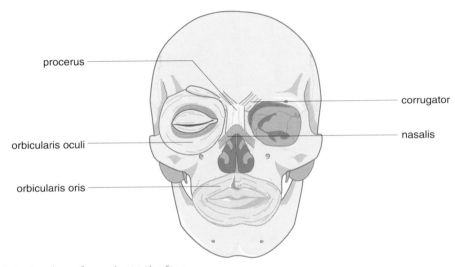

procerus

corrugator

nasalis

orbicularis oculi

orbicularis oris

Figure 14.8 *Anterior view of muscles to the face*

Name of the Muscle	Position of the Muscle	Action of the Muscle
Orbicularis oris	Surrounds the opening of the mouth occupying the entire width of the lips.	Closes or narrows the lips, used to press the teeth against the teeth and to purse the lips as in whistling.
Labitis of the upper lip	Towards the inner cheek beside the nose, attached to the maxillae and the skin of the corners of the mouth and upper lip.	Raises the corner of the mouth to create a snarling expression.
Buccinator	Main muscle of the cheek, attached to both the maxilla and mandible. Forms a muscular plate between the teeth.	To keep the cheek stretched during all phases of opening and closing the mouth. Also to compress the cheeks when blowing.
Depressors of the lower lip	Under the corners of the mouth and lower lip, from the mandible to the skin of them both.	Draws down the corners of the mouth to give a sad expression.

The face muscles *(Continued)*

Related anatomy and physiology

Name of the Muscle	Position of the Muscle	Action of the Muscle
Mentalis	Located at the point of the chin, attached to the mandible and the skin of the lower lip.	Lifts and wrinkles the skin of the chin and turns the lower lip outwards creating a pouting expression.
Masseter	Found at the outer cheek in front of the ear, attached to the zygomatic arch and the mandible.	Raises the lower jaw, exerting pressure on the teeth when chewing.
Risorius	Lies above the buccinator, attached to above the angle of the mandible and the skin at the corner of the mouth.	Pulls the corner of the mouth sideways to create a grinning expression.
Zygomaticus	Lies across the inner cheek, attached to the zygomatic bone and the corners of the mouth.	Lifts the corners of the mouth upwards and sideways to create a smiling expression.

The face muscles

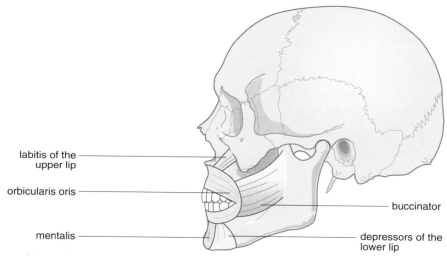

Figure 14.9 *Lateral view of muscles to the face 2*

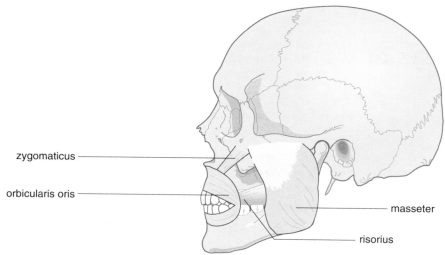

Figure 14.10 *Lateral view of muscles to the face 3*

The muscles of the neck and chest

Name of the Muscle	Position of the Muscle	Action of the Muscle
Sternocleidomastoid	Lies across the side of the neck, attached to the clavicle and sternum and the mastoid process of the temporal bone.	Contraction of one muscle turns the head in the opposite direction and when contracted together the chin is pulled down towards the head (nodding).
Platysma	Extends down the front of the neck from the sides of the chin to the clavicle, either side of the throat.	Depresses the mandible and lower lip causing wrinkling in the skin of the neck especially when yawning.
Pectoralis major (Pectorals)	In the chest, attached to the clavicle, sternum across the ribs to the humerus.	Brings the arm forward and across the chest, used in pushing.

The neck and chest muscles

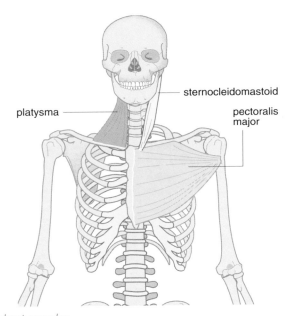

Figure 14.11 *The neck and chest muscles*

The muscles of the neck and shoulder

Name of the Muscle	Position of the Muscle	Action of the Muscle
Trapezius	Diamond-shaped muscle at the upper back, neck and shoulder, attached to the occipital bone and the vertebrae of the thorax to the scapula and outer end of the clavicle.	Raises the shoulder to the ear, holds the scapula and shoulder still during arm movements and extends the neck.
Deltoid	Forms a cap over the shoulder. The front is attached to the clavicle and the back, to the scapula, and the two heads meet to attach to the humerus.	The front brings the arm forward, the back takes it backwards and together they take the arm out to the side.

The neck and shoulder muscles

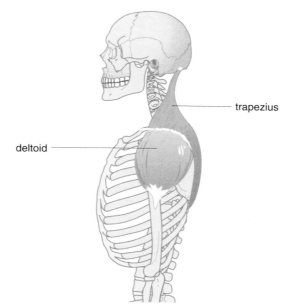

Figure 14.12 *The neck and shoulder muscles*

The muscles of the upper arm

Name of the Muscle	Position of the Muscle	Action of the Muscle
Biceps	Found at the anterior aspect of the upper arm above the elbow, attached to the scapula and the radius.	Flexes the elbow and supinates forearm and hand.

The upper arm muscles   *(Continued)*

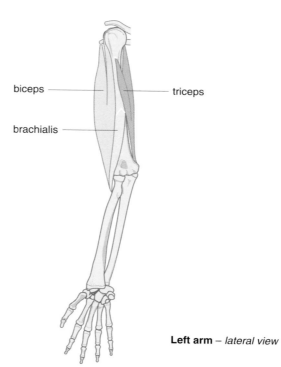

Left arm – *lateral view*

Figure 14.13 *The upper arm muscles*

Name of the Muscle	Position of the Muscle	Action of the Muscle
Brachialis	Across the elbow, attached to the humerus and the ulna.	Flexes the elbow.
Triceps	Found at the posterior aspect of the upper arm, attached to the scapula and humerus and the ulna.	Extends the elbow.

The upper arm muscles

The muscles of the forearm and hand

Name of the Muscle	Position of the Muscle	Action of the Muscle
Supinator	A muscle attached to the lateral aspect of the lower humerus and the radius, under the extensors of the digits.	Supinates the forearm and hand.
Extensors	A group of muscles found at the lateral aspect of the forearm attached to the lower humerus, radius and ulna and the metacarpals and phalanges of the fingers.	Extend the wrist, fingers and thumb.
Pronators	Two muscles attached to the medial aspect of the lower humerus and the radius.	Pronates the forearm and hand.
Flexors	A group of muscles found at the medial aspect of the forearm, attached to the lower humerus, radius and ulna and the metacarpals and phalanges of the fingers.	Flex the wrist, fingers and thumb.

The forearm and hand muscles   *(Continued)*

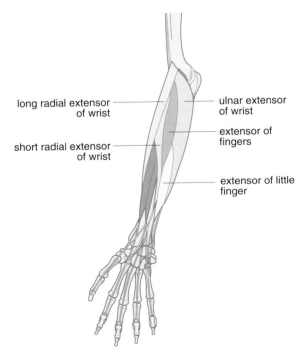

long radial extensor of wrist

short radial extensor of wrist

ulnar extensor of wrist

extensor of fingers

extensor of little finger

Figure 14.14 *Muscles of the forearm and hand 1*

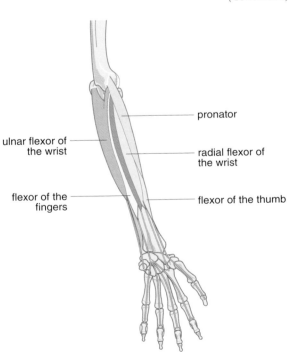

ulnar flexor of the wrist

flexor of the fingers

pronator

radial flexor of the wrist

flexor of the thumb

Figure 14.15 *Muscles of the forearm and hand 2*

Related anatomy and physiology

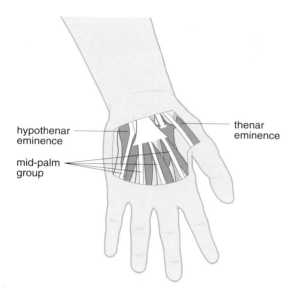

hypothenar
eminence

thenar
eminence

mid-palm
group

Figure 14.16 *Muscles of the hand*

Name of the Muscle	Position of the Muscle	Action of the Muscle
Hypothenar eminence	In the palm of the hand below the little finger, attached to the carpals, metacarpals and phalanges of the little finger.	Abducts, adducts and flexes the little finger.
Thenar eminence	In the palm below the thumb, attached to the carpals, metacarpals and phalanges of the thumb.	Abducts, adducts and flexes the thumb and draws it towards the palm.
Mid-palm group	Centre of the palm below the middle three fingers, attached to the carpals, metacarpals and phalanges of those fingers.	Abducts, adducts and flexes the middle three fingers.

The forearm and hand muscles

The muscles of the thigh

The muscles of the thigh and buttocks are listed as group names.

Name of the Muscle	Position of the Muscle	Action of the Muscle
Quadriceps	A group of four muscles found at the front of the thigh, attached to the pelvic girdle and femur, passing over the knee to the tibia bone.	Flex the hip and extend the knee.
Adductors	A group of muscles found on the inside of the thigh, attached to the pelvic girdle, femur and the tibia.	Adduct and rotate the femur laterally.
Sartorius	Runs across the front of the thigh diagonally from the lateral aspect of the pelvis to the medial aspect of the tibia.	Flexes both the hip and the knee, abducts and rotates the femur laterally.
Hamstrings	A group of three muscles at the posterior aspect of the thigh, attached to the pelvic girdle passing over the hip and knee to the tibia bone.	Extend the hip and flex the knee.

The thigh muscles

(Continued)

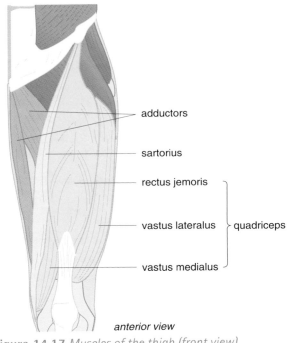

Figure 14.17 *Muscles of the thigh (front view)*

anterior view

adductors

sartorius

rectus jemoris

vastus lateralus

vastus medialus

quadriceps

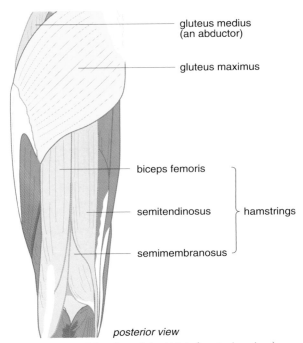

Figure 14.18 *Muscles of the thigh (posterior view)*

posterior view

gluteus medius (an abductor)

gluteus maximus

biceps femoris

semitendinosus

semimembranosus

hamstrings

Name of the Muscle	Position of the Muscle	Action of the Muscle
Gluteus maximus	Forms the buttocks, attached to the pelvic girdle and the posterior aspect of the femur.	Extends the hip.
Abductors	A group of muscles, including the gluteus medius and minimus, found at the lateral aspect of the thigh and hip, attached to the upper part of the pelvic girdle and the upper femur.	Abduct the hip and rotate the femur medially.

The thigh muscles

The muscles of the lower leg and foot

Name of the Muscle	Position of the Muscle	Action of the Muscle
Tibialis anterior	Anterior aspect of the lower leg, attached to the tibia and the middle cuneiform and first metatarsal.	Dorsiflexes the ankle and inverts the foot.
Extensors of the toes	Anterior and lateral aspect of the lower leg, attached to the tibia and fibula and the phalanges of the toes.	Extend the toes and help dorsiflex the ankle.
Gastrocnemius	Posterior aspect of the lower leg, main muscle forming the calf. Attached to the lower part of the femur across the back of the knee and ankle to the calcaneum.	Flexes the knee and plantar-flexes the ankle.
Soleus	Under the gastrocnemius, attached to the tibia and fibula across the ankle to the calcaneum.	Plantar-flexes the ankle, an important action for propelling the body forward in walking and running.

The lower leg and foot muscles

(Continued)

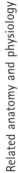

Related anatomy and physiology

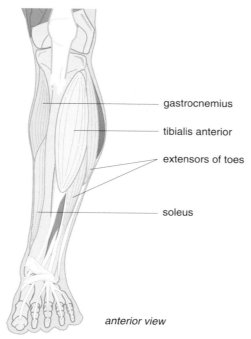

gastrocnemius

tibialis anterior

extensors of toes

soleus

anterior view

Figure 14.19 *Muscles of the lower leg and foot (front view)*

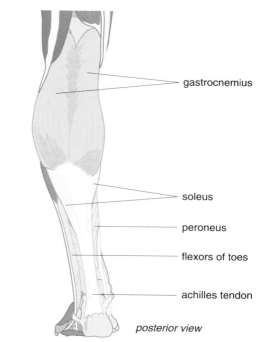

gastrocnemius

soleus

peroneus

flexors of toes

achilles tendon

posterior view

Figure 14.20 *Muscles of the lower leg and foot (posterior view)*

Name of the Muscle	Position of the Muscle	Action of the Muscle
Tibialis posterior (not shown on diagram)	Very deep in the calf, attached to the tibia and fibula across the ankle to the navicular bone.	Inverts the foot.
Peroneus	A group of three muscles found laterally and posterior in the calf, attached to the fibula across the ankle to the underneath of the first and fifth metatarsals.	Everts the foot.
Flexors of the toes	Muscles deep in the posterior aspect of the lower leg, attached to the tibia and fibula and the phalanges of the toes.	Flexes the toes and helps to plantar-flex the ankle.

The lower leg and foot muscles

The skin

This section includes:

■ functions of the skin

■ structure of the skin

■ skin diseases and disorders.

The skin is the most important organ that a therapist will consider. It forms part of the excretory system, protects the body from harm and disease and has an integral sensory role in the functioning of the body. Almost all beauty therapy treatments have an affect on the skin or its appendages (the nails and hair). For this reason a sound knowledge of the skin is required and the topics discussed here should be considered with the relevant chapters of this book relating to treatments.

The functions of the skin

Sensation

The skin is equipped with many **sensory nerve endings**, making it sensitive to touch, differences in temperature, pain, itching and pressure. When the nerve endings are stimulated, the information is relayed along a sensory nerve to the central nervous system where it is acted upon. For example, in the case of an increase in temperature, the action will be to send a message along the motor nerve to the sweat glands to stimulate them into producing more sweat to cool the body.

Heat regulation

The body must maintain a temperature of 37°C in order to be healthy and the skin plays an important role in this. When the body temperature rises, the sweat glands in the skin produce sweat. This cools the body down by using the heat to evaporate the sweat from the skin surface. The skin also becomes red (**erythema**). This is caused by the blood vessels near the surface of the skin **dilating** (widening) to allow more blood to come to the surface. As it does so, the heat is lost to the atmosphere, a little like a central heating system losing heat to a room through a radiator.

When the body is cold, the skin stops or slows down the sweating process and the blood vessels **constrict** (narrow) to keep in the warmth. 'Goose bumps' occur as a result of each **arrector pili muscle** contracting and lifting the hairs away from the skin to trap a layer of air next to it as insulation. As we have very little hair on our bodies this does not work well in humans but is effective in animals. The adipose tissue contained in the subcutaneous layer of the skin helps to keep us warm by insulating the body from the cold.

Absorption

The skin is able to absorb very little as its main job is to prevent the entry of harmful substances. Certain substances, however, can pass through the epidermis such as oils, sunlight and small quantities of water. The epidermis can absorb cosmetic preparations containing oils, and sunlight can penetrate to the dermis if not properly protected. Other substances that are known to penetrate the skin are drugs, for example those used in hormone replacement therapy patches, anaesthetics and essential oils.

Excretion

This is the removal of waste products and the skin is one of three excretory organs of the body, the lungs and kidneys being the others. The skin assists in this role by sweating, which removes excess water and salts from the body. The other 'waste product' the skin eliminates is heat and this is done as described earlier.

Secretion

Sebum is an natural oil produced by the **sebaceous glands** found in the dermis. The oil flows from the glands onto the skin surface, lubricating and maintaining the skin's softness and pliability and rendering it waterproof. When sebum mixes with sweat on the skin surface the **acid mantle** is formed, which protects the skin from micro-organism invasion. The face, chest and back have numerous sebaceous glands and can often appear oily with a shiny appearance.

If the glands are overactive the skin is known as an oily or greasy skin type and the formation of blocked pores, **comedones** (blackheads) and **pustules** (spots) are likely. When underactive the skin is rough to touch and may appear flaky and is known as dry skin.

Protection

The skin protects the body from injury and invasion by foreign bodies such as micro-organisms. The uppermost layers of the epidermis thicken with pressure and are able to quickly replace themselves if damaged. The protective function of the acid mantle has already been described. Sebum contributes

Related anatomy and physiology

275

to this and provides a waterproof layer that controls water loss through the epidermis. Specialised cells called **melanocytes** present in the bottom-most layer of the epidermis produce **melanin**, a pigment that colours the skin to absorb sunlight and prevent its harmful rays from damaging the dermis and its structures.

Vitamin D production

Vitamin D is formed by the action of sunlight on a fatty substance present in the skin. It is absorbed into the blood vessels and used with calcium and phosphorus for the formation and maintenance of bones. Excess is stored in the liver.

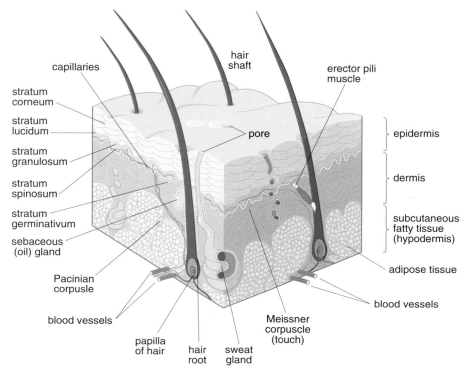

Figure 14.21 *Structure of the skin*

Structure of the skin

The epidermis

The epidermis is the outermost layer of the skin nearest the surface. It is made up of five distinct layers and varies in thickness, being thinnest on the lips and eyelids and thickest on the soles of the feet and the palms of the hands. The epidermis is affected by beauty therapy treatments and the application of products although it consists mainly of dead cells, which are constantly being shed and replaced by new cells from underneath.

The five layers are:

Figure 14.22 *The epidermis*

■ The **stratum germinativum** (basal layer). The cells are cube shaped, with each cell having a nucleus. They are moist and obtain nutrients and oxygen from the tissue fluid that seeps from the blood vessels in the dermis. The nutrients and oxygen is used for cell division or **mitosis**, when the nucleus divides to form new cells. As new cells are formed, the old ones are pushed towards the surface, undergoing change as they do so. One in four to ten cells are specialised cells called melanocytes that produce a pigment called melanin. This contributes to the skin's colour and darkens when exposed to ultraviolet light from the sun, protecting the underlying dermis and all its structures from the harmful effects. Light and dark skins have the same number of melanocytes, but the darker the skin colour, the more active melanocytes there are, explaining why a fair skin burns more easily in the sun.

■ The **stratum spinosum** (prickle layer) is formed from cells from the stratum germinativum. The cells appear to grow spines or 'prickles', giving rise to their name. It is here that melanin passes into the cells from the melanocytes. Some cells have nuclei and mitosis still continues.

■ The **stratum granulosum** (granular layer) is the site of **keratinisation** where the cells from the stratum spinosum form a protein called **keratin**. The cells begin to die, losing their moisture and hardening. The nuclei and the cell walls break down resulting in the death of the cells as they work upwards towards the surface.

■ The **stratum lucidum** (clear layer) is not present over the entire body and appears clear under a microscope due to the absence of nuclei and cell walls. An enzyme has destroyed the melanin and the cells are flat, dry and keratinised giving a semi-transparent appearance. Present at this area of the epidermis is the 'rheins barrier', a layer of a thick mucus-like substance formed as the cells of the stratum granulosum expel water and mix with the fatty acids present in the skin. The barrier prevents water, products and micro-organisms from penetrating into the sterile dermis.

■ The **stratum corneum** (horny layer) consists of dead, flat keratinised cells that are shed from the surface by natural rubbing from clothing, etc. or by special skin products containing granules that slough off the dead skin. This process is called **desquamation**.

The dermis

The dermis lies beneath the epidermis and is known as the true skin, as all the living and functioning structures are present here. It has the same thickness over the entire body of approximately 3 mm and can be divided into two areas.

■ The **papillary layer** is the uppermost portion of the dermis and lies directly under the epidermis. Its name is derived from the projections that point upwards into the epidermis, called **papillae**. Many of these papillae are supplied with blood vessels, providing nutrients and oxygen to the cells of the stratum germinativum, while others contain sensory nerve endings, giving rise to the skin's function of sensation.

■ The **reticular layer** lies beneath the papillary layer and contains a dense network of collagen and elastin fibres running parallel to the skin surface. Together these fibres give the skin its elasticity and when damaged, by ultraviolet light for example, premature ageing results.

The dermis contains glands and other structures that enable the skin to perform its functions. These structures include:

■ The **blood supply** of the skin is a network of arteries that run parallel to the skin's surface under the dermis. Smaller vessels branch off upwards to form capillary networks around the hair follicles, sweat and sebaceous glands and arrector pili muscles and the dermal papillae in the papillary layer. The capillaries provide fresh blood containing nutrients and oxygen necessary for mitosis, muscle contraction and the formation of sweat and sebum. Deoxygenated blood passes downwards in small vessels to the main venous network in the dermis. The amount of blood flowing to the surface is controlled by the motor nerve supply to the artery walls, which bring about vasodilation or vasoconstriction.

■ The **lymph capillaries** form a fine network of vessels throughout the dermis, which act as a waste disposal system. The capillaries drain away excess tissue fluid containing waste products from cell activity and foreign bodies such as micro-organisms that may have entered during an injury.

■ The **nerve supply** of the skin provides the skin with sensations of **touch**, **pain**, **pressure** and **temperature**. This is possible due to the network of **sensory nerve endings** or **receptors** present. Most lie deep in the dermis but others that register pain and temperature can be found in the lower epidermis. All are stimulated by external influences such as heat and the message is taken along the sensory nerve to the central nervous system where the brain decides how to act upon the information. If necessary another message is sent to bring about the action. This happens everywhere in the body but a common example in the skin is the response to changes in temperature. When the sensory nerve ending is stimulated by heat, the return message from the brain will travel along a **motor nerve** to the blood capillary walls and vasodilation results. At the same time a message to the sweat glands increases their activity, cooling of the body.

- The **sweat glands** are made up of a coiled tube deep in the dermis and a long tube or duct that reaches up through the epidermis to the skin surface. There are two types of gland but both produce sweat almost constantly to regulate the body temperature. The difference comes in the type of sweat they produce. The **eccrine glands** are found in abundance over the entire body and excrete water and salts. The **apocrine glands** are found in the armpits and genital area and open out into hair follicles rather than the skin surface. They excrete water, salts, urea and fats. It is the breakdown of this type of sweat by bacteria that causes body odour.

- The **hair follicle** is formed by a depression of epidermal cells downwards, deep into the dermis. It is responsible for the production of a keratinised structure called **hair** from the **bulb** at the base. The necessary nutrients and oxygen required for hair growth are supplied by the blood vessels in the **dermal papilla**. Connected to the follicle is the arrector pili muscle, which, when it contracts, pulls the follicle and therefore the hair into an upright position causing 'goose bumps' and trapping an insulating layer of air next to the skin to keep the body warm.

- The **sebaceous glands** are found all over the body except the soles of the feet and the palms of the hands. They are more numerous on the scalp, face, chest and back, with few being found at the knees or elbows. They commonly open out into hair follicles but some open onto the skin surface. The glands produce an oil called sebum, which lubricates the skin keeping it soft and pliable and preventing moisture loss from the dermis. Together the sweat and sebum form an invisible layer over the skin called the **acid mantle**, which prevents invasion from harmful micro-organisms.

Skin diseases and disorders

The following charts of skin conditions include treatable conditions such as milia and comedones as well as those listed as contraindications. Refer to each treatment in the relevant chapter for clarification of the relevant contraindications.

Some useful terms

- A **macule** is a small coloured area of skin that can be lighter or darker than the surrounding skin. It can be seen rather than felt. An **ephelides** (freckle) is an example.
- A **papule** is a small, solid, raised painful lump, red in colour and often develops into a pustule.
- A **pustule** develops from a papule and pus (which indicates infection is present) forms a yellow centre.
- A **vesicle** is a small, raised blister containing a watery substance called **serum**. It may be surrounded by an area of red skin and irritation.
- A **bulla** is a vesicle larger than 0.5 cm, commonly called a **blister**.
- A **nodule** is a small, rounded swelling either above or below the skin surface, also known as a **cyst**.
- A **tumour** is larger than a nodule and can be formed from hard or soft tissue.
- A **weal** appears as a white, raised area of indistinguishable shape surrounded by a red area. It may appear and disappear quickly, for example **hives**.
- **Scales** are used to describe flakes of easily detached skin seen in conditions such as **psoriasis**.
- **Fissures** are cracks in the epidermis exposing the dermis.
- A **crust** results from the drying out of fluid from a lesion. Serum forms a yellow crust and blood forms a brown crust, called a **scab**.

- An **excoriation** results from the removal of the epidermis by friction also known as an **abrasion.**
- An **ulcer** is an extensive open sore with the resulting pus formation. It involves the epidermis and the dermis and healing results in scar formation.
- A **scar** is the replacement tissue formed during the healing of a wound.
- A **keloid** is an overgrown scar caused by the overdevelopment of collagen, common in black skins.

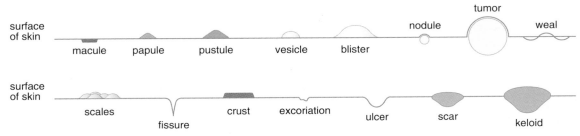

Figure 14.23 *Skin blemishes and lesions*

Other terms that are useful to know are:

- **Erythema** – redness caused by the dilation of blood capillaries in the skin.
- **Hyperaemia** – an increase in blood flow to an area resulting in erythema.
- **Weeping** – a watery discharge from broken skin.
- **Oedema** – swelling of the tissue due to an accumulation of fluid.
- **Inflammation** – appears as red, painful swelling, warm to touch and followed by the formation of pus. Usually the result of bacterial invasion of the skin.
- **Bruising** – is an area of unbroken skin discoloured by blood from the damaged blood vessels in the dermis, usually as a result of a physical blow.

Skin blemishes and lesions

Blemishes may be present as a result of:

1. **Congenital malformation,** in other words, those existing at or from birth.
2. **Abnormal functioning** of the skin structures, those associated with the sebaceous glands, the sweat glands, pigmentation or with skin growth.
3. **Skin disease** by micro-organisms: bacteria, fungi or viruses and parasites.
4. **Damage** by external agents such as the sun, chemical trauma or physical trauma.

Congenital malformation

Malformations of structures within the skin at birth or shortly after will result in blemishes such as **birthmarks**, which persist throughout life. These conditions are skin abnormalities.

Skin disease

Micro-organisms in the salon

Micro-organisms can be transmitted in the salon environment. They require warmth, moisture and nutrients to multiply, all of which can be found in the salon. It is the therapist's duty to control the salon environment to prevent bacterial growth and cross infection. This involves hygiene and **sterilising procedures** and good **ventilation** through the salon. These measures ensure that the health of both the therapist and client is maintained. More details of suitable methods of sterilisation can be found in chapter 1.

Related anatomy and physiology

Abnormalities of the sebaceous gland

Condition	Description	Appearance	Cause	Treatment
Seborrhoea	apparent in areas where sebaceous glands are prominent: the face, chest and back	excessive oiliness on the skin, pores become enlarged and blocked with sebum with the formation of blackheads – leads to dull, congested skin or acne	hormonal changes at puberty lead to overactive sebaceous glands	cleanse with the appropriate products, exfoliate and recommend the client has regular professional facials and uses appropriate products at home
Comedones (blackheads)	associated with seborrhoea	small dark or black blockage in a pore	hardened, keratinised sebum blocks the hair follicle or pore, darkens due to the oxidation of the sebum in the air, can become inflamed leading to papules and pustules	soften with steam and massage before extraction, advise client to cleanse with appropriate products, exfoliate and have regular professional facials
Milia	commonly found on fine skins in the cheek and eye area	white, pearl-like nodules	sebum is trapped under the epidermis due to the pore or follicle opening being overgrown by the stratum corneum	newly formed milia disperse with massage; if well established, can be removed with the help of a sterile probe or lance
Acne	there are various grades of acne some of which require medical attention – a doctor's approval must be sought before beginning treatment; commonly found in teenagers due to the hormone imbalance occurring at the time of puberty, but not limited to them alone; may affect the face, chest and back	excessive oil, comedones, papules, pustules and scarring may be present depending on the severity	the pore or follicle becomes blocked with sebum and skin cells and the sebaceous gland continues to produce sebum which cannot escape; anaerobic bacteria within the pore or follicle multiply and the structure becomes infected leading to the formation of pus; the contents of the follicle may be pushed deeper into the dermis forming a cyst	if the client has sought medical attention, this will usually involve the use of antibiotics and the drugs Retin A or Accutane; these drugs cause a variety of side effects such as dryness and sensitivity and so treatment by a therapist should be minimal at this time – after medical treatment the therapist can treat the skin with caution as seborrhoeic and in consultation with the physician; cystic acne should not be treated in the salon
Steatoma	commonly known as sebaceous cysts	soft or hard cyst varying in size from a pea to an egg	sebum is trapped within the gland due to a tightened or small opening into the follicle	steatoma are harmless and cosmetic treatments may be given unless there is infection present; medical attention is necessary for surgical removal

Condition	Description	Cause	Treatment
Rosacea	this condition seldom appears before the age of 30	inflammatory condition affecting the cheeks and nose, appears as temporary erythema and later flushing, becoming permanent; seborrhoea, papules and pustules are present in the area	unknown but is thought to relate to earlier seborrhoeic conditions in youth	medical referral is advisable; camouflage make-up can ease distress; advise client to avoid effectors of vasodilation such as spicy foods, heat and alcohol
Asteatosis	very dry skin, which can be uncomfortable	flaky, dry skin with itching and cracking	underactive sebaceous glands associated with the thyroid gland or old age	advise the use of emollient creams

Abnormalities of the sweat glands

Condition	Description	Appearance	Cause	Treatment
Hyperidrosis	excessive perspiration affecting the hands, feet and underarms where these glands are prolific	skin in the area is wet; the moisture may run down the skin in severe cases	can be congenital but usually follows an emotional problem since the glands are controlled by the nervous system	frequent bathing, use of astringents and antiperspirant
Prickly heat	heat-induced rash	small, red vesicles accompanied by itching and inflammation of the sweat glands	exposure to excessive heat such as the sun or sunbeds; sweat ducts get blocked by plugs of keratinised cells	frequent bathing in cool bath or shower; keep away from further heat; astringents can help

Abnormalities associated with pigmentation

Condition	Description	Appearance	Cause	Treatment
Ephelides (freckles)	affect fair-skinned people, found in abundance all over the body	small, brown macules that darken in sunlight and fade during the winter	congenital condition, inherited with the natural colouring	advise the use of a sunblock during exposure to sun; if disfiguring, can successfully be camouflaged with make-up
Lentigines	larger than a freckle	an area of brown pigmentation that does not darken in sunlight	congenital defect of the skin	camouflage make-up
Chloasma (hyper-pigmentation)	common in women	light brown patches of pigmentation that darken with exposure to sunlight, vary in shape and size and can appear anywhere on the body but mainly the face, nipples and pubic area	melanocytes are stimulated by the increase in the hormone oestrogen during pregnancy and sometimes as a result of taking the contraceptive pill	the condition fades considerably after the birth or finishing the pill but a sunblock is advisable to avoid darkening; camouflage make-up is useful for facial cases; desquamation treatment can help

(Continued)

Related anatomy and physiology

Beauty Therapy: The Basics for NVQ 1 and 2

Condition	Description	Appearance	Cause	Treatment
Vitiligo (hypo-pigmentation)	condition that is most obvious on dark skin sometimes referred to as leucoderma	area of no pigmentation affecting the body or face and hair leaving white misshapen patches	the melanocytes are destroyed so no melanin is produced; can be congenital	use a sunblock on the affected areas; skin has a normal texture so camouflage make-up is successful
Pigmented naevi	birthmark	large or small areas of light to dark brown pigmentation affecting any part of the body or face	congenital malformation	if on the face and causing distress camouflage make-up will help; raised naevi can be removed surgically if troublesome
Moles	very common type of blemish	vary in size, colour, and vascular appearance, can be raised or flat, found on the face or body, hair may grow from the mole	congenital malformation	can be surgically removed if troublesome; if any changes occur to moles the client should be advised to see a physician
Albinism		pigment is absent throughout the body so an albino will have fair skin, white hair including the eyebrows and lashes and no colour to the eye	congenital defect where melanocytes are present but do not produce melanin	avoid sunlight and use a sunblock
Port wine stain	haemangioma disorders relate to vascular abnormalities	large, flat, red or purple area of permanently dilated capillaries, commonly found on the face	congenital defect that persists throughout life and does not fade	very effective results can be obtained with camouflage make-up and recently laser therapy has been developed that fades the blemish considerably; only available through a physician
Strawberry mark	another vascular condition	bright red area seen at birth or shortly afterwards; soft to the touch and raised	multiplication of blood capillaries in the dermis	usually fades or disappears before adulthood, otherwise camouflage make-up is successful
Spider naevi	vascular abnormality	a centrally dilated vessel with others radiating from it	associated with rise in oestrogen levels in pregnancy or liver disease	advise camouflage make-up techniques or diathermy coagulation by a trained electrologist
Dermatosis papulosa nigra	occurs in black skinned men and women of African descent	brown or black raised spots across the cheeks and nose sometimes referred to as flesh moles	a natural characteristic in some black skin (they are benign)	specialist foundation products can help to even out the darker colour of the spots

Abnormalities associated with skin growth

Condition	Description	Appearance	Cause	Treatment
Psoriasis	fairly common non-infectious skin condition	oval- or round-shaped patches, raised and with the presence of silvery scales; patches have a distinct red outline and there may be some irritation if scratched, and if the scales are removed then there will be bleeding; commonly found on the knees, elbows, face and scalp but can appear anywhere on the body	faulty keratinisation of the skin cells and increased mitosis in the stratum germinativum; stress and anxiety worsen the condition	responds well to relaxation treatment such as massage and exposure to sunlight; medical attention is required in some cases depending on the severity; creams containing Vitamin A and/or steroids may be used; if no infection is present and the skin is unbroken normal cosmetic treatments can go ahead
Skin tags	small growths	fibrous growth of skin tissue commonly found in the neck area, common in elderly clients and can be pigmented making them more obvious	excessive growth of the skin thought to be related to friction in the area	the attachment to the skin can be treated with diathermy under medical supervision but this does not prevent others from arising
Keloids	common on black skins	an overgrowth of scar tissue at the site of an injury	skin cells divide more fervently to compensate for the injured site	there is no treatment of this condition although surgery has been performed in severe cases and drugs administered to slow down skin growth; cosmetic treatments can go ahead as long as they do not aggravate the site of the blemish

Infections caused by bacteria

Condition	Description	Appearance	Cause	Treatment
Pseudo-folliculitis	small pus-filled spots	infection of a hair follicle with subsequent inflammation and pus formation	streptococci bacterial invasion of the follicle caused by infected implements such as razors or infected cosmetics	treatment cannot be carried out until the condition has cleared, treated by thorough cleansing and application of antiseptic
Furuncle	boil	acute pus formation involving the epidermis, dermis, subcutaneous tissue, hair follicles and sebaceous gland, with swelling, redness and pain as well as pus formation	staphylococci invasion through a papule or abrasion of the skin	requires medical attention if large and painful, probably the administration of antibiotics and lancing; do not perform cosmetic treatments in the affected area

(Continued)

Related anatomy and physiology

Condition	Description	Appearance	Cause	Treatment
Carbuncle	similar to a furuncle but more deep-seated found on the neck or back	a very painful central sore appears, can leave serious scarring	bacterial infection	requires medical attention
Impetigo	highly contagious, found around mouth and nose, common in children	vesicles that readily rupture to form a yellow crust	bacterial infection, poor hygiene	medical attention is required; do not perform treatments
Conjunctivitis	highly contagious eye infection	the mucous membrane of the eye becomes inflamed and the eye appears red, puffy, weeping and feels gritty	bacterial infection of the membrane of the eye	medical attention is required; do not perform treatments; advise separate towels and flannels to avoid cross infection in the home
Stye		red swelling on the upper or lower eyelid at eyelash level; the eye may weep and pus is formed	the eyelash follicle becomes infected with streptococci bacteria	medical attention is required, usually antibiotics and lancing if serious

Infections caused by fungi

All types of fungal infection of the skin and nails are types of ringworm (tinea). All types of ringworm are saprophytic (that is, they live on dead or decaying matter).

Condition	Description	Appearance	Cause	Treatment
Tinea corporis	ringworm of the body	red, scaly, circular patches occurring on the trunk or limbs, spreading outwards, healing from the centre to give the ring appearance; vesicles and pustules can be present	common in pet owners as cats and dogs pick up the condition and easily transfer it to the arms and legs of their owners; highly contagious	medical attention is required involving the administration of a cream or tablets containing griseofulvin; do not perform treatments

Infections caused by viruses

Condition	Description	Appearance	Cause	Treatment
Herpes simplex	cold sores	first sign is itching or burning of the skin around the mouth or nose area, followed by vesicle formation; these weep or burst to form a crust that can	viral infection transmitted by contact either directly (e.g. kissing) or indirectly (e.g. drinking from the same glass); infection can reoccur as	medical attention can be sought for bad attacks but treatment is available over the counter in the form of antiviral creams; do not

				perform treatments if present
Herpes zoster	commonly known as shingles; very painful	vesicles appear following nerve pathways	the virus lies dormant in the body until the body's resistance is low; some people say that the sun and wind can trigger an attack	infectious; seek urgent medical attention; do not treat a client with this infection
			chickenpox virus	
Warts	highly contagious condition, which can appear in different forms	common warts – firm, raised, rough nodules of varying size, can have dark spots within the body of nodule; flat warts – smooth, pearly elevations about pinhead in size, found in groups on the hands and feet	viral infection passed on through contact	creams and lotions that contain salicylic acid can be bought over the counter; best removed under medical supervision; treatment can go ahead if the wart is covered with a waterproof dressing
	easily split causing bleeding and scab formation; complete healing takes 10–14 days			

Infections caused by parasites

Condition	Description	Appearance	Cause	Treatment
Pediculosis	found on body hair but commonly on the head	lice and eggs (nits) adhere to hair shaft; may be itching	infestation by lice	highly contagious; do not treat the client
Scabies	commonly known as 'itch mites', which burrow into the skin to lay their eggs	red, irritating lines or spots between fingers or other folds of skin	infestation by Acarus scabiei	contagious; do not treat the client

Skin damage by external agents
The sun

Condition	Description	Appearance	Cause	Treatment
Ageing	hereditary factors influence rate of ageing; the sun can speed up the processes	the skin appears leathery and will have many fine lines and wrinkles; elasticity is weak with the skin being slow to return to normal when stretched	ultraviolet light penetrates the epidermis and the dermis to the collagen and elastin fibres, which are destroyed	exfoliate to remove the thickened epidermis and promote blood circulation, encourage growth of the collagen and elastin fibres with facials and suitable products; suggest specialist facials such as

(Continued)

Related anatomy and physiology

Beauty Therapy: The Basics for NVQ 1 and 2

Condition	Description	Appearance	Cause	Treatment
				non-surgical facelift, galvanic and faradic treatments and encourage the client to use moisturisers and foundation containing sun protection factors at all times
Sunburn	skin can suffer long-term damage following sunburn	the skin becomes red (erythema) with accompanying irritation and blistering, depending on the severity	ultraviolet light penetrates the epidermis to the level of the blood capillaries causing them to dilate; the longer the exposure the longer the capillaries remain dilated and so the erythema can last from several hours to days	soothe and cool the skin with cold water, rose water or a mask made from calamine mixed with rose water; if severe seek medical attention
Skin cancer	serious condition requiring urgent medical attention	begins as a pale lesion, red patch or a mole that changes its appearance, for example getting larger, darker or becoming raised	it is not fully understood why cells become cancerous but it is known that the sun is the main cause of skin cancer, especially in areas of the world where the sun is at its strongest	medical attention is required immediately; the client should seek a doctor's approval before any cosmetic treatment

Chemical trauma

Condition	Description	Appearance	Cause	Treatment
Dermatitis	allergic reaction to an irritant such as continuous use of strong chemicals, particularly alkaline e.g. detergents	red, dry, itchy area with the presence of papules and vesicles in severe cases; skin may crack and bleed leaving it open to infection by micro-organisms	prolonged contact with irritants such as detergents which break down the acid mantle, leaving the skin open to sensitivity	the condition is not contagious or infectious, so cosmetic treatment can go ahead; if infection is present the client should seek medical attention and should also avoid contact with the irritant
Eczema	inherited allergic condition; perfumed products can cause condition to worsen	similar to dermatitis in appearance but reoccurs throughout life	contact with an irritant can trigger an attack as can stress; thought to be a congenital condition, common in those who have a family history of hay fever or asthma	advise the client as for dermatitis, but in addition suggest stress-relieving massage if there is no infection present

| Allergies | an allergic reaction can occur to many external and internal agents; the list includes cosmetics, washing powder and foods such as strawberries, heat and drugs | may begin as erythema, irritation or a burning feeling; if left untreated may develop into swelling or even blisters and weeping | which **allergen** triggers the reaction is dependent on the individual so it is important to ask the client if they have any known allergies; it is possible that a client may develop an allergic reaction to an unknown substance during or after a treatment; to avoid this, it is wise not to treat clients with several known allergens, in other words, one who is **hypersensitive**; it is the therapist's duty to know the active ingredients of their treatment range | remove products from the area immediately with water only; continue to splash the area with cool water until symptoms subside; if they do not, the client should see a doctor as soon as possible |

Physical trauma

Condition	Description	Appearance	Cause	Treatment
Broken capillaries	common in fine and delicate skin types on the inner cheek and nose areas	fine, red lines in the skin surface	extremes in temperature, incorrect skincare, sunburn or physical pressure such as during extraction	protect the skin from the elements with moisturisers and foundation, treat gently during cosmetic treatment and camouflage using green corrective concealer; diathermy coagulation by a professional electrologist can be recommended
Urticaria	hives or nettle rash	red, itchy weal that can be localised or widespread; can appear and disappear within hours	allergic reaction to a foreign body causing the skin cells to release histamine; the allergen can be a food such as strawberries, an insect bite, pollen or drugs	the condition usually corrects itself within a few hours but may require medical attention if severe; do not perform treatments that may worsen the condition
Dark circles under the eyes	darkness under or around the eyes		thought to be caused by a lack of sleep, but can be an inherited condition, can also be an indication of illness or oedema	a light covering of concealer can disguise the problem but the cause needs to be addressed if a cure is required

Related anatomy and physiology

Hair structure and growth

This section includes:

- types of hair
- hair structure
- the structure of the hair follicle
- growth cycle of hair.

Hair is a dead keratinised structure protruding out of an indentation in the skin called a **follicle**. This is a downward growth of epidermal cells into the dermis from which the hair gains its nutrients for growth. The hair can be divided into two portions:

1. The **hair shaft** – the portion extending above the skin surface.

2. The **hair root** – the portion below the surface of the skin.

Types of hair

There are two main classifications of hair:

1. **Vellus hair** is the soft, downy hair found all over the body except the eyelids, lips, palms of hands and soles of the feet. This type of hair originates from a lobe of a sebaceous gland and so has a shallow follicle. When the follicle is stimulated, for example, there is an increase in blood circulation, by hormonal changes during puberty, pregnancy or menopause. It is possible for a vellus hair to become a coarse, dark terminal hair.

2. **Terminal hair** is deep-seated and extends from a deeper follicle. These hairs are found on the scalp, underarms, eyebrows, pubic regions, arms and legs.

Hair structure

The structure of each hair is divided into three layers:

- cuticle
- cortex
- medulla.

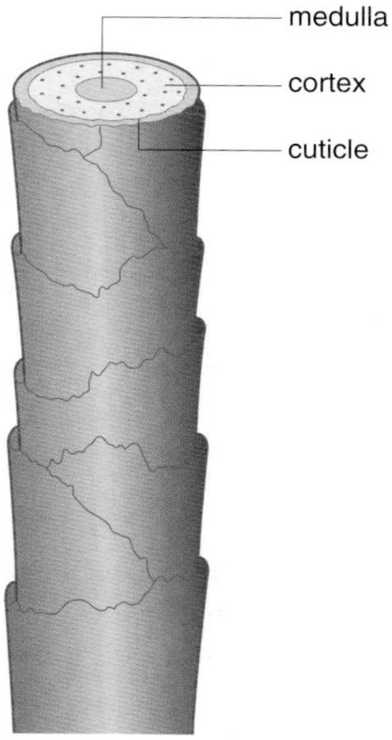

Figure 14.24 *Structure of a hair*

The cuticle

The outermost layer is composed of overlapping transparent scales. The cuticle of hair protects the layers that lie underneath. When substances such as lash tint come into contact with the cuticle, the scales become raised due to the alkalinity of the chemicals. This allows the chemicals to enter into the cortex of the hair.

The cortex

Made of many **micro-fibrils** arranged into bunches to form elongated cells, the cortex makes up the bulk of the hair and gives it strength and elasticity. It is within the cells of this layer that granules of pigment can be found. This gives the hair its colour: melanin produces the brown-black shades and pheomelanin gives the red-yellow shades.

The medulla

This layer is not always present, particularly in fine hair. When seen it lies in the centre of the cortex and its function is unclear.

The structure of the hair follicle

The hair follicle is formed by a depression of the epidermis downwards into the dermis to form a tube-like structure. It is from this that the hair grows. The lower portion of the follicle is called the **bulb**. Approximately two-thirds of the way up the follicle are the sebaceous glands, which produce sebum, a natural oil. This lubricates the neck of the follicle, the skin surface and the hair.

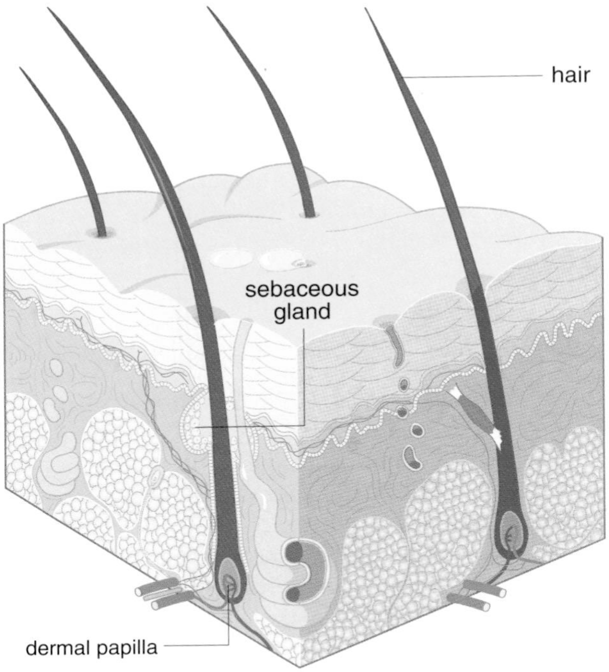

The bulb

The lower portion of the bulb is called the dermal papilla or matrix. This has a rich blood supply and is where the cells grow and divide by a process called mitosis. New cells are pushed upwards, changing shape and becoming keratinised as they do so, until they enter the upper bulb or **keratogenous zone**. Here they harden and form the layers of the hair.

The dermal papilla

This is an elevation into the base of the bulb, which contains a rich blood supply. It is from here that the cells receive the nutrients and oxygen necessary for mitosis to occur. While the follicle is in contact with the dermal papilla it will be active, in other words, capable of producing cells to form a growing hair.

Figure 14.25 *Structure of the hair follicle*

hair

sebaceous gland

dermal papilla

The inner root sheath

The inner root sheath is made up of similar cells to the cuticle of the hair. They lie in the opposite direction, facing down towards the dermal papilla. This allows the two cuticles to interlock, helping to secure the hair in its follicle.

The outer root sheath

The outer root sheath is continuous with the stratum germinativum of the epidermis and is therefore made up of growing cells. This enables the follicle to grow and renew cells during the life cycle. The root sheath can be clearly seen as a silver sheath on some hairs when they are plucked from the follicle.

Growth cycle of hair

A hair follicle actively produces hair for distinct periods of time, before going through stages of change and then rest. There are three stages that a follicle goes through:

1. **Anagen** – the active, growing stage.
2. **Catagen** – the changing stage.
3. **Telogen** – the resting stage.

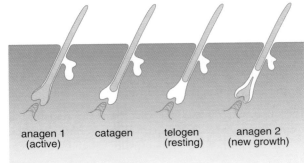

anagen 1 (active) catagen telogen (resting) anagen 2 (new growth)

Figure 14.26 *Three stages in the life cycle of a hair*

Related anatomy and physiology

Anagen

At the onset of anagen, the hair germ cells in the outer root sheath are stimulated into activity by hormones. This results in the formation of the **dermal cord**. The cells of the dermal cord undergo mitosis and a new follicle is produced. This grows in length and width, the food and oxygen being obtained from the connective tissue sheath. The newer follicle extends downwards to the dermal papilla, which enlarges and the bulb is formed around it. The bulb begins production of new hair cells, receiving the necessary nourishment from the dermal papilla. These cells form the inner root sheath and then a new hair. As the new hair grows up the follicle, it may push the old hair out (if it has not fallen out already) and eventually the new hair appears at the surface. The hair continues to grow while the follicle is active. The time varies according to the area of the body but can be as long as six years. Towards the end of anagen, melanin production begins to slow down and eventually ceases as the follicle enters the next stage.

Catagen

This stage is also known as the transitional stage where the dermal papilla breaks down and the hair detaches itself from the base of the follicle and the bulb. The hair is known as a **club hair** because of its appearance. When plucked it has a black blob on the end. Club hairs are only attached to the follicle by the inner root sheath. The hair continues to rise up the follicle to just below the sebaceous gland until it is no longer attached by the inner root sheath. At this time the hair can be removed from the follicle just by brushing. The follicle below the hair shrinks and breaks away from the dermal papilla but the remaining cells are already organising themselves to form the new matrix and hair germ cells. All this takes place over a period of a few days.

Telogen

Known as the resting stage, the follicle remains at approximately half of its normal length for a few weeks before anagen begins again.

Knowledge of the hair growth cycle is important to a beauty therapist for waxing. It can explain the premature appearance of hairs after waxing and the difference in time between treatments as well as being able to judge the effectiveness of an epilation treatment.

The structure of the nail

This section includes:

- nail structure
- nail growth
- nail diseases and disorders.

The nail is made of layers of dead cells containing a protein called **keratin**, also found in skin and hair. The layers are held together by a substance called **lamellae**. The nail is divided into three main parts:

1. The **free edge** – the part that protrudes over the fingertip.
2. The **nail plate** – forming most of the visible portion of the nail.
3. The **nail root** – the part of the nail buried into the skin.

The upper part of the nail root forms the **nail fold** and the lower part forms the **matrix**. This is part of the germinating layer (stratum germinativum) of the epidermis and is the region from which the nail grows. The matrix receives the nutrients and oxygen for growth from a network of blood vessels in the **nail bed**.

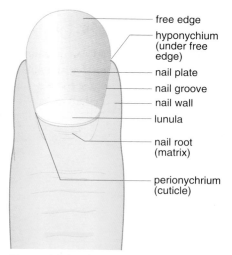

free edge
hyponychium (under free edge)
nail plate
nail groove
nail wall
lunula
nail root (matrix)
perionychrium (cuticle)

Figure 14.27 *A cross-section through the end of a finger and nail*

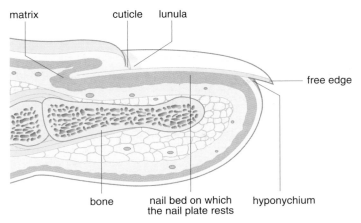

matrix   cuticle   lunula

free edge

bone   nail bed on which   hyponychium
the nail plate rests

Figure 14.28 *A nail in its bed*

Nail structure

Part of Nail	Description	Function
Free edge	the part of the nail plate that protrudes over the fingertip, likened to the claws of an animal	protects the fingertips from physical harm; improves the appearance of the hands when manicured
Hyponychium	a layer of epidermis found under the free edge	prevents bacteria and dirt from getting under the nail plate and infecting the nail bed
Nail plate	the main part of the nail, made up of layers of dead keratinised cells	protects the tips of the fingers and toes, which have a network of sensory nerve endings
Lunula	also known as the half-moon, it is the visible portion of the matrix and appears pale due to a reduced blood supply	as the upper part of the matrix, it is part of the growing area for the nail – the nail plate and the nail bed are formed here
Cuticle	a layer of epidermis that overlaps the base of the nail plate	prevents bacteria and dirt from entering the nail fold
Eponychium	part of the cuticle at the base of the nail over the lunula, which moves forward with the nail plate as it grows	protects the growing part of the nail
Matrix	lies beneath the nail fold – an injury to the matrix can cause deformity in the nail plate or the plate can be shed completely from the nail bed	the matrix has a rich blood supply, which enables it to produce the nail plate and bed
Nail bed	this is the portion on which the nail plate rests; it has a plentiful blood supply when healthy and so gives the nail its pink colour	the blood supply provides the food and oxygen to the matrix and the ridges anchor the nail plate to prevent lifting; it also has a nerve supply making the nail bed sensitive to pain and pressure
Nail wall	the folds of skin running up the sides of the nail plate	forms the frame to the nail and provides protection from physical harm
Lateral nail fold	either side of the nail plate the skin folds over to enclose the nail plate	guides the nail to grow straight

Related anatomy and physiology

Nail growth

Nail formation

The nail originates from the cells of the stratum germinativum within the nail fold and the matrix. As the cells divide they push old ones up towards the free edge. The cells keratinise, die and form the nail plate in layers held together by water from the cells and the fatty acids present called lamellae. The nail bed is formed at the same time but the keratinisation process is not completed so the cells remain living until they reach the hyponychium where they dry out and die to form this protective strip under the free edge.

Healthy nails

Healthy nails appear firm but flexible, smooth and slightly pink in colour. The surrounding cuticle should be unbroken, flexible and should not be stuck to the nail plate.

A healthy nail will grow approximately 3–4 mm per month and will grow faster in the summer, and in children and pregnant women. Children and pregnant women have higher levels of nutrients in the blood. In summer, due to the increase in temperature blood circulation is faster. Toenails grow more slowly than fingernails (about 2 mm per month) and are often thicker and harder.

To produce healthy nails the vitamins A, B complex and D are needed together with the minerals calcium and iron.

ACTIVITY

Try to find the words listed below in the wordsearch.

Eponychium   Free edge   Hyponychium   Nail plate   Matrix   Mantle   Lunula   Nail fold   Nail bed   Nail wall   Cuticle

Z	X	O	L	G	M	A	C	J	N	L	N	O	E	A	D
X	W	Y	J	K	A	D	F	G	A	M	P	R	T	S	U
C	C	A	B	W	T	X	Z	T	I	S	P	J	I	L	M
A	D	F	H	I	R	N	A	I	L	F	O	L	D	N	V
P	P	R	R	O	I	L	M	T	W	V	X	Z	W	I	L
N	B	N	D	E	X	I	R	T	A	M	A	N	T	L	E
A	F	A	G	H	E	J	D	K	L	U	A	L	O	U	R
S	T	I	R	P	U	E	C	E	L	I	G	H	V	N	W
Z	X	L	Y	W	B	O	D	D	L	H	A	C	B	U	J
E	O	P	A	L	U	P	S	G	T	C	U	R	V	L	W
X	U	L	I	Z	W	S	R	T	E	Y	I	V	H	A	I
L	M	A	O	N	P	O	J	B	D	N	E	T	C	Q	R
Z	N	T	Q	R	O	U	V	W	T	O	V	Q	U	B	C
D	L	E	U	V	Z	K	I	M	Q	P	X	M	R	C	Q
A	I	M	E	B	W	O	H	D	F	Y	V	H	T	V	X
F	G	O	T	E	P	O	N	Y	C	H	I	U	M	W	B

The effects of nail care treatment

Nail treatments such as buffing and massage benefit nail growth by increasing the blood supply to the nail bed. In doing so, more nutrients and oxygen are available for the cells to grow and divide. This means that the nails will grow more quickly and stronger.

The effects of illness

Systemic illness, in other words disease or illness affecting a system of the body, can influence the rate of growth and appearance of the nails, as well as the skin and hair. Poor health or poor diet can cause the nails to be brittle or very soft, flexible, pale, discoloured or blue in colour and the cuticles to be dry, split and hardened.

Damage to the nail

Physical and chemical agents can cause nail damage.

Physical damage

Nail bed

A knock or blow that is hard enough to damage the nail bed will appear as a bruise under the nail. The blood vessels in the nail bed break, allowing blood to flow out under the nail plate. After a little time the blood vessels mend, leaving some under the nail plate. This dries, sticks to the underside and grows up with the nail plate until it reaches the free edge where it can be removed.

Matrix

Damage to the matrix can result in temporary loss of the nail or permanent damage to the nail plate. When the matrix is damaged by a severe knock or blow, some of the cells die. This results in a temporary halt in the production of the nail plate and nail bed. This can appear as a ridge in the nail or, if a lot of the matrix is damaged, the loss of the nail plate.

The dead cells need to be replaced and are made by the matrix itself. When fully healed, the matrix will begin to make the nail plate and nail bed again. If, however, the damage is severe enough, the matrix may not heal completely, leaving scar tissue. This will appear as a permanent condition in the nail such as a vertical ridge or split.

Chemical damage

Strong chemicals such as detergents or even nail polish remover, with continuous use, will cause the nail and cuticle to dry out. The nail may appear brittle, discoloured (usually yellow), flaky and ridged. The cuticle will be dry, white in colour and inflexible.

Nail diseases and disorders

The presence of some conditions may contraindicate nailcare treatment. A therapist must be able to recognise conditions in order to make the decision as to whether a nail care treatment can be performed or not. The therapist must never make a diagnosis but should refer the client to a specialist as appropriate. The signs of infection or inflammation are:

- redness
- swelling
- pain
- pus formation.

Contraindications

These can be divided into three types of condition:

1. Those that need medical referral.
2. Those that prevent treatment.
3. Those that restrict treatment.

1 Conditions requiring medical referral

Common diseases caused by micro-organisms may require treatment by a medical practitioner. When referring a client to their GP, it is important to do so without causing alarm or embarrassment.

Ringworm (tinea)

Not a 'worm' as the name implies, but a fungal infection which can affect the nails and the skin. The disease is highly contagious and is often passed on by pets. Do not touch the area but tell the client to see a doctor as soon as possible for suitable treatment.

Look out for:

- Yellow or white streaks and thickening of the nail plate. Sometimes the top layers of the nail will peel off. This is known as onychomycosis.
- Red, slightly raised patches of skin in the shape of a ring.
- On the feet, it appears as white, moist flaking or peeling between and around the bottom of the toes. Commonly called 'athlete's foot', it often spreads to the toenails.

Warts and verrucae

These are contagious conditions caused by a virus affecting the skin of the hands or feet (see Figure 14.34). Do not touch. If minor, they can be covered with a dressing and the treatment can be performed. If severe, the client should see a doctor. Look out for raised, horny lumps with black dots on the hands and horny lumps in an uneven shape which grow into the skin on the soles of the feet, characteristic of verrucae.

Whitlow (paronychia/onychia)

A contagious infection of the skin, cuticle or nail bed, caused by bacteria entering through an opening in the skin or cuticle (see Figure 14.35). It can be caused by bad nail care techniques but is usually associated with nail biting. Severe cases may need lancing or a course of antibiotics, so advise the client to see a doctor. Look out for red painful swelling and the formation of pus.

2 Conditions preventing treatment

These conditions may need medical referral if severe. Mild cases can restrict treatment.

Eczema

An inflamed, red skin condition that is not contagious. It can be stress-related or the result of an allergy, for example to metals, chemicals, drugs, clothing or products such as nail enamels. If severe or with open sores, treatment would be contraindicated. When mild, however, treatment can go ahead, avoiding the area affected. Look out for redness, swelling, blisters, flaking, weeping and cracking of the skin. Eczema can give rise to changes in the nail such as ridging and pitting.

Dermatitis

It is a term used to describe any inflammation of the skin caused by an external irritant such as detergent. Care should be taken not to irritate the skin by using chemicals and perfumed products.

Psoriasis

An inherited condition aggravated by stress, drugs or infection. Commonly found on knees and elbows, it is not infectious so treatment can go ahead but with restrictions. Some nail care treatments such as massage are thought to benefit the condition. However, if severe or open, cracked or infected, it is wise to refer the client to a doctor. Look out for:

- severe ridging or pitting of the nail plate
- raised, red, silvery, scaly skin patches, circular or oval in shape with a definite outline.

Onycholysis

This term means the separation of the nail plate from the nail bed caused by systemic illness, injury, nail disease or infection, circulatory problems or as a reaction to drugs. It appears as a white area of the nail plate due to loss of blood supply. In severe cases, the nail plate may be shed completely or discoloration can be caused by the invasion of fungi or bacteria. If severe and of systemic or disease origin, the client should be referred to a doctor. Mild cases restrict treatment in that the affected finger should be omitted.

Bruised nail

Bruised nails are caused by injury to the nail bed with bleeding under the nail plate. There is dark purple, blue or black discoloration. Perform nail treatments with care, avoiding pressure. If severe, involving the loss of the nail plate, refer the client to a doctor. If mild, miss the finger out from the treatment. Cover with a dark-coloured enamel if appropriate.

Chilblains

Caused by poor blood circulation and, therefore, common on fingers and toes. The condition appears in cold weather. When severe, refer the client or delay treatment until the condition has improved. If mild, avoid the affected area. Look out for red, itchy swellings that become painful in the cold.

Ingrowing toenails (onychocryptosis)

Can affect the fingers, but most common on the toes. The edges of the nail cut into the nail wall, which then can become infected by bacteria. The problem is caused by restrictive footwear, by clipping the corners of the nail too low at the nail wall or it can be a congenital defect. If inflammation or infection is present, the client should be referred to a doctor; if not, the condition should be referred to a chiropodist and the nail omitted from the nail care treatment.

3 Conditions restricting treatment

Corns

These are similar to calluses in that they are formed by an increase in pressure or overuse. A corn, however, develops a root-like structure that penetrates into the skin and when it presses on a nerve it causes pain. A client with a deep, developed corn needs referral to a chiropodist. Soft, new corns can be treated in the same way as calluses.

Bunions (hallus vulgus)

This is a condition where the big toe is forced towards and under the other toes due to pressure and friction from tight or pointed footwear. This causes the joint to swell and become inflamed causing pain. Another cause may be an inherited weakness in the arches of the foot. The therapist can assist with massage when the bunion is newly formed but in most cases the condition needs to be treated by a chiropodist or by referral to a doctor for surgery. During pedicure, take care with the area as pressure may be painful. Filing and cuticle work can be performed with care although enamelling may be difficult if the toe is severely affected.

Arthritis

There are two types of arthritis. Osteoarthritis is the wear and tear of the joints and is more common in elderly clients. Rheumatoid arthritis is a disease that can affect a person at any age. Both involve painful joints, especially with movement or weight bearing. The conditions are usually treated with drugs and physiotherapy but, when under control, gentle massage can mobilise joints and eliminate fluid, reducing swelling. Such treatment should only be performed by a therapist with medical permission. The heat associated with paraffin wax treatments can give relief to painful joints.

The following table details common nail disorders, their causes and the relevant treatment required.

Condition	Cause	Appearance	Treatment
Corrugations	Vertical ridging can be hereditary or caused by damage of the matrix with age, indicating dryness. Horizontal ridging, if present on all nails, indicates a temporary pause in growth due to illness such as measles. If present on only one nail, the ridge may be caused by damage to the matrix.	Vertical or horizontal ridges or furrows within the nail plate.	If the ridging is mild, use a buffer with paste polish to buff the nails. Horizontal ridges grow out with the nail but avoid the use of coloured enamel as it is difficult to remove from the ridge. If ridging is severe treat the nails as fragile.
Bitten nails (onychophagy) See figure 14.29	Nervous or stress-induced habit.	The free edge, nail plate and cuticle are bitten to leave the hyponychium exposed and the cuticle and surrounding skin ragged. Nail biting is the most common causes of deformed nails, due to the increased risk of infection.	Regular manicures help to overcome the habit. File the nails smooth to remove ragged edges, remove ragged cuticle, skin and hangnails with nippers to avoid temptation to bite. Give attention to the cuticles, massaging with oil or cream.
Hangnails (agnail) See figure 14.30	Dryness, cutting off too much cuticle during manicure or the habit of chewing the cuticle.	Hard, dry pieces of nail or cuticle found in the nail groove or wall. If pulled, can result in torn tissue and subsequent infection.	Remove with cuticle nippers and suggest regular oil manicures, which will prevent dryness.
Split nails (onychorrhexis)	Injury, filing too deeply into the nail wall, excessive use of solvents such as polish remover, chemicals and alkalines, pressure on very long nails.	Horizontal or vertical splits in the free edge, often at flesh level or below. When associated with dry hair and skin, this suggests a glandular disorder.	Perform oil manicures, use only the fine side of an emery board when filing, regular application of cuticle cream.
Brittle nails (fragilitas unguium)	Dehydration of the nail plate due to overexposure to alkaline, solvents or immersion in water. Can also indicate an iron deficiency or anaemia.	Yellow, thick nails that break easily.	Avoid contact with chemicals and solvents, wear rubber gloves and use barrier creams. Regular use of cuticle cream, especially at night.
Flaky nails See figure 14.31	Dryness caused by exposure to solvents and chemicals.	The layers of the nail plate separate at the free edge.	Protect with gloves and barrier creams, regular use of nail strengtheners and cuticle cream, especially at night. File with the fine side of an emery board only and use polish remover containing oil.
Blue nails See figure 14.32	Poor circulation due to cold, hereditary defect or heart disorder.	Nail plate appears blue instead of pink. May cause ridging of the nail plate.	Increase the circulation by exercise, massage and buffing.

Condition	Description	Treatment
White spots (leuconychia)	Mild injury to the base of the nail.	White spots within the nail plate. The injury causes the layers of the nail to separate.	They grow out with the nail plate. Avoid pressure on the cuticle during nail care treatment. Use the fine side of an emery board when present in the free edge.
Pterygium	It is either hereditary or can be caused by infrequent attention to the cuticle.	The cuticle is often dry, split and grows in excess. Grows forward and sticks to the nail plate.	Careful use of the cuticle knife and nippers to remove the excess cuticle. Oil manicures help prevent the regrowth from sticking back down to the nail and keeps the cuticle soft and supple.
Excess perspiration (hyperhydrosis)	Can be hereditary or caused by a stressful situation.	Hands or feet are damp and clammy. feet can suffer from odour as they are confined within shoes.	Sweaty hands are difficult to treat, but a light dusting of talc can help. Feet should be washed daily and antiperspirant sprays or powders can be used. Socks or tights should always be worn and synthetic shoes should be avoided. Leather allows air to circulate around the feet. Special odour-absorbing inner soles can also be used in footwear.
Hard skin (callous)	Thickening of the stratum corneum due to pressure and/or overuse, formed to protect the affected area.	Dry, hard, inflexible overgrowth over a bony prominence such as knuckles or joints.	Mild calluses may be removed by softening in warm water before the use of corn plane or chemical hard skin remover. Severe calluses need referral to a chiropodist.

Related anatomy and physiology

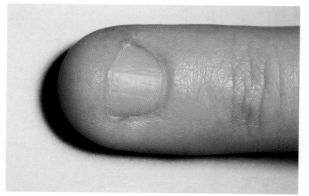

Figure 14.29 *Bitten nails*

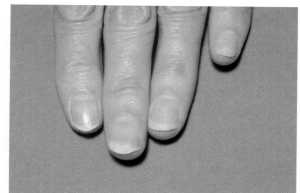

Figure 14.30 *Flaky nails*

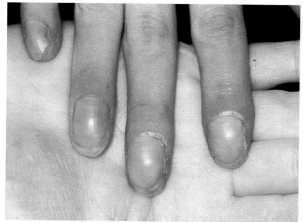

Figure 14.31 *Blue nails*

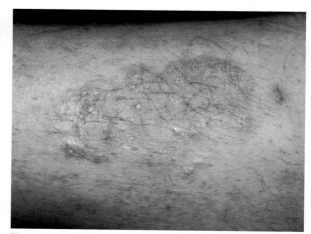

Figure 14.32 *Ringworm*

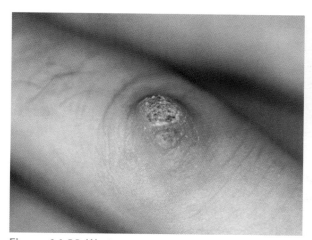

Figure 14.33 *Warts*

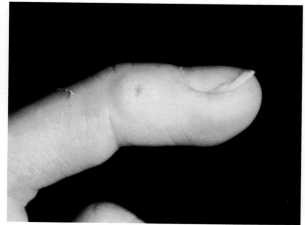

Figure 14.34 *Whitlow*

Blood

This section includes:

- composition of blood
- functions of blood
- blood circulation
- blood supply to head and neck
- blood supply to arm and hand
- blood supply to leg and foot.

Blood is a liquid that travels inside vessels called:

- arteries
- arterioles
- veins
- venules
- capillaries.

The blood moves along arteries due to the pumping action of the heart, which is made of a muscle tissue called **cardiac muscle**.

The blood moves along the veins through a series of valves that control the flow.

Composition of blood

Blood is composed of a fluid called **plasma,** which is mostly water with salts, nutrients and waste products dissolved in it. Within the plasma are red blood cells or **erythrocytes**, which carry oxygen to the tissues and give blood its red colour. **Leucocytes** or white blood cells have a defensive function as they fight disease and prevent infection whilst **platelets** and **blood proteins** such as **fibrinogen** help the blood to clot, preventing micro-organism invasion and blood loss.

Functions of blood

Transport

- Oxygen is carried from the lungs to all living tissues.
- Carbon dioxide is carried from the tissues to the lungs to be exhaled.
- Nutrients from the digestive system are carried to the tissues.
- Excess water is taken from the tissues to the kidneys for excretion.
- Waste products from cell activity are taken to the kidneys or skin for excretion.
- Hormones released from endocrine glands are carried to their target organs.

Defence

- White blood cells are taken to a site of injury to fight invading bacteria and so stop infection.
- Other white blood cells produce **antibodies** that fight diseases that have entered the bloodstream.
- Blood proteins and platelets combine at the site of injury or damage to form a clot that plugs the wound, preventing blood loss and the invasion of bacteria. The clot hardens to form a scab which protects the area while new tissue grows underneath.

Related anatomy and physiology

Heat distribution and regulation

■ Body heat produced in the organs and muscles of the body is distributed around the body to maintain a temperature of 37°C.

■ The dilation of the blood capillaries in the skin allows excess heat to be lost to the atmosphere. When the temperature of the body needs to be maintained, the blood capillaries constrict, preventing blood from nearing the surface of the skin.

Blood circulation

As mentioned previously, blood is moved along the vessels by the pumping action of the heart. The heart has four chambers: **right atrium, right ventricle, left atrium** and **left ventricle**. A wall separates the left and right sides and valves that open and close separate the top chambers from the bottom.

The valves allow blood to flow from the top atria into the bottom ventricles. When the heart contracts or beats, the right side beats just before the left and this pushes blood out of the **ventricles** into the blood vessels. Other valves in the vessels prevent the blood from reversing back into the heart so that when it relaxes blood is drawn into the **atrium**. The vessels from the lower right ventricle carry blood to the lungs where it gives up carbon dioxide and takes on fresh oxygen. It then returns to the heart, entering the top left atrium. The blood passes through the valve into the bottom left ventricle where it is pumped out along a large vessel called the **aorta**, which supplies the whole body with blood. To complete the journey, blood returns from the areas of the body through the inferior and superior venae cavae to the top right chamber to begin the cycle again.

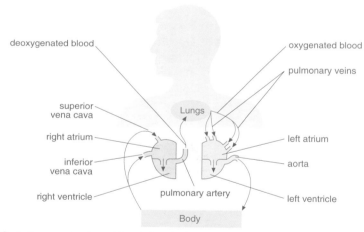

Figure 14.35 *A simplified diagram to show blood circulation*

Blood supply to the head and neck

Oxygenated blood leaves the heart through the aorta. This large vessel stretches upwards in front of the heart and then arches over to run down behind it. As it does so two smaller arteries branch off and travel upwards on either side of the neck. Once in the neck area they are called the **common carotid arteries** and as they near the head they divide to form the **external and internal carotid arteries**. At the level of the ear, the internal carotid disappears through a hole in the skull to supply blood to the brain and eyes. The external carotid artery splits further to supply blood to the skin and muscles of the face and scalp. There are three main branches, called the **facial artery**, the **temporal artery** and the **occipital artery** and they supply blood to the areas after which they were named.

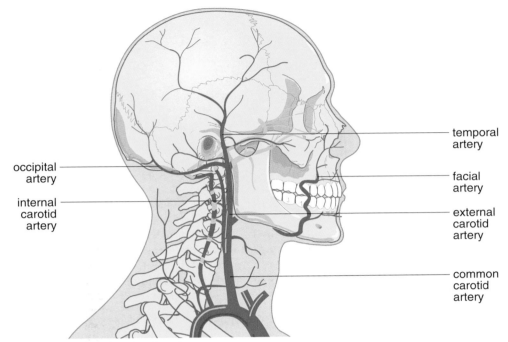

occipital
artery

internal
carotid
artery

temporal
artery

facial
artery

external
carotid
artery

common
carotid
artery

Figure 14.36 *Arteries of the head and neck*

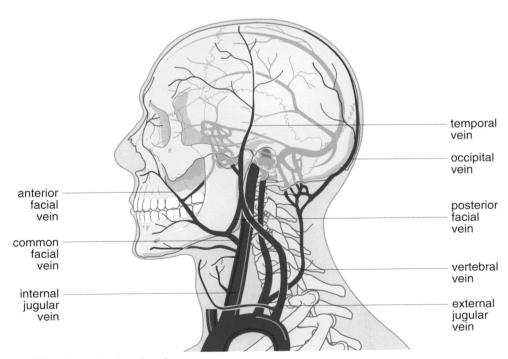

anterior
facial
vein

common
facial
vein

internal
jugular
vein

temporal
vein

occipital
vein

posterior
facial
vein

vertebral
vein

external
jugular
vein

Figure 14.37 *Veins of the head and neck*

As arteries become smaller they are known as **arterioles**. These become smaller still until they are the thickness of a hair, when they are known as **capillaries**. The walls of a capillary are very thin, just one cell thick. This allows the food and oxygen contained within the blood to be lost to the surrounding tissues and the waste products of cell activity to be collected by the blood. This process is called **capillary**

exchange. Once this has happened the blood begins its journey back to the heart. The capillaries join to form small vessels called **venules**, which in turn join up to form **veins**. The veins returning the blood back to the heart from the head and neck are called the **internal and external jugular veins**. The former exits the skull through a hole near the ear as before and the external jugular vein drains blood from the **facial, temporal** and **occipital veins**.

The internal and external jugular veins do not join together but run down the neck independently to join a large vein called the superior vena cava, which eventually returns the blood to the heart.

Blood supply to the arm and hand

The blood supply to the arm begins with the **subclavian artery**, which has branched off the **aorta**. The subclavian artery becomes the **axillary artery** and then the **brachial artery**, which runs down the inner aspect of the upper arm to about 1 cm below the elbow, where it divides into the **radial** and **ulnar arteries**. The radial artery runs down the forearm next to the radius bone to the wrist where it nears the surface and can be felt as the **radial pulse**. It continues over the carpals to pass between the first and second metacarpals into the palm. The ulnar artery runs down the forearm next to the ulna bone, across the carpals into the palm of the hand. Together they form two arches in the hand, the **deep** and **superficial palmar arches**. From all these arteries branch others to supply blood to the structures of the upper arm, forearm, hand and fingers.

The venous return of blood from the hand begins with the **palmar arch** and **plexus**, which is a network of capillaries present in the palm. Three veins carry the deoxygenated blood up the forearm: the **radial vein**, the **ulnar vein** and the **median vein**. The former two run parallel to the bones of the same name, the latter runs up the middle. Just above the elbow, the radial and ulnar veins join to become the **brachial**

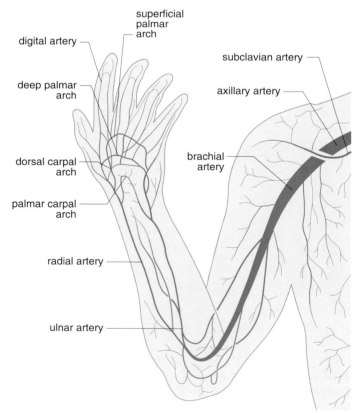

Figure 14.38 *Arteries of the arm and hand*

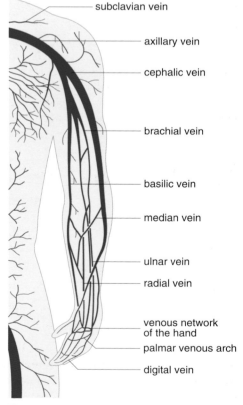

Figure 14.39 *Veins of the arm and hand*

vein, and the median vein joins the **basilic vein**, which originated just below the elbow along with the **cephalic vein**. As the veins continue over the elbow they link to form a network that eventually divides, with the basilic vein joining the brachial vein, which then becomes the **axillary vein**. The cephalic vein travels up the arm separately and becomes the **subclavian vein** in the upper chest.

Blood supply to the leg and foot

The aorta travels down the length of the trunk to the lower abdomen where it divides into two arteries which supply either leg. The artery in the thigh is called the **femoral artery**, named after the bone of the thigh. At the knee the femoral artery becomes the **popliteal artery**, which divides into two below the knee. One of these arteries runs down the front of the lower leg and is called the **anterior tibial artery**, while the other runs down the back and is known as the **posterior tibial artery**. This artery divides at the inside of the ankle becoming the **medial plantar artery** on the inside of the foot and the **plantar arch** on the sole of the foot. The anterior tibial artery becomes the **dorsal metatarsal artery** on top of the foot.

There is a network of veins in the foot that become the **dorsal venous arch** on top of the foot. This travels the inside of the foot to the ankle where it becomes the **small saphenous vein**. It continues up the back of the whole leg to the thigh where it is known as the **great saphenous vein**. Two small veins called the **anterior tibial veins** travel up the front of the lower leg while two veins, the **posterior tibial veins**, run up the back. These four veins converge just below the knee to become the **popliteal vein** at the back of the knee and then eventually the **femoral vein** in the thigh. The great saphenous vein and the femoral vein join at the groin and return to the heart via the inferior vena cava.

The lymphatic system

This section includes:

- composition of lymph
- functions of lymph
- lymph drainage and structures
- lymph drainage from the head and neck
- lymph drainage from the arm and hand
- lymph drainage from the leg and foot.

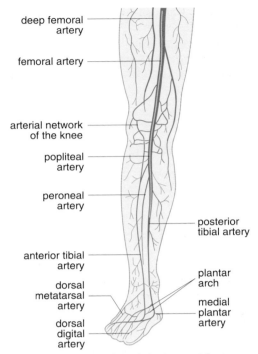

Figure 14.40 *Arteries of the leg and foot*

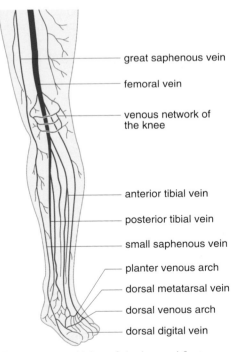

Figure 14.41 *Veins of the leg and foot*

The lymphatic system defends the body from infection and works as a waste disposal system. It consists of fine tubes or **lymph capillaries** present within all tissues. These collect the tissue fluid containing waste products, toxins and micro-organisms. Once inside the capillaries the fluid is known as **lymph**. The capillaries join to form a network of vessels running alongside the blood vessels with the lymph travelling in the same direction as the venous flow, towards the heart. This is known as **lymph drainage**.

Related anatomy and physiology

Composition of lymph

The composition of lymph is similar to that of blood plasma only it contains no erythrocytes, so it appears straw coloured instead of red. It also has fewer blood proteins and nutrients but has a larger number of white blood cells, fats and waste materials.

Functions of lymph

1. To fight infection.
2. To return nutrients and blood proteins from the tissues to the blood circulatory system.
3. To transport white blood cells to the blood circulatory system.
4. To transport fats from the small intestine to the liver.
5. To prevent oedema (swelling) by draining excess tissue fluid from the tissues.
6. To produce lymphocytes (a type of white blood cell).

Lymph drainage and structures

Introduction

The lymphatic system defends the body from infection and works as a waste disposal system. It consists of fine tubes or **lymph capillaries** present within the tissues. These collect the **tissue fluid** containing waste products, toxins and micro-organisms. Once inside the lymph capillaries the fluid is known as **lymph**. The composition of lymph is similar to that of blood plasma but it contains less blood proteins and food materials and more waste material. White blood cells are numerous in the lymph. The lymph capillaries join to form a network of vessels running alongside the blood vessels with the lymph travelling in the same direction as the venous flow, towards the heart. This is known as **lymph drainage**.

Lymph capillaries

These are fine, blind-ended tubes about the size of a human hair. They are present between the cells of all tissues but are found in large numbers in the areas of the body most likely to become infected or where micro-organisms can enter easily such as the toes, fingers, around the stomach and small intestine, the mouth, ears, eyes and nose.

Lymph vessels

The lymph capillaries form a network that join to form larger **lymph vessels**. These are similar to veins in structure and in the direction in which they run. They have thin, weak muscular walls and valves to prevent the backflow of lymph.

The lymphatic system relies on the pumping action of surrounding muscles to move the lymph along these vessels. As the muscles contract they become shorter and fatter, which squeezes the lymph vessels and pushes the lymph along, the valves preventing its return. This causes a vacuum below the valve, which is filled from lymph further down the vessel. This reaction reoccurs as far as the lymph capillaries, which causes more tissue fluid to be drawn into them.

Lymph nodes

Lymph nodes are areas where the lymph is cleansed by first being filtered and then by the action of special white blood cells present in the node. These cells destroy micro-organisms and other unwanted material so that when the lymph leaves the node it consists of mainly white blood cells and food materials. The nodes are found in groups in order for the lymph to be cleansed several times before being deposited back in the bloodstream.

Lymph ducts

Once the lymph has been cleansed it travels along vessels to the chest area where it is deposited back into the bloodstream through tubes called **lymph ducts**. Lymph collected from the right side of the head, chest and the right arm drains into the **right lymphatic duct** while lymph from the rest of the body drains into the **thoracic duct**. These ducts deposit the lymph into the subclavian veins.

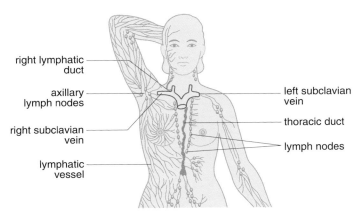

Figure 14.42 *Lymph ducts*

Factors affecting lymph drainage

1. **General blood circulation** – if the heart works well there will be good lymph drainage due to capillary exchange in the tissues; if not **oedema** (swelling) will occur.
2. **Exercise** – the action of the muscles on the lymph vessels speeds up lymph drainage and improves the performance of the heart.
3. **Massage** – deep movements press on the lymph vessels forcing the lymph along them. These movements are always performed towards the heart, that is in the direction of lymph flow. See page 130 for further information on these massage techniques.

The effects of lymph drainage on skin and muscle tissue

Good lymph drainage benefits the function and appearance of the skin and enhances the performance of muscle tissue by improving the internal environment through the removal of waste material. The removal of the waste allows further capillary exchange to occur with the local blood capillaries, hence more food and oxygen is provided for the cells.

Lymph drainage from the head and neck

The lymph capillaries collect the fluid from the tissues of all the organs and structures within the head and neck. It flows downwards towards the chest, passing through the lymph nodes shown in Figure 14.44. Numerous nodes are present due to the large number of openings, the ears, nose and mouth, through which micro-organisms could potentially enter the body. Swelling is unlikely in this area due to the effect of gravity assisting lymph flow, although 'puffiness' around the eyes caused by blocked sinuses can be improved by lymph drainage massage techniques. The right lymphatic duct before passing collects lymph from the head and neck into the blood circulatory system.

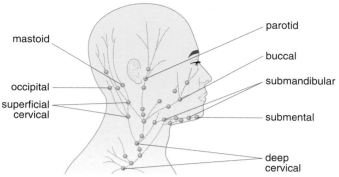

Figure 14.43 *Lymph nodes of the head and neck*

Lymph drainage from the arm and hand

The lymph drainage from the arm and hand follows the venous blood flow up the arm towards the chest. The major lymph nodes are found in the inner part of the elbow and the armpit (axillary). The cleansed lymph from the right arm and hand is collected by the right lymphatic duct and that from the left arm by the thoracic duct.

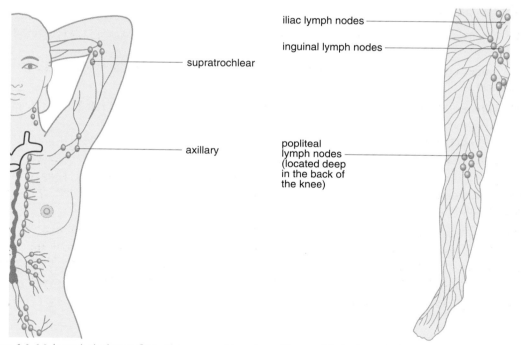

Figure 14.44 *Lymph drainage from the arm and hand* Figure 14.45 *Lymph drainage from the leg and foot*

Lymph drainage from the leg and foot

Lymph drainage in the leg works against gravity. Tissue fluid can collect in the feet and ankles causing **oedema** (swelling). This is more likely in someone who stands still for long periods of time. The major lymph nodes are found at the back of the knee and in the front of the groin. The lymph from both legs and feet are collected by the thoracic duct to be emptied into the blood circulatory system at the chest.

The nervous system

This section includes:

- the central nervous system
- the peripheral nervous system
- the autonomic nervous system
- the nerves of the head and neck
- the nerves of the arm and leg.

The nervous system consists of special cells called **neurones** that make up the brain, spinal cord and pairs of nerves. Its function is to receive and transmit impulses or messages to and from organs and muscles. In doing so the nervous system integrates and controls all the functions of the body. The nervous system is divided into two parts. These are the **central** and the **peripheral** systems.

The central nervous system (CNS)

The brain and the spinal cord make up the CNS. These important organs are protected by bone that completely surrounds them. In the case of the brain, it is the **cranium**, and the spinal cord is protected by the **vertebrae** of the spine. From the brain and spinal cord come pairs of nerves that make up the peripheral nervous system.

The peripheral nervous system

There are 12 pairs of nerves from the brain called **cranial** nerves and 31 pairs from the spinal cord called **spinal nerves**. Each pair can contain either **motor** or **sensory** neurones or both.

- Sensory neurones take messages from the sense organs, such as those in the skin, to the central nervous system.
- Motor neurones take messages from the CNS to muscles or glands such as the sweat glands in the skin.

The autonomic nervous system

The autonomic nervous system is a specialised part of the peripheral nervous system and is **involuntary**, in other words under subconscious control. It is responsible for controlling involuntary actions of the body such as heartbeat, breathing rate, pupil dilation and the involuntary muscles that make up the blood vessels and digestive tract. There are two parts:

1. **The parasympathetic system** helps to create the conditions needed for rest, sleep and digestion.
2. **The sympathetic system** works antagonistically with the parasympathetic system to create the conditions needed for physical activity. It works with the hormone **adrenaline** to prepare the body for 'fight or flight' and is responsible for the conditions associated with 'stress' in modern-day living.

The effects of the autonomic system are summarised in the table below:

Part of Body Affected	Sympathetic	Parasympathetic
Pupils	dilate	constrict
Blood vessels	of digestive trace – constrict giving the feeling of 'butterflies'; of skeletal muscles – dilate; tone is increased in walls of larger vessels leading to high blood pressure	of glands – dilate
Heartbeat	quick and strong	slow and weak

(Continued)

Part of Body Affected	Sympathetic	Parasympathetic
Breathing	quick and deep	slow and shallow
Sweat glands	activity increased	activity decreased
Action within digestive tract	decreased	increased
Digestive glands	decreased	increased

The 31 pairs of spinal nerves are numbered according to the section of the spinal column from which they arise:

- 8 pairs of **cervical** nerves (neck region)
- 12 pairs of **thoracic** nerves (chest region)
- 5 pairs of **lumbar** nerves (lower back region)
- 5 pairs of **sacral** nerves (bottom region)
- 1 pair of **coccygeal** nerves (tail region).

Each nerve serves an area of the body according to its position.

The nerves of the head and neck

The fifth and seventh cranial nerves are responsible for the sensations and movement of the facial muscles.

The fifth cranial nerve or trigeminal nerve

This is mainly a sensory nerve carrying information to the brain from the skin of the face, the teeth and the membranes of the nose and mouth. There is also a motor branch to the muscles of mastication. The main branches are the mandibular, maxillary and ophthalmic branches.

1. **The mandibular branch**
   - **Sensory** – for the teeth of the lower jaw, membranes of mouth and cheeks, and the skin of the lower part of the face.
   - **Motor** – to the masseter and temporalis (the muscles of chewing).

2. **The maxillary branch**
   - **Sensory** – for the upper jaw, the skin on the temples, sides of forehead and upper cheeks.

3. **The ophthalmic branch**
   - **Sensory** – for tear glands and the skin of forehead, nose and upper eyelids.

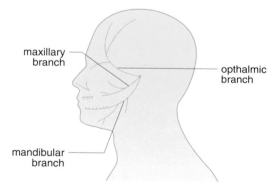

Figure 14.46 *Branches of the fifth cranial or trigeminal nerve*

The seventh cranial nerve or facial nerve

This is mainly a motor nerve serving the muscles of facial expression, but has a small sensory branch for the sensation of taste from the front of the tongue. There are five main branches.

1. **The temporal branch**
   - **Motor** – leads to the muscles of the ear, the orbicularis oculi and the frontalis.

2. **The zygomatic branch**
   - ■ **Motor** – leads to the orbicularis oculi.
3. **The buccal branch**
   - ■ **Motor** – leads to the buccinator, the upper lip, and sides of the nose.
4. **The mandibular branch**
   - ■ **Motor** – leads to the lower lip and the mentalis muscle.
   - ■ **Sensory** – from the front of the tongue.
5. **The cervical branch**
   - ■ **Motor** – leads to the platysma muscle in the neck.

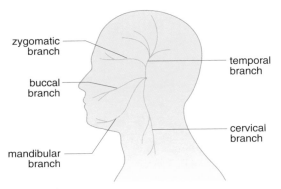

Figure 14.47 *Branches of the seventh cranial or facial nerve*

The nerves of the arm and leg

> **!** The sternomastoid and the trapezius muscles are served by the eleventh cranial nerve or accessory nerve.

The Arm		The Leg	
Muscle	Nerve	Muscle	Nerve
Deltoid	C5 and 6	Gluteus maximus	L5, S1 and 2
Biceps	C5 and 6	Quadriceps	L3, 4 and 5 and S1
Brachialis	C5 and 6	Hamstrings	L4 and 5 and S1 and 2
Triceps	C7	Adductors	L2, 3 and 4
Flexors	C6, 7 and 8	Abductors	L4 and 5
		Sartorius	L2 and 3
Extensors	C6 and 7	Gastrocnemius	L5 and S1
Supinator	C5 and 6	Soleus	L5, S1 and 2
Pronators	C6 and 8	Anterior tibialis	L2, 3 and 4
		Extensors of toes	L5 and S1
		Flexors of toes	L5, S1 and 2
		Peroneus	L5 and S1
		Posterior tibialis	L4 and 5

The fifth to eighth cervical nerves (C) serve the arm and the second to fifth lumbar (L) and first to second sacral (S) nerves, the leg. Due to the size of the muscles of the limbs, a large muscle may be served by more than one nerve. It is easier, therefore, to list the nerves according to the muscles they serve.

GLOSSARY

Abduct away from the body

Access and egress terms used in health and safety legislation, refers to the way in and way out of an area

Acid mantle the protective film formed on the skin composed of sebum and sweat

Adduct towards the body

Aerobic with oxygen

Aftercare advice to the client regarding things she must do or not do to preserve and maintain the effects of a particular treatment

Ampoule A sealed glass or plastic phial containing active ingredients beneficial to the skin. Applied to the face under special masks

Anaerobic without oxygen

Anterior towards the front

Confidentiality private information which the client has trusted you with

Consultation a discussion with the client to gain important details and give advice prior to treatment

Contra-actions reactions to the treatment, such as excessive erythema, allergic reaction

Contraindications any signs which indicate that a particular treatment should not be carried out, e.g. infection, open wounds in the area to be treated

COSHH control of substances hazardous to health regulations, legislation concerned with the safe handling, storage and use of chemicals and other products which are used or sold in the salon

Cosmetics preparations used to enhance the skin and hair

Couperose skin redness caused by broken capillaries usually found on the cheeks

Cross infection infection which passes from one person to another by direct contact or from articles or implements

Dehydrated lacking in moisture

Demal papilla a rich supply of blood vessels providing nutrients and oxygen for the growth of hair, found at the root of the hair follicle.

Dermatosis papulosa nigra lesions that develop through defects in the philosebasceous follicle. Small lumps appear at the mouth of the follicle and are dark in colour

Desquamation natural shedding of surface skin cells (stratum corneum)

Dorsiflexes moves the top of the foot towards the shin

E-mail electronic mail which links computers across the world to relay information

Emollient an ingredient in skin creams which softens

Environmental Health Officer (EHO) an employee of the local council responsible for inspecting and implementing standards of health and safety in the work place

Erythema redness of the skin brought about by physical or chemical stimulus which dilates the capillaries in the skin

Everts lifts the outside of the foot

Exfoliate the removal of dead cells from the surface of the skin (epidermis) using either special cosmetics or implements

Extension Increasing the angle of two bones (e.g. straightening the arm)

Fax facsimile, a means of transmitting paper information using telephone lines

Flexion decreasing the angle of two bones (e.g. bending the arm)

Florid skin redness caused by a mass of broken capillaries in the skin, usually found on the cheeks and nose

Health and Safety Executive (HSE) the governing body which regulates the law relating to health and safety

Histamine reaction a chemical in the body tissues that causes an allergic reaction such as, itching, blisters, erythema, etc.

Home care advice recommendations given to the client at the end of treatment relating to home care regime, lifestyle, use of products and contractions

House style images such as logos or practice which gives a business its individual identity

Humectant a substance which attracts water

Hypo-allergenic cosmetics which are designed for sensitive skin that do not contain perfume or additives

Inferior below; front of body

Ingrowing hair when the hair is prevented from emerging from the follicle so by a layer of epidermal cells causing the hair to turn back on itself. This results in infection at the mouth of the follicle

Inverts lifts the inside of the foot

Job description written details of an employee's specific work role, duties and responsibilities

Keloid overgrown tissue at the site of a scar

Keratin the protein found in skin, hair and nails

Key skills skills which have been identified as those

which are needed to be effective at work and throughout life, e.g. communication

Lateral to the side of the midline of the body

Legislation the laws which govern the country. In business these relate to health, safety, the environment and working with people

Limits of own authority the extent of your responsibility as determined by your own job description and work place policies

Litigation legal action, such as suing a salon for negligence

Lymph straw coloured liquid found in the lymphatic system

Medial towards the midline of the body

Medical referral any condition which requires the client to consult a doctor or other medical practitioner such as a chiropodist

Menopause the stage in woman's life when there are major changes in the production of reproductive hormones

Moisturisers products which help to hydrate the skin by replacing or retaining the water found in the epidermis

Nutrients chemical and compound elements essential for life i.e. food for metabolism and growth

Overlay a thin coating applied to the natural nail or over a nail tip

Petty cash a small sum of money available for items such as coffee, paying the window cleaner etc.

Pigmentation the colour of the skin and hair is determined by the natural pigment called melanin which is produced by cells called melanocytes

Plantar flexes pointing the toes

Posterior back of the body

Pronate rotating the forearm inwards

Risk assessment any risk associated with chemicals or processes used in the salon is assessed, usually by the manager, and training or guidance given to staff

Sallow skin yellowish coloured skin associated with an oily skin

Salon services the treatments available to the client and are printed on the salon price list

Sanitisation cleansing or washing to an antiseptic level so as to inhibit bacteria

Secondary infection where an open wound becomes infected

Skin analysis assessment of the clients skin to ascertain skin type, skin disorders or imperfections

Skin test products which are known to cause allergic reaction in some people are tested on the skin prior to treatment. A positive result will show as irritation and redness at the site of the test and treatment with that product must not be carried out. A negative result will show that there is no adverse reaction and treatment can continue

Smile line a curve on the nail that is appears naturally as the hyponychium shows through the nail plate or may be emphasised by a coloured overlay or nail polish

Sun Protection Factor (SPF) a number which gives a guide to the effectiveness of a sun-screening product

Sunscreen products used on the skin to filter out harmful rays from the sun – UVA and UVB

Superfluous hair normal hair growth that is unwanted i.e. regarded as unfashionable or unsightly, e.g. underarm hair

Superior above

Supinate rotating the forearm outwards

Systemic medical condition a medical condition found in the internal organs of the body, e.g. heart

Technical skills the practical activities the therapist carries out in treating clients

Terminal hair course dark hair found on the scalp, under the arms and pubic area

Translucent allows light to pass through – associated with face powder

Treatment plan the stages you intend to follow in carrying out a particular treatment or course of treatments, includes evaluating the progress and success of the treatment

Vasoconstriction narrowing of the blood vessel so that a decrease in flow occurs

Vasodilation enlargement in diameter of the blood vessels so that an increase in flow occurs

Vellus hair fine downy hair found on most areas of the body

Wrap fibreglass or silk used to overlay the nail

KEY SKILLS/CORE SKILLS TASKS

Introduction

Key skills are a range of essential skills that are part of everyday life and underpin success in training, employment, personal development and future learning. They are important in learning because they help us to focus on how and what we learn. They are also important in our personal life because they enable people to manage their lives and develop their career and their relationships with others.

In this section of the book we have provided tasks and examples of where evidence can be collected towards qualifications in key skills/core skills.

Chapter 1 – Health and safety

The beauty therapy salon requires a team approach to ensure that the business runs smoothly, profitably and meets health and safety requirements. The salon duties activity found on page 16 requires you to take responsibility for the allocation of salon duties to the staff team and to monitor performance. Evidence produced by carrying out this activity will go towards assessment of key skills.

Working with others

Evidence   Duties rota

Evidence   Feedback from colleagues on how well you worked with the team in allocating and monitoring salon duties

Information Technology

Evidence   Compiling a duties rota using appropriate software

Problem solving

Evidence   Identify where the duties rota had to be changed due to staff absence or heavy workload, explain how you handled the situation and decided on an alternative strategy

Communication

Evidence   Discussions with the staff team to decide upon the needs of the salon and to ensure that tasks are completed

Evidence   Produce a report for a senior member of staff to inform them about health and safety matters or the way in which staff carry out salon roles for their appraisals

Chapter 2 – Salon reception duties

An important part of the beauty therapist's job is to handle the many tasks of the salon reception. It is usually only large organisations that have full-time receptionists. Evidence produced by carrying out this activity will go towards the assessment of key skills.

1. Put together a weekly diary or log of all the jobs you undertake each day and keep together copies of information and materials which you use throughout the week. This could include messages, faxes, e-mails, samples of treatment dockets, cash sheets which you have added up and till receipts. It is important that you collect only materials which you have worked with and those should be authenticated by your supervisor on the day of the activity.

2. Keep a list of all the visitors to the reception (other than clients). Briefly describe how you handled different types of people, their business with the salon (example of a log can be found on page 32) and any problems you encountered. Include how you maintained security procedures with regard to visitors.

3. Keep a record of appointments you have made during the week using the salon appointment book. Clearly identify where you have handled cancellations, taken telephone appointments, informed staff about client delays or cancellations.

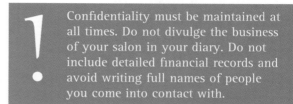

Confidentiality must be maintained at all times. Do not divulge the business of your salon in your diary. Do not include detailed financial records and avoid writing full names of people you come into contact with.

4. Maintain and update as necessary the client records file.

Working with others

Evidence   Keeping an appointment book, receiving visitors and keeping a register of visitors

Communication

Evidence   Dealing with clients

Evidence   Written messages, keeping client records

Evidence   Receiving faxes, e-mails, written instructions

Application of number

Evidence   Keeping records of takings throughout the day

Evidence   Dealing with discrepancies, working out treatment cost

Problem solving

Evidence   Extracts from the diary or log showing problems and how they were handled

Chapter 3 – Promoting products and services to clients

Collecting clients' comments on a client questionnaire can be an effective way of evaluating how successfully the business provides a service to its clients and to find out if the salon is meeting the needs of its clientele. You can also use client comments to help you to establish how successful you are in your treatments. These should be collected in your log or diary as well as through evaluation sheets after you have completed a course of treatment.

Information Technology

Evidence Design a questionnaire to gain information from your clients on a range of treatment, client care and service, and issue the questionnaire to as many clients as possible

Evidence Evaluate the responses

Evidence Produce a table or graph of findings

Communication

Evidence Issuing evaluation sheets or questionnaires to the clients with an appropriate explanation

Application of number

Evidence Data from the questionnaire

Chapter 4 – Personal performance and teamwork

Planning for activities such as a holiday, a birthday party or a shopping trip requires some organisation and planning to ensure that everything runs smoothly. You will need to take account of what needs to happen (**target**) and by when (**time**). When the event is over you will look back on what happened (**review**) and perhaps decide to do some things differently.

On page 57, under Appraisal, a process of action planning is discussed in relation to your job role. You may begin by identifying your strengths and weaknesses. Using a similar process of planning prepare an action plan for your personal development over a two-year period. This should relate to your future career.

If you have undergone an appraisal in your salon you may present the appraisal action plan as evidence. You may also have a National Record of Achievement (NRA) from when you were at school. This will also contain evidence of planning for your future career.

Reviewing your action plan and amending your targets is an important part of the continuous cycle.

Communication

Evidence Appraisal interview or tutorial

Improving own learning and performance

Evidence Action plan for your future development

Evidence reviewing the action plan to see if targets are being met

Chapter 5 – Preparation for treatments and client care

1. Collect information to show that you have carried out consultations with different clients for a range of treatments. This could include:
   - client feedback in your diary or log
   - observation records by your beauty therapy assessor
   - client record cards and treatment plans.

You will need to think about the following range of treatments:

- Make-up – chapter 6
- Facial treatments – chapter 7
- Lash and brow treatments – chapter 8
- Depilatory waxing – chapter 9
- Manicure and pedicure – chapter 10
- Nail extensions and nail art – chapter 11
- Ear-piercing – chapter 12
- Spa treatments – chapter 13.

2. Choose two clients, one of whom should be new to you, and write a summary on how you carried out the consultation. Include examples of the questions you asked and what information you gained from the questioning.

3. Calculate the cost of a course of:
   - six pedicure treatments
   - four lash tints.

   Use your salon price list to make the calculation and take account of VAT at the present rate.

Application of number

Evidence Calculating the cost of treatments to include VAT

Problem solving

Evidence Make decisions about contraindications and appropriate treatment based on information gained from the client

Communication

Evidence Discussion with a client during the consultation

Evidence Produce a range of completed record cards and treatment plans

Evidence Using the ongoing information contained in record cards to adapt treatment plans

Working with others

Evidence Treatment plan agreed with the client

Evidence Written feedback provided by clients in your log/diary or on the record card on the success of the series of treatments

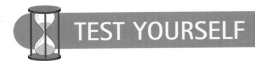
Chapter 1 – Health and safety

1. The act that covers local by-laws for hygiene procedures in the salon is the:
   a) Workplace (Health, Safety and Welfare) Regulations
   b) Personal Protective Equipment at Work Regulations
   c) Local Government (Miscellaneous Provision) Act
   d) Control of Substances Hazardous to Health Act.

2. The Electricity at Work Regulations require the therapist to:
   a) switch on an electrical heater at the start of the day
   b) ensure that all electrical equipment in the salon is in safe working order
   c) wear rubber gloves
   d) know the symbols on fire extinguishers.

3. When making a visual check on electrical equipment before switching a machine on, you must look at:
   a) the red indicator light that tells you the machine has mains power
   b) the manufacturer's instructions
   c) all the dials and switches
   d) the cables and flexes for loose wires or exposed wires.

4. Give two ways of avoiding straining your back when picking up a heavy object.

5. State three precautions which should be taken before starting treatment to avoid cross infection.

6. What are the signs of bacterial infection on the skin?

7. Give two reasons why salon dress/overall should be worn when working in the salon.

8. The most efficient method of sterilising small metal tools, such as eyebrow tweezers, is by:
   a) placing in a UV cabinet
   b) rinsing under the tap
   c) wiping with an antiseptic
   d) using an autoclave.

Chapter 2 – Salon reception duties

1. When accepting a credit card as payment, always check:
   a) the name of the bank that issued the card
   b) the account number
   c) the signature
   d) the hologram.

2. Good communication is an essential part of the receptionist's job. Give three examples of communication skills the therapist should use to deal with a client at the reception desk.

3. When handling enquiries on the telephone, you must:
   a) smile
   b) speak clearly

    c)   make eye contact

    d)   talk about the weather.

4. Which Act governs the way a salon handles a client's personal information?

5. Give three important details that must be recorded in the appointment book when making an appointment for a client.

6. If a client makes a complaint to the receptionist, it should be handled by:

    a)   listening attentively and not making judgements

    b)   becoming angry

    c)   ignoring the client

    d)   offering a free cleanser.

Chapter 3 – Promoting products and services to clients

1. The standard of goods and services sold to consumers is governed by the:

    a)   Employers' Liability Compulsory Insurance Act

    b)   Consumer Protection Act

    c)   Health and Safety at Work Act

    d)   Local Government (Miscellaneous Provisions) Act.

2. Give one reason for promoting salon services.

3. The best way to promote the salon is by ....?

4. Give three ways of advertising a new treatment being introduced to the salon.

5. When selling a product to your client for home use, you should:

    a)   never tell the client the price

    b)   link the product to the salon treatment

    c)   sell products that you want to get rid of

    d)   tell the client that it will make her/him look 10 years younger.

6. Give one reason why the client should be recommended to buy products from the salon rather than the supermarket.

Chapter 4 – Personal performance and teamwork

1. Communication is an important part of teamwork. Give three ways that staff can communicate with each other in the salon.

2. Give three ways of ensuring that you are an effective member of a team.

3. Providing support for other members of the team in the salon is important because:

    a)   you will make friends

    b)   the others do not like doing the laundry

    c)   the salon will work more efficiently

    d)   you will comply with the Health and Safety at Work Act.

4. Give two ways that you can demonstrate reliability.

5. Give three questions you could ask yourself when considering your future development.

6. Give three ways that you can ensure that you keep up to date with new products and treatments.

Chapter 5 – Preparation for treatments and client care

1. A facial examination must be carried out to assess:
   a) contraindications
   b) skin type
   c) blemishes
   d) all of the above.

2. The treatment couch should be prepared with clean laundry for every client. Is this true or false?

3. What procedure should be followed if a piece of electrical equipment is found to be faulty?

4. Why is it important to read and follow manufacturers' instructions?

5. It is important to cleanse the hands before starting treatment by:
   a) rinsing hands under cold water
   b) wiping the hands with a flannel
   c) washing with soap and hot water
   d) rubbing hands on overalls.

6. The client should always sign the record card:
   a) to meet the requirements of the Data Protection Act
   b) to meet the requirements of the Health and Safety at Work Act
   c) to make the client feel involved in the treatment
   d) to check for mistakes.

7. Give two facial expressions that would indicate that you are interested in what your client is saying.

8. Give three ways in which you can start a conversation with your client.

9. Give an example of:
   a) a closed question
   b) an open question.

10. Give two ways that you can ensure that you show courtesy and respect when greeting your client.

11. When caring for your client you should ensure that:
    a) they are comfortable during the treatment
    b) they make another appointment before they leave the salon
    c) you are on time for your lunch break
    d) you work as quickly as possible.

12. How should a client be informed that their appointment is delayed by 30 minutes?
    a) send a junior member of staff to say you are running late
    b) do not say anything
    c) go yourself and explain why you are unable to start the treatment on time
    d) offer the client a coffee.

Chapter 6 – Make-up

1. How should day make-up be adapted for the evening?

2. What steps should you take to avoid the risk of cross infection when using mascara?

3. What consideration should be given when selecting lipstick colour for black skin?

4. Eyeshadow should be applied with a disposable applicator:
   a) because it is easy to apply
   b) to avoid infection
   c) it makes the eyeshadow stay on longer
   d) it does not stretch the delicate skin round the eyes.

5. Why must the skin be kept cool during a make-up application session?

6. Why should a bride be recommended to visit the salon for a practice make-up before her wedding day?

7. Give two reasons for applying face powder.

Chapter 7 – Facial treatments

1. Give three reasons why it is important to keep client records.

2. Describe the characteristics of oily, dry and combination skin.

3. Name four contraindications to a facial treatment.

4. Why should you analyse the skin accurately prior to treatment?

5. Which statement is correct?
   a) Moisturiser should be applied lightly to leave a film on the surface of the skin.
   b) Moisturiser should be massaged into the skin.

6. Name two benefits of mask application.

7. What is the purpose of home care advice?

8. State the reason for using each of the following products:
   a) cleanser for an oily skin
   b) exfoliating product for dry skin
   c) mask for a mature skin
   d) moisturiser for a mature skin.

9. Which cleanser would be most efficient for removing heavy make-up?
   a) soap
   b) cleansing lotion
   c) cleansing gel
   d) cleansing cream.

10. An oily skin can be recognised by:
    a) flaky patches
    b) shine on the skin

    c)   client complaining that skin feels tight

    d)   the appearance of fine lines.

11. List four characteristics of a mature skin.

12. How do the following lifestyle considerations affect a client's skin type?

    a)   diet

    b)   water intake

    c)   smoking.

Chapter 8 – Lash and brow treatments

1. Why is a patch test important before lash and brow tinting?

2. How can you minimise discomfort during eyebrow shaping?

3. Give two benefits of lash tinting to a client who wears contact lenses.

4. How can a natural effect be achieved when applying strip lashes?

5. Lash tint colours the eyelashes by a process called:

    a)   hydration

    b)   pigmentation

    c)   exfoliation

    d)   oxidation.

6. Give three contraindications to eye treatments.

Chapter 9 – Depilatory waxing

1. State two safety measures that must be carried out before applying wax to a client's skin.

2. Give two contraindications to waxing the:

    a)   eyebrows

    b)   top lip

    c)   legs.

3. What PPE should be worn for waxing?

4. What is erythema?

5. What are the ingredients of cold and hot wax?

6. What are the alternative methods of hair removal to waxing?

7. What are the advantages of sugaring over other waxing methods?

8. Explain why shaving leaves the area feeling bristly.

Chapter 10 – Manicure and pedicure

1. What is the main reason for using buffing paste when buffing?

    a)   to stimulate nail growth

    b)   to condition the nails

c) to improve the colour of the nails

d) to give the nails shine.

2. Nitrocellulose is an ingredient found in:
   a) cuticle remover
   b) buffing paste
   c) nail varnish
   d) hand cream.

3. When shaping the nail the emery board should be used:
   a) with a sawing action across the top of the free edge
   b) in one direction towards the centre of the free edge
   c) across the surface of the nail plate
   d) by pulling back the nail wall and filing the free edge to a point.

4. Which product contains a solvent?
   a) hand cream
   b) buffing paste
   c) cuticle remover
   d) varnish remover.

5. Which is the correct way to hold a cuticle knife, to ensure that the blade and not the point is used?
   a) in an upright position between the thumb and first finger
   b) like a pen
   c) flat in the palm of the hand with the thumb and first finger guiding the implement
   d) between the thumb and middle finger.

6. Hot water is essential during the manicure:
   a) to soak the client's nails and cuticles
   b) to wash the towels
   c) to clean the manicure implements
   d) to wipe up any spillages.

7. Give two contraindications to manicure.

Chapter 11 – Nail extensions and nail art

1. Nail primer contains a fungicide to:
   a) harden the nail
   b) help the artificial nail to stick
   c) prevent disease
   d) soften the nail plate.

2. The nail plate is buffed with an abrasive file to:
   a) smooth the nail plate
   b) reduce the length of the nail plate
   c) help the false nail stick to the nail plate
   d) clean the nail plate.

3. Fibreglass nail extensions provide the most natural effect because:
   a) they are strong and flexible
   b) they are thick and heavy
   c) they are a natural colour
   d) they are easy to apply.

4. Give three contraindications to artificial nails.

5. The hands should not be soaked in water before applying artificial nails because:
   a) it will soften the nail plate
   b) it will soften the cuticle
   c) the adhesive will be diluted
   d) a fungal infection could occur.

6. What is a dappen dish?

Chapter 12 – Ear-piercing

1. Which piece of legislation provides guidelines on hygiene practice for ear-piercing?

2. Why is only the soft tissue of the ear lobe suitable for piercing?

3. Why is it important to gain parental or guardian's consent when piercing the ears of a client under 16 years of age?

4. How often should the ears be cleaned by the client after piercing?
   a) once a day
   b) twice a day
   c) once a week
   d) twice a week.

5. How long should the studs that are applied during piercing be kept in the ears?
   a) 2 weeks
   b) 4 weeks
   c) 6 weeks
   d) 8 weeks.

6. Which of these hygiene precautions must the therapist take when piercing ears?
   a) wash hands
   b) wear disposable gloves
   c) cover cuts and abrasions on the hands
   d) all of the above.

Chapter 13 – Spa treatments

1. Modern saunas are made of:
   a) logs
   b) pine
   c) fibreglass
   d) plastic.

2. Steam baths are usually made of:
   a) wood
   b) enamel
   c) fibreglass
   d) plastic.

3. What are commonly found in steam rooms to cool clients down?
   a) swimming pools
   b) plunge pools
   c) spa pools
   d) cold towels.

4. The humidity level in a steam bath is:
   a) higher than a sauna
   b) lower than a sauna
   c) the same as a sauna
   d) the same as a spa pool.

5. The jets within a spa have a similar effect on the body tissues as:
   a) massage
   b) sauna
   c) a steam room
   d) a flotation pool.

6. The area around a spa should be:
   a) wet
   b) open and airy
   c) non-slip
   d) dry.

7. Before a client uses spa treatment equipment they should:
   a) shower and remove jewellery
   b) have a pedicure
   c) have a leg wax
   d) sit and rest.

8. Spa treatments can affect the muscles by:
   a) relaxing muscles
   b) building muscle tone
   c) strengthening muscle fibres
   d) building muscle bulk.

9. The chemical added to a communal spa is:
   a) surgical spirit
   b) chlorine
   c) cidex
   d) alcohol.

10. Aftercare advice for spa treatments should recommend which of the following:

   a) exercise and more heat treatments

   b) always follow with a cup of tea

   c) rest and drink plenty of water

   d) exercise.

Chapter 14 – Related anatomy and physiology

The skin

1. The process by which epidermal cells are shed from the surface of the skin is called:

   a) mitosis

   b) pigmentation

   c) desquamation

   d) oxidation.

2. Sweat is produced by:

   a) the sebaceous gland

   b) the endocrine gland

   c) hair follicles

   d) the sudoriferous gland.

3. Give four functions of the skin.

4. The function of sebum is to:

   a) lubricate

   b) stimulate

   c) irritate

   d) desquamate.

5. Cell division is called:

   a) mitosis

   b) lordosis

   c) kyphosis

   d) cellosis.

6. A healthy skin is slightly acid. Is this statement true or false?

7. The papilla at the base of the hair follicle is:

   a) nerve fibres

   b) growing cells

   c) a type of hair

   d) blood vessels.

The nails

8. What is leuconychia?

9. On which part of the nail is the hyponychium found?

10. What is the correct name for the half-moon?

11. What four words best describe when infection is present?

12. What is onychophagy?

13. What is pterygium?

Muscles

14. The buccinator is found:
    a) on the forehead
    b) on the cheek
    c) on the neck
    d) around the mouth.

15. The action of the orbicularis occuli is to:
    a) open the mouth
    b) close the eyes
    c) wrinkle the nose
    d) chew.

16. The sternocleidomastoid is found in the:
    a) face
    b) arm
    c) shoulder
    d) neck.

17. The gastrocnemius is found in the:
    a) calf
    b) ankle
    c) upper leg
    d) arm.

18. The biceps is found in the:
    a) back of the arm
    b) lower arm
    c) front of the arm
    d) wrist.

Bones

19. Name the two bones of the forearm.

20. What is the difference between a ligament and a tendon?

21. The metacarpals are found in the:
    a) foot
    b) knee
    c) hand
    d) neck.

22. Name three bones of the cranium.

23. Name the bone that forms the cheekbone.

24. The bone of the lower jaw is called the:

   a) lacrimal

   b) turbinate

   c) mandible

   d) vomer.

Circulation

25. Give two functions of the blood.

26. The main artery of the body is:

   a) pulmonary

   b) carotid

   c) temporal

   d) aorta.

27. Name the vessel that carries oxygenated blood away from the heart.

28. The function of the lymph nodes is to:

   a) fight infection

   b) produce white blood cells

   c) drain tissue fluids

   d) all of the above.

29. Oxygenated blood is carried through the veins. Is this statement true or false?

30. The main lymph nodes in the neck are the:

   a) carotid nodes

   b) cervical nodes

   c) occipital nodes

   d) thoracic nodes.

Nerves

31. The central nervous system is made up of the:

   a) brain and spinal cord

   b) brain

   c) cranium and spine

   d) nerves.

32. The autonomic nervous system controls:

   a) moving the arms

   b) nodding the head

   c) the heartbeat

   d) rubbing the hands.

TEST YOURSELF ANSWERS

Chapter 1 – Health and safety

1. c

2. b

3. d

4. Bend the knees; keep back straight; keep feet apart and flat to the floor

5. Wash hands; sterilise equipment; disinfect working surfaces; use clean towels; check for contraindications

6. Redness, swelling, pain and pus

7. To project a professional image; protect the therapist's clothing; a fresh clean overall demonstrates high standards of personal hygiene

8. d

Chapter 2 – Salon reception duties

1. c

2. Understanding; listening; speaking clearly; eye contact; positive body language

3. b

4. The Data Protection Act

5. Full name; telephone number; service required

6. a

Chapter 3 – Promoting products and services to clients

1. b

2. Ensure profitability of the salon

3. Word of mouth

4. Local newspaper, leaflets issued to clients, free samples. Promotion or demonstration in the salon

5. b

6. So that professional advice can be given regarding the suitability of the products for the client's skin

Chapter 4 – Personal performance and teamwork

1. Staff meetings; notice board; internal telephones; e-mail; verbally

2. Taking a share of salon responsibilities and tasks; help others when they are busy or running late; sharing good practice; good communication

3. c

Test yourself answers

329

4. Punctuality; not take unnecessary time off work; carry out treatments in commercially recommended time scale

5. Where am I now? Where do I want to be? How will I get there?

6. Trade shows; trade magazines; training courses; manufacturer's videos

Chapter 5 – Preparation for treatments and client care

1. d

2. True

3. Take out of use and label 'out of order'

4. For safety reasons, you must be sure that you are using products and equipment to their recommendations

5. c

6. a

7. Eye contact; nodding the head

8. Discuss the treatment; ask about home care routine; remember some topic from the client's last visit e.g. holiday

9. Closed – Do you use a cleanser Mrs Smith?
   Open – Can you tell me how you cleanse your skin at home Mrs Smith?

10. Use the client's name; show the client to the treatment room; offer to take the client's coat; smile and make eye contact

11. a

12. c

Chapter 6 – Make-up

1. By intensifying the colours of the make-up; by applying heavier make-up

2. Use disposable mascara applicators; use block mascara; use applicator for each eye to avoid spreading infection from one eye to the other

3. Choose strong and bright colours

4. d

5. Perspiration can cause the make-up to change colour and the foundation will not adhere to the skin

6. To enable the therapist to experiment with a range of 'looks'; to ensure the bride is completely happy with the make-up

7. To remove shine; hide blemishes

Chapter 7 – Facial treatments

1. Identify individual clients; identify the services they received and products used/purchased; any contraindications problems or difficulties that may have occurred; to keep records up to date

2. **Oily skin** may have enlarged pores, thick coarse epidermis, shiny appearance and sallow colour – comedones, pustules, papules and milia may be present; **dry skin** has small tight pores, moisture content is poor and there are patches of flaky skin – is prone to sensitivity, milia and broken capillaries; **combination skin** has an oily 'T' zone with enlarged pores, dry cheeks and neck – comedones, pustules and papules may be present in the oily areas and milia and broken capillaries may be present in the dry areas

3. Cold sores; conjunctivitis; eczema; cuts; abrasions; redness; swelling; rashes; blood shot and watery eyes

4. By analysing the skin accurately you will be able to provide the most effective treatment and skincare advice to your client

5. a

6. Deep cleanse the skin; soften and nourish the skin; tighten and tone the skin; soothe and calm the skin

7. The purpose of home care advice is to ensure the ongoing effectiveness of the salon treatment by: encouraging the client to use the correct products; follow a daily regime; be aware of their life style and how it can affect their skin.

8. a) to remove surface oil, grime and make-up
   b) to slough off skin scales from the surface of the skin
   c) to hydrate and firm the skin
   d) to hydrate the skin and help to reduce loss of moisture

9. d

10. b

11. Skin is often dry and thin; loss of elasticity causing expression lines to form; loss of muscle tone causing loss of contours of the face; crepey skin; broken capillaries

12. a) Poor diet is reflected in poor general health which causes changes in skin condition
    b) Low water intake is reflected in a dehydrated skin
    c) Smoking causes premature lines to appear around the mouth, the skin becomes dry and discoloured

Chapter 8 – Lash and brow treatments

1. To check that the client is not allergic to the products used for tinting

2. Warm the skin with hot cotton-wool pads to open the hair follicle, use quick movements to pluck the hair

3. Mascara can cause irritation to contact lens users, however with tinting mascara does not need to be worn; a client can have difficulty applying mascara without lenses in place

4. Trimming the lashes to suit the shape of the eye and trimming to produce natural length of the lashes

5. d

6. Conjunctivitis, watery eyes, allergies, stye

Chapter 9 – Depilatory waxing

1. Look at the consistency of the wax; aarry out a skin sensitivity test

2. a) Conjunctivitis; stye; watery eyes
   b) Cold sore (herpes simplex); hairy moles; impetigo
   c) Varicose veins; sun burn; skin infection e.g. folliculitis

3. Disposable gloves and aprons should be worn for waxing

4. Erythema is a reddening of the skin due to a dilation of the capillaries

5. The ingredients in cold wax are rubber latex solution and solvents or substances, such as honey. The ingredients in hot wax are beeswax and resins.

6. Other methods of hair removal are: shaving; plucking /tweezing; threading; abrasive mitts; electrical depilatory

7. The advantages of sugaring are: the beauty therapist has the paste in her hand first and so cannot burn the client; the paste is water soluble therefore easy to remove after treatment; the sugar paste is entirely natural and hypoallergenic

8. Shaving leaves a blunt end to the hair just at the surface of the skin which feels bristly

Chapter 10 – Manicure and pedicure

1. d

2. c

3. b

4. d

5. c

6. a

7. Redness, swelling, pain and pus, bitten nails, over growth of the cuticle, ringworm (tinea), dermatitis, severe eczema, whitlow (onychia)

Chapter 11 – Nail extensions and nail art

1. c

2. c

3. a

4. Severely bitten nails; thin flaky nails; any sign of infection e.g. bacteria or fungal; allergy to nails products

5. d

6. A small glass or plastic dish used for products during treatment. This avoids product contamination caused by using products straight from their container

Chapter 12 – Ear-piercing

1. Local Government (Miscellaneous Provisions) Act

2. Piercing the cartilage can cause overgrowth of the tissue, resulting in a condition known as cauliflower ear

3. The law regards those under 16 year olds to be minors and therefore as a means of protecting young people the parent should give permission for the treatment to be carried out

4. a

5. c

6. d

Chapter 13 – Spa treatments

1. b

2. c

3. b

4. a

5. a

6. c

7. a

8. a

9. b

10. c

Chapter 14 – Related anatomy and physiology

The skin

1. c

2. d

3. Protection; heat regulation; sensation; secretion; excretion; absorption

4. a

5. a

6. True

7. b

The nails

8. White spots in the nail

9. Under the free edge

10. Lanula

11. Redness, swelling, pain and puss

12. Bitten nails

13. Over growth of the cuticle

Muscles

14. b

15. b

16. d

17. a

18. c

Bones

19. Radius; ulna

20. A ligament attaches a bone to bone; a tendon attaches a muscle to a bone

21. c

22. Frontal; parietal; occipital; temporal

23. Zygomatic

24. c

Circulation

25. Heat regulation; transportation; fights infection

26. d

27. Pulmonary vein

28. d

29. False

30. b

Nerves

31. a

32. c

INDEX